SKIN REVOLUTION

SKIN REVOLUTION

Authentic Beauty from the Living Matrix

LESLIE KENTON

with Jesse Kenton-Smith BSc (Hons), MBBS, FRCS

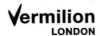

Vermilion
LONDON

10

First published in the United Kingdom in 2003 by
Vermilion, an imprint of Ebury Press
Random House UK Ltd
Random House
20 Vauxhall Bridge Road,
London SW1V 2SA

www.randomhouse.co.uk

Addresses for companies within
The Random House Group Limited can be found at:
www.randomhouse.co.uk/offices.htm

The Random House Group Limited Reg. No. 954009

A CIP catalogue record for this book
is available from the British Library

Penguin Random House is committed to a sustainable future for our business, our readers and our planet. This book is made from Forest Stewardship Council® certified paper.

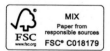

ISBN 9780091889661

Typeset by Palimpsest Book Production Limited,
Polmont, Stirlingshire

Printed and bound in Great Britain by Clays Ltd, St Ives plc

For Leonard Lauder
with admiration and much affection

The material in this book is intended for informational purposes only. None of the suggestions, advice or information is meant in any way to be treated as prescribing a treatment. Any attempt to treat a medical condition should always come under the direction of a competent physician. Neither the publisher nor we accept responsibility for injuries or illness arising out of suggestions, advice or information contained in this book so far as the law of England and Wales permits. I am only a reporter but one who has worked in the beauty and health industry for thirty years. I have a profound interest in helping myself and others to maximise the potentials for positive health which include being able to live at a high level of energy, intelligence and creativity. For all three are expressions of harmony within a living organic system and all play a vital part in deep beauty – the full expression of the unique nature of a man or woman.

Leslie Kenton
London 2003

CONTENTS

REVOLUTIONISE YOUR SKIN . . . RESHAPE YOUR LIFE

PART ONE:

THE LIVING MATRIX

dive into it . . . transform your skin forever

MY LIFE IN BEAUTY

a tale of obsession

I am a sucker for beauty. I always have been. It dazzles me, whether in the form of a man, a woman, a sunrise, or tiny shoots poking their heads through encrusted mud after a devastating flood. One way or another I have spent more than thirty years of my life working with beauty, writing about it, researching for product formulation and helping create skin-care ranges in the beauty industry.

For years I had a recurring dream: I am walking through a wood and come upon a tree so magnificent I cannot bare to look upon it. I never understood what the dream was telling me. Then one day I got it: true beauty – the dazzling uniqueness of a tree or a wonderful piece of music or a woman – be she 18 or 80 – in some way annihilates us. It takes us beyond what we feel comfortable with – to what physicists call *zero point* – a realm of no thoughts, no opinions, just a sense that we are at that moment in the presence of something wondrous.

'The absence of flaw in beauty is itself a flaw.'

Havelock Ellis

The Cave Of Beauty

To me there is nothing more beautiful than the unique nature of a human being – that 'seed power' within each of us which carries the genetic potentials of what we can become. Each man or woman boasts her own brand of seed power – a unique collection of physical characteristics, passions, needs, quirks and agendas. Like a stalk of bamboo in a Zen painting, the seed power of a human being is absolutely unique, yet carries with it a magnificent sense of the universal. The more freely and fully a person's seed power gets expressed in how they speak, think, look and live, the more beautiful they become. This is what I call *deep* beauty.

Real beauty is about authenticity coupled with the energy that comes from living your own truth instead of buying into somebody else's rules. The mythologist Joseph Campbell used to say that the best way

3

to live your life is to 'follow your bliss'. I think he's right. When you live this way, your eyes shine, your body grows stronger and your skin glows, no matter what your age. So much for inner beauty.

'to be nobody but yourself, in a world which is doing its best to make you everybody else, means to fight the hardest battle which any human being can fight . . .'

e.e.cummings

A Passion For Adornment

I also love the trappings and trimmings – the glory and glamour of lotions and potions, sparkling eyeshadows and shimmering lip-glosses. Since I was a teenager, my dressing table has been littered with colours and brushes, hair clips, bottles and sprays. They are my playthings for adornment and exaggeration. Like the ribbons nineteenth century women wove into their hair and bodices – mmm . . . sheer delight. The one thing beneath it all that every woman has longed for since the dawn of time is wonderful skin. We have long needed a real skin revolution.

I had a beautiful mother. She looked like a cross between a golden-haired fairy godmother and a Hitchcock blonde. Always impeccably dressed, my mother could walk through a barnyard in a white suit and emerge without a speck. Not me. I am a walking advertisement for what I ate for lunch, since most of it ends up down my shirt.

Cool Beauty

My mother was a cool beauty. She never shared with us her clothes, her jewellery, her cosmetics. Even to walk through her dressing room and touch them was a crime punishable by banishment. But she did share some important advice: first she taught me that beautiful skin matters. To maintain it, she insisted, you need just the right amount of sunlight – half an hour early or late in the day – *no more ever*. She was adamant I needed to eat natural foods and to supplement my diet with some judiciously chosen vitamins and minerals as well. Stay away from sugar and breads and pizzas, she insisted. Never go to bed without cleansing your face first, and nourish your skin to keep it soft and smooth with something really active – be it fresh papaya or an absurdly expensive but irresistible French night cream – to help repair cell damage that occurs during the day. It was she who taught me to fall in love with the ritual of nurturing my skin.

At first I balked at the idea. Then, in my mid-twenties I decided she was right. I began to make a little time each day to look after myself. I came to realise that the time a woman spends at her dressing table (this can be as simple an affair as a cardboard box covered with cloth at which you sit on a cushion) is a time of silence, solitude, and renewal. It is even better than meditation. And it's a lot more fun. I believe it to this day.

The Beauty Business

My involvement with skin beauty began in a big way when I was 32. I became the first Health and Beauty Editor for Harpers & Queen magazine in London. For that matter, I was the first 'health and beauty editor' anywhere. Why *health* and *beauty*? Because I figured these two aspects of a woman's life are so dependent on each other, that they cannot be separated.

'Beauty is power; a smile is its sword.'

Charles Reade

I was blessed with a remarkable Editor as my boss: Willie Landels, a man of vision, humour, intelligence and the best kind of sophistication. Willie gazed benignly upon my naïve American enthusiasm and my obsession with getting to the bottom of whatever I was investigating. He decided to place his trust in me. We worked together for almost fifteen years. Right from the first month he provided me with the freedom to write whatever I thought was important, and to say whatever I found to be true about it. In the decade and a half I worked with Harpers & Queen, only once did Willie question anything I wanted to write. It was a piece on outward bound for women. He insisted it was 'too downmarket'. Nobody ever changed anything in my copy – except to correct my abysmall [sic] spelling. Nor, after the first few weeks did anyone attempt to influence or control what I wrote.

Such freedom is a great blessing. It enabled me to delve deep into whatever fascinated me – from writing about how Lancôme formulated their first liposome to exposing the way plutonium, with its radioactive half life of 2,300 years, was being irresponsibly dumped into the Irish Sea from Britain's nuclear fuel reprocessing plant in Cumberland. (That was kind of scary. After the article appeared my telephones were tapped for more than a year and my London flat broken into although nothing was stolen.)

Commercial Pressures

In the magazine world, a beauty editor (nowadays most hold the far grander title of 'Beauty Director') is continually bombarded by the publisher and advertising director at the magazine to write about products from cosmetic companies who have bought advertising. Harpers and Queen was no exception. Within the first fortnight, I was approached by its Advertising Director, Terry Mansfield – who later became Managing Director and Chairman of the National Magazine Group in Britain. Terry told me that one of the cosmetic giants had just bought an expensive double paged spread to promote some new skin cream. Would I please make sure I wrote glowing words of praise about the product in our next issue, he requested.

With puritanical American blood surging through my veins, I was shocked. (I suspect, a wee bit self righteous too.) 'But Terry,' I whined, 'I can't do that. I can only write about what *I believe* in. If I wrote that kind of stuff, our readers would never come to trust me. Your advertisers don't want to buy space in a magazine its readers can't trust. Do they?' I think Terry was so stunned by my naïvete that he didn't quite know what to say. When Willie, the editor, learned about my response to Terry's request, he smiled a secret smile. A year later Harper's beauty advertising had doubled. Soon after it tripled. Terry never brought up the subject again.

Gradually my articles on health and beauty – some of which, I suspect were too technical for anybody (including me) to fathom – attracted a wide audience. An 'inside joke' began to circulate. It was said that the reason why my stuff was so widely read was that, although nobody understood a word of it, nobody wanted to admit this so they just kept on buying the magazine.

Enter The Professionals

As my audience grew, big cosmetic companies in the United States, France and Japan began to approach me asking if I would help them develop and market their skincare products. Leonard Lauder, Estée Lauder's son, head of the Lauder companies, was one of them. Leonard, a remarkable man for whom I have enormous respect and affection to this day, asked me if I would create a range of products for him and then run the new company. It was to be called 'Prescriptives'.

'Beauty is its own excuse for being.'

Proverb

It sounded fun, but I am such a bloody-minded, independent creature that I could not imagine myself working for Estée Lauder or any other any corporation. After all, I even carried out my work for Harpers & Queen as a self-employed woman, free to come and go as I pleased. I turned down Leonard's offer.

I have only had one job in my life. It lasted three days. At the age of seventeen, between my freshman and sophomore year at Stanford University in California, I landed myself a summer job, working in the collating and duplicating department of Capitol Records in Hollywood. I loved it – stapling documents, stuffing envelopes. Trouble was I would finish my work by 11 in the morning. And although they had no more work to give me they wouldn't let me read my novel. It turned out I was supposed to *pretend* to be working – something I couldn't manage. So I quit. That was the beginning and the end of my work experience. I have never had another job. I don't even have a CV. Just as well. I wouldn't know how to write one.

Beauty Of Body And Soul

In the early eighties, instead of formulating cosmetics, I wrote my first book – *The Joy of Beauty*. It was (still *is* for that matter – since in one incarnation or another, it has remained in print ever since) a 'monster' of a book. It was commissioned by Hodder & Stoughton. On receiving the manuscript, Eric Major, Hodder's managing director, horrified by the size of what I'd written, decided they could not afford to publish it. A year later it was published, first by Doubleday in the United States and soon after by Century – now Random House – in the United Kingdom.

The Joy of Beauty looks at beauty not only as totally dependent on high level health, but as nothing less than the *full expression of the individual nature of a woman.* To be beautiful, I believe, you must dare to be who you *are*, not try to fit in with somebody else's idea of what you 'should' be.

'. . . and then the day came when the risk to remain tight in a bud was more painful than the risk it took to blossom.'

Anaïs Nin

What Lies Beneath

Fifteen years ago I became disgruntled over the hypocrisy surrounding 'natural' skincare and toiletry ranges. High Street shops are full of them as are pharmacies and worldwide franchises which blow their own horns about all the good they are supposed to be doing for people and planet. Most of the products they sell are anything *but* natural. Yes, they have the odd chamomile extract or peppermint promise, but these so-called 'naturals' are chock-full of chemical preservatives, colourings, sequestering agents and fragrances to pollute the body and undermine health and beauty. Most of the time the companies who market and the people who sell such products don't even know themselves that they speak 'with forked tongue' as they sing the praises of the 'natural' lotions and creams they sell.

Private Labels

Few cosmetic companies manufacture their own products. Private label manufacturers do the work for them. Manufacturers are inclined to tell the companies they make for whatever story fits with the marketing brief they have been given. Seldom do they reveal the whole truth about what lies within the formulations they produce.

Eventually, the widespread sham endemic in the natural skincare market made me feel that I wanted to do something different. I made up my mind I would create an *authentic* natural range which would take the best that nature has to offer – from properly extracted, pure organic essential oils to truly active herbal extracts – and create something of real power with them. I wanted to be free to tell the truth about what was and was not present in products sold. If we needed, for instance, to use a paraben to preserve a product (99.9 per cent of all skincare products still do), I figured we should be honest about it. Then, once we worked out a more natural way to prevent contamination, I figured we would switch over to that instead. I wanted to create a *genuinely* natural range. And I wanted to call it 'Origins'.

New Ethos

My vision for the range was this: let's take power from the earth to enhance the health and beauty of human beings who can then return power to the planet and each other by living out more of their own beauty and authenticity. I wanted to make a range which would not only *tell* the truth, but *be* the truth. I went to see Leonard Lauder and told him about my intention. 'This is what I want to do' I said. 'Do you want to do it with me?' Leonard became as excited about the project as I was. Standing in the midst of a mountain stream in Aspen Colorado we agreed: I would conceive and create the Origins range.

'I discovered the secret of the sea in meditation upon a dewdrop.'
Kahlil Gibran

It was both enormously challenging and great fun. I had done product development before as a consultant, but this time it was different – this was *my baby*. I travelled the world seeking the best of everything – organic essential oil suppliers in southern France, a wonderful little ink bottle in Germany which we used to package a precious eye serum. I wanted the range to be fresh, new and completely different from traditional Lauder brands. It had to have its own ethos, its own spirit, its own style. Leonard, whose expertise in marketing is matched only by his respect for vision and invention and his skill at finding creative people then giving them their head, virtually gave me carte blanche to do what I believed in.

I knew Origins needed its own space, so we found a big loft at 250 Park Avenue South, in Manhattan. Rejecting the Lauder designer's proposed office designs (they reminded me of overstuffed hotel lounges), I insisted we fill our offices with rainforest plants, tiled floors and slab doors for desks. That done, we set to work to create the Origins range.

Now worldwide, Origins has long since grown up. It is a lovely range, although by no means everything I had wanted it to be: I wanted also to provide *internal* nutritional support for skin, as well as skincare and makeup products. I wanted the products to be completely without chemicals (none of the cosmetic giants have worked out how to manage this one yet). And I wanted to create even more products to uplift, relax and strengthen people on a psychological and spiritual level than we did in the end. But still Origins was a source of great satisfaction. It was wonderful to see my first dream of a unique range of cosmetics come to birth.

After I finished work on Origins – I was no longer associated with the range after that – I became Beauty Director of Mirabella magazine, still nurturing the idea that to do the best for skin you need effective internal products as well as creams and lotions. They need to be easy to use, effective and able to enhance the looks and functioning of skin in medically measurable ways.

Skincare From Inside Out

In the early 90s, a biochemist whom I had known for several years (it was he who launched Efamol evening primrose oil in the UK), told me about 'the world's first internal supplement for skin that really works'. Made from protein fractions and glycosaminoglycans (mucopolysaccharides) taken from marine cartilage, it had been created by two Swedish scientists, Ake and Atti-la Dahlgren. It was called Imedeen. He suggested that we form a company together and introduce Imedeen to Britain.

'The only tyrant I accept in this world is the "still small voice" within me.'
Henry David Thoreau

I never believe anything until I experience it or see it happen before my eyes. Marine cartilage sounded pretty fishy to me. My biochemist friend was quick to counter my scepticism. He told me that the formula had been extensively researched for several years, then tested by scientists and dermatologists in Holland and elsewhere. He showed me papers of studies done in European hospitals. I said, 'Well, let me try it and see what I think.' Several weeks later, pleased with my results, I rang him and said, 'OK. Let's have a go.'

Together we formed a company. A few months later we launched the product. I wanted to tell only the right person in the press about it – someone who had brains and integrity – a good investigative journalist. So I approached Newby Hands. Newby was then writing for the Daily Mail. Soon after, she left the Mail to become Health and Beauty Director for Harpers & Queen. There she has remained – doing a far better job for them than I ever did.

Newby was as excited as I about the new technology. She gave Imedeen a full page spread in the Mail. Several national television programmes were keen to know about the world's first, hospital tested, internal treatment for skin too. The product took off like a rocket. The success of Imedeen surprised even me. In two and a half years, without advertising, we took sales from zero to £2.6 million a year. But I was still obsessed with the idea that there is more that can be done to help us realise our skin's full potential for health and beauty. I just did not know what.

Hounded Into Writing
Meanwhile, for several years my publisher at Random House, Amelia Thorpe, had been hounding me to write another book on ageing. Under the onslaught, I finally gave in. I began to research the subject in a way I had not done since *Ageless Ageing* – fifteen years before. I soon became excited by what I was finding out. I saw that, as yet little known, late-twentieth century discoveries had been made about human

health, which were of major importance to skin beauty and preventing skin ageing: the Human Genome Project and the influence of good *gene expression* on skin, Stanford endocrinologist Gerald Reaven's identification of the *Syndrome X* epidemic and its relationship to degenerative conditions, a number of quantum leaps in clinical understanding of how to enhance the cellular energy on which skin radiance depends, and knowledge about how to prevent excess glucose in the body from combining with collagen proteins, causing skin to wrinkle and sag.

'True progress quietly and persistently moves along without notice.'
St. Francis de Sales

Having written two books as a result of my research, *The X Factor Diet* and *Age Power*, my passion to find deeper, more powerful ways of preventing and reversing age damage to skin was greater than ever. I began to experiment with the possibilities.

Come The Revolution

I was amazed at what I found. Although as yet little applauded, a revolution is taking place in skincare. What can now be done to protect skin from damage, to transform its look, to improve how it functions and feels, bears little resemblance to what was possible even ten years ago. I learned how each of us, armed with new knowledge, can take action ourselves to reverse signs of ageing, by making simple changes in the way we eat, live and care for our skin.

This is how *Skin Revolution* came to be written. This book is the culmination of years of on-going research into the nuts and bolts of beauty on every level. Working on it has been an exciting journey for me – one which has taken me from investigating the skin enhancing properties of a cream made in Chile from the slime of snails, to learning paradigm breaking discoveries about how light energy behaves in living skin. I uncovered hidden truths about sunscreens, skin cancer and the build up of ubiquitous chemicals in our environment, and why and how the skincare products we use can seriously undermine both health and beauty. Even more important, I learned simple, efficient ways of eliminating the toxic burden skin carries, allowing its own metabolic functions to take over, and bring about natural regeneration and rejuvenation. All of these things and more have opened a new universe of possibilities for enhancing skin beauty. I hope you will be as surprised and excited as I am by what you will find here.

Living Matrix – The Next Challenge

As a result of the research I did for *Age Power* and for this book, my love affair with beauty and my passion to work with it at its cutting edge, have brought me to something else too – something brand new and equally exciting.

For years cosmetic company executives in Europe, America, as well as Japan have asked me why have I never formulated my *own* skincare range. My answer is always the same: 'there are lots of good skincare products on the market, why should I create yet another one?' I have insisted that I never would unless I came up with an approach to transforming skin so unique, powerful, and natural – something which works so well on skin that anyone who uses it decides they would be crazy to go without it – that it *had* to be made.

Well, it has happened. Out of my research, and with the inspiration and help of the scientists and physicians I have worked with and learned from, I have created a unique skin product based on an approach to skin health and beauty at the deepest metabolic, energetic and architectural levels. Worthy of the name 'revolutionary', it is called Living Matrix Mist™.

Synergistic Skin Support

Its name comes from the body's living matrix itself – a multi-dimensional continuum of cellular activities on which the skin is utterly dependent to maintain a high degree of dynamic order, energy and structure on which skin health and beauty depend. Living Matrix Mist™ is designed to be used by every skin type, sex and age, from 15 to 115. You spray it on your face at the same time as you brush your teeth – morning and night. You can also use it during the day whenever you need uplifting or your skin feels in need of help. Even over makeup it does the job.

The purpose of Living Matrix Mist™ is simple: to provide skin with a synergistic composite of everything it needs – in natural, biologically active form – both to protect it from damage and to enable it to reach its highest potential for health, beauty and order on a cellular and molecular level regardless of its age or condition. Living Matrix Mist™ provides the natural nuts and bolts skin needs to function optimally. It is skin's own natural metabolic processes that work the wonders.

'Order is the shape upon which beauty depends.'

Pearl Buck

A Passion For Beauty

This is the story of how my obsession with beauty led me to *Skin Revolution*. I hope what you find in the pages that follow will inspire your own personal revolution. May it help you to take control of your own skin health and raise your skin to new heights of beauty whatever your age, sex or challenges right now. As my personal skin revolution has been, your own skin revolution is likely to be, sometimes fascinating, sometimes challenging, yet incredibly rewarding. More than a few 'sacred cows' may have to be sacrificed along the way. But then that's part of the fun of making powerful changes and learning to do things in new, more powerful and effective ways. Enjoy it.

LESLIE'S FIVE DAY
FACELIFT DIET

activate your living matrix

When it comes to skin – how it looks, feels and behaves – the quickest way to improve it is my Five Day Facelift Diet. It can firm contours and soften lines. It brings a glow to your eyes and radiance to your face. Most people also feel a new vitality, and experience freedom from cravings for sweets and renewed emotional balance. it's a great way for a quick face, body and energy makeover when you feel you need one.

Based on cutting-edge scientific information about the kind of foods our bodies have been programmed to thrive on for over one million years of human evolution, as well as the *biophoton* – light carrying – power of fresh raw vegetables, Five Day Facelift is a powerful programme to counter slackness, quell inflammation, and ameliorate bags and sags. It can bring you a quick taste of the kind of long lasting skin transformation which is possible from inside out.

'Whatever you can do, or dream you can, begin it. Boldness has genius, power and magic in it. Begin it now.'

Johan Wolfgang von Goethe

FAST RESULTS YOU CAN SEE

The Diet Helps:

- ❑ Firm skin.
- ❑ Detoxify skin.
- ❑ Clear puffiness.
- ❑ Smooth fine lines.
- ❑ Counter cross linking which causes wrinkles to form.
- ❑ Prevent irregular pigmentation.
- ❑ Enhance skin's immune functions.

- ❑ Reduce inflammation.
- ❑ Increase radiance.
- ❑ Make eyes shine and spirits soar.

'We all have big changes in our lives that are more or less a second chance.'

Harrison Ford

Help When You Need It

'I spent a fortune on cosmetics, last year,' a friend told me recently. 'Nothing seems to help. My daughter is getting married in two weeks, what should I do?' I suggested she see what my Five Day Facelift Diet could do for her. Sceptical, but having run out of alternatives, she decided to give it a go. That was a Saturday night. She gathered together all the foods she would need on the Sunday, cleared the coffee, sugar and breakfast cereals from the cupboard, and dived in on Monday.

When I saw her a week later she looked great – a good ten years younger – with shining eyes, improved contours and a great glow. I asked her if she was pleased. 'Pleased? I am over the moon,' she said. 'This morning someone asked me if I had fallen in love I looked so good. Oh and by the way, I've lost six pounds. Why did you never tell me about this?'

Let's just look at the diet itself so you can get started right away. Then we'll explore how and why it works so well.

YOUR OWN FIVE DAY FACELIFT

You will be eating delicious foods. Always take something raw at the start of each meal. This will not only supply your body with high levels of antioxidant-rich phytonutrients and enzymes for efficient digestion, it also helps protect from mucus-producing immune reactions which can lead to water retention and make skin puffy. The food choices are simple. You can even eat the same thing each day if you like so it's easy to remember. Or you can try some of the alternative meals from the Living Matrix 21 Day Turnaround (see page 201) if you want more variety.

HERE'S WHAT THE MENU LOOKS LIKE

ON RISING
- 200ml spring or purified water with juice of ½ lemon squeezed into it.

BREAKFAST
- 2 cups porridge made with steel cut oats (not 'instant oats' as they shunt too much sugar into your bloodstream too fast, and make it with water not milk).
- 1 grated or chopped apple or a handful of berries (strawberries, blueberries, raspberries, loganberries, blackberries – fresh or frozen).
- 1–2 tablespoons walnuts – preferably chopped but whole is OK (optional).
- 1–2 tablespoons almonds – preferably chopped (optional).
- 1 tablespoon cold pressed flaxseed added *after* the porridge has been removed from the stove.
- a dash of cinnamon (optional).
- 1 cup of green tea and/or 200ml of spring or purified water.

EVERY HOUR OR TWO
- 200ml spring or purified water.

LUNCH
- Raw Powerhouse Salad – an inspiring medley of brightly coloured crunchy vegetables – (see page 227 for How To) dressed with extra virgin olive oil and fresh lemon juice, garlic, herbs and seasoning. Eat it with . . .
- 100g to 200g of omega-3-rich fish (wild salmon, tuna – fresh or tinned – mackerel, sardines, herring etc.).
- a slice of melon (any kind but watermelon which is too high in sugar) or a handful of any kind of berries.
- 1 cup of green tea and/or 200ml of spring or purified water.

EVERY HOUR OR TWO
- 200ml spring or purified water.

DINNER

- 100g to 200g of any kind of fish, organic lamb's liver or tofu or an omelette.
- Large mixed green salad dressed with avocado, herbs, garlic, extra virgin olive oil and flaxseed oil, and fresh lemon juice or cider or balsamic vinegar.
- slice of melon (any kind except watermelon which is too rich in sugar) together with a handful of berries – fresh or frozen.
- 1 cup of green tea and/or 200ml of spring or purified water.

EVENING

- 200ml spring or purified water.

SNACKS (OPTIONAL)

If you want a snack, one of the following can be eaten twice a day either between breakfast and lunch, lunch and dinner or at bedtime:

- 50g chicken or turkey breast.
- 1 kiwi fruit or a small pear or apple.
- a handful of macadamias or walnuts.
- 200ml spring or purified water.

Lunch and dinner are interchangeable.

WHAT YOU WILL EAT

Protocol is simple. Foods are delicious and easy to prepare. For the next five days, you will eat and drink:

- ❑ Three meals a day.
- ❑ At least half of your foods fresh and raw.
- ❑ As many non-starchy vegetables as you like.
- ❑ As many top quality proteins at each meal as you like.
- ❑ 1 to 3 pieces of non sweet fruit.
- ❑ 1½ to 2 litres or more of pure water a day.
- ❑ A good balance of essential fatty acids – omega-6s and omega-3s.
- ❑ Two protein-rich snacks each day if you want them.

'Things do not change; we change them.'

Henry David Thoreau

THAT'S IT!

What could be simpler? If you're at home all day it's a cinch. (See page 248 for how to make – and dress in the same bowl – a protein rich salad – from start to table in five to ten minutes.) If you work in an office, make your Powerhouse Salad either the night before or while your porridge is cooking, put it in a container and take it with you. If you eat in restaurants, familiarise yourself with the myriad possibilities which can go into a Powerhouse Salad and tell the waiter what you want. Good restaurants are happy to oblige.

'We cannot become what we need to be by remaining who we are.'

Max Depree

The Penny Drops

I first became aware of what dietary change could do for skin more than thirty years ago. It happened before my very eyes. I was suffering from *endogenous depression* – where you feel blue and dejected all the time with no apparent reason. Three doctor friends taught me the natural way to detoxify my body and restore good enzyme function naturally using a high raw diet. Not only did the depression clear, my skin glowed.

Later, I learned how powerful a rejuvenator adequate quantities of the right kind of clean, pure water can be for skin. Only during the last three years spent researching the ageing process have the final pieces to the puzzle of how to use diet to regenerate and rejuvenate skin fallen into place. I learned about, and began to work with, new research into how sugar affects the body for good or ill and how our evolutionary inheritance governs the skin's response to what we eat, as it does that of the whole organism.

Stop Premature Ageing

Most skin ages long before its time. The fundamental processes behind premature ageing occur for reasons which, until now, skin scientists have tended to overlook: a starchy diet of convenience foods on which we have been living in the twentieth century – and which we are *still* being urged to eat – all those breakfast cereals, breads, pastas, dairy products and junk fats, undermines our health and predisposes us to degeneration. Why? Because such foods – recent twentieth century inventions – can wreak havoc with the skin. They are far removed from what our genes need to allow skin and body to thrive. In over a million years of evolution, we human beings have never had to handle anything like them. They don't match our genetic programming. Our bodies are unable to cope with them in quantity long-term. In time, the biological functions – on which beautiful skin and health depend – begin to falter and skin beauty breaks down.

The high-carbs-low-fat diet governments are still urging us to eat screws up our energy, makes us grow fat, tired and ill over the years and creates high levels of toxicity in the body. It encourages free radical damage, and undermines youthful skin functions destroying the contours of a face, making skin puffy, dehydrated, highly prone to allergic reactions and slack. Too much carbohydrate-rich food from grains and sugars raises blood sugar levels and screws up the way the hormone insulin behaves, flooding your body with excess glucose. Skin's collagen proteins react with sugar in destructive ways, making collagen fibres – on which the very architecture of skin relies – bunch up and crosslink. Crosslinking of collagen produces deep expression lines and loss of firmness. Enough of the bad news.

'The bond between the sugar and collagen generates a large number of free radicals leading to more inflammation. When glycation occurs in the skin, the ultimate effect is not unlike tanning a hide. Over time, skin begins to resemble a cross between beef jerky and an old boot, unevenly discoloured and heavily striated with deep lines and grooves.'

Nicholas V. Perricone MD

Major Turnaround Starts Here

The good news is that five days of dietary changes can not only trigger a major turnaround in how your skin looks, feels and functions. It can enhance over-all health and beauty and begin to reverse many visible signs of ageing. Even more important: seeing for yourself what the Five Day Facelift can do to change your skin whets your appetite for the deeper long term regeneration that comes later. You will learn in depth about why and how such changes happen, and how to make them a part of your own life in later chapters. Right now, see for yourself. Try it.

Biochemical Benefits

My Five Day Facelift brings specific benefits to the skin's living matrix on which beauty depends. (More about this amazing matrix, guardian of your skin's beauty, in chapters to come.) It enhances enzyme functions, eliminates wastes and provides the nuts and bolts – phytochemicals, minerals, trace elements and vitamins – which your skin needs for optimal health and beauty.

My five day diet is especially rich in omega-3 fats found in fatty fish and in flax oil. These vital nutrients – which few of us get enough of – counter inflammation. Inflammation is one of four major issues involved in skin ageing (see Sugar Baby or Lean Machine). Together with the omega-6 fatty acids from avocados, seeds, sprouts and nuts, these essential fats make available half of what skin needs to build and repair its cell membranes. The other half comes from plenty of good quality protein. A combination of the two is essential for your skin to manufacture strong, fluid, healthy cell membranes. When its cell membranes are well constructed, skin retains moisture well and the process of intra-cellular exchange of nutrients and oxygen, as well as the elimination of wastes, takes place as it is meant to.

Easily assimilated protein foods help your body's metabolic processes to balance the way it handles insulin. Insulin is not just a hormone important for diabetics. It is the most important hormone of all when it comes to how quick or slow your body ages. Protein in the foods you eat also provides the essential amino acids from which your skin's special fibroblast cells can manufacture new, fresh collagen.

Finally, don't forget pure water. Drink *at least* 1200ml a day. Double that if you can manage it. The water you drink performs several trans-formative functions for skin: fresh, clear water detoxifies wastes and clears puffiness. It carries to skin cells the nutrients and (this may surprise you) makes available the hydroelectric energy they need for peak performance. Water makes high levels of energy available to the whole of your body.

'Still around the corner there may wait, a new road or a secret gate.'

J. R. R. Tolkein

Energy Matters

The energetic aspects of internal and external skincare are at last begin-ning to be acknowledged by forward-thinking cosmetic chemists and a rapidly growing number of scientific researchers and doctors. We have too long been taught to think of skin only in *chemical* terms.

Emerging paradigm scientists are now turning to *biophysics* for answers as well. They are busy exploring why, for instance, a particular cream or lotion, or a diet high in fresh living foods, can alter dramatically the look and health of skin. Meanwhile, cutting edge energy medicine is advancing viable theories to explain many things which, in chemical terms, remain mysterious.

Energy matters. One of the developing world's largest cosmetic corporations discovered this for themselves when they purchased a company which, at the time had created one of the most effective (and expensive) creams in the world. They found – at first to their dismay – that they were obliged to play specific music, which enabled micro-organisms used in the production of this skincare product, to do the work of making the product effective. They still can't explain exactly why, when they did not do this, the cream they produced had lost much of its potency. Now, when the product gets made, the music gets played.

Life Energy For Skin

Energy is in no small part what makes a predominately raw diet the quickest and most powerful way to transform the look and feel of skin. When more than half the foods you eat consists of low or medium *glycaemic* bright coloured fruits and vegetables – the non-starchy, non-sugary kinds which don't raise the levels of sugar in your blood too far or too fast – you not only provide your skin with the best possible combinations of potent plant-based antioxidants, you supply your whole body with enzymes it requires to metabolise what you eat well.

Intrinsic to living foods, enzymes are essential to the beauty and vitality of skin. They are about as close as you can get to being carriers of 'life force' itself. Because the natural enzymes in our foods are destroyed when they are cooked or processed, the average modern diet is virtually devoid of enzymes. Your skin needs an abundance of good quality enzymes to digest your foods effectively, to assimilate nutrients, and to help direct metabolic processes on which health and beauty depend. Skin even relies on enzymes to dissolve away wastes and break down old cells and tissues, so fresh new ones can be made to take their place. Research shows that enzymes we take in from living foods support our body's own enzymic functions.

'. . . we know that there are mechanisms even in the human machinery that allow for the reversal of ageing, through correction of diet, through antioxidants, through removal of toxins from the body . . .'

Lydia M. Child

Forced to live on the average diet of too many cooked and processed foods, anyone's skin eventually becomes depleted of enzymes needed for building and repair. It loses vitality at a cellular level, and becomes prone to early ageing. Living foods help counter this.

Go For Colours

So do the newly-discovered *phytonutrients* they contain – plant factors such as sulphoraphane in broccoli, carotenoids in spinach and carrots, flavonoids in fruits. These bright coloured plant chemicals are even more powerful in their anti-ageing actions than the famous free radical scavenger vitamins and minerals we have been told we need more of in the past twenty years: vitamins A, E and C and the minerals zinc and selenium. Each plant-based wonder-worker brings its own cocktail of antioxidant, anti-ageing compounds to your skin, protecting it from free radical damage and enhancing its functioning. Some are powerfully anti-inflammatory. Others improve the way your immune system functions. A few – such as alpha lipoic acid (ALA) and the *proanthocyanidins* found in grape seeds – are almost universal in their anti-ageing effects on skin.

Drink Light

Raw foods also carry what German scientist Fritz-Albert Popp – a world expert on energy measurement in living systems – describes as *biophoton* radiation. He is talking about light – what the famous Swiss physician Max Bircher-Benner called *sunlight quanta*. By this, Bircher-Benner meant the energy from the sun on which all life depends. Biophoton energy is collected by plants during the process of photosynthesis. Such light-based energy is not only necessary for plants to live, but for animals, like us, who feed on them, to maintain high-level health. This is why Bircher-Benner in Switzerland, Max Gerson in Germany, and scores of other nature-oriented physicians throughout the world have used a high-raw or all raw diet for more than two centuries to help the body heal a wide variety of serious illnesses from *cancer* to *systemic lupus* as well as to reverse degeneration.

Like enzymes, biophotons are disrupted, disordered and destroyed when we cook our foods. No wonder living foods play a major role in skin regeneration and rejuvenation. My Five Day Facelift Diet and The Living Matrix 21 Day Turnaround Programme which follows make the best possible use of raw power to help you create lasting skin beauty.

Drink Order

When we consume *living* cells of plants in a raw state, the highly ordered *biophoton* radiation they carry becomes part of our own body. There it stimulates vitality, helps rebalance our own energies and optimises the functioning of skin. In no small part it is thanks to these phenomena that a woman who goes to a good spa or health farm is put onto a diet of raw foods and juices. (She is usually charged a small fortune for the privilege, as well.) After a week of such eating, a woman returns home looking five to ten years younger.

'One is not born a woman, one becomes one.'

Simone de Beauvoir

A Dead Giveaway

Human skin is one of the most highly developed organs in any living system. It even has its own 'immune system' as well as a network of neurological connections with the brain and body which makes it highly sensitive and responsive, both to external stimuli and to your emotions and biochemistry from within. When something goes wrong in your body or your life, your skin is a dead giveaway. If you have been binge eating or even eating in a way that is less than optimal (as all of us do from time to time) your skin shows it. When the body is a bit toxic, skin can become puffy, jowly, lined and lacklustre. When you are tired, skin loses its translucency and its surface becomes uneven. If your skin has a tendency to oiliness, this only gets worse. If it leans toward the dry, it can come to look and feel like that of an Australian crocodile. As your body goes, so goes your skin.

'Women have to harness their power – it's absolutely true . . . And if you can't go straight ahead, you go around the corner.'

Cher

KEY ELEMENTS FOR RENEWAL

DRINK LIKE A FISH

Why water? Water detoxifies skin and increases its bioenergy and radiance. Keep a bottle of spring or purified water with you throughout the day. This way it is an easy matter to get at least 1200ml of water a day – more if you can. (I swallow two or more litres a day as a matter of habit.) Ironically, water is essential in relieving skin puffiness. Puffiness comes because your skin retains water when it is attempting to dilute any toxicity present. Toxic skin is poor skin. It has poor colour, texture and form. Drinking purified or spring water helps clear it.

OMEGA-3 MAGIC

Major natural anti-inflammatories, omega-3 essential fatty acids are hard to come by when eating the standard Western diet. Inflammation is a major factor in undermining skin beauty and premature ageing. Flaxseed oil, oily fish, and walnuts – all good sources of omega-3 fats – help quell it. Your skin thirsts for them. They too play a central role in my Five Day Facelift Diet.

PROTEIN MATTERS

Few of us get enough good quality protein. In part this is because too many people – especially women – avoid protein foods, munching on carbohydrates instead. Protein is essential for strong healthy collagen and the formation of new cell walls which in turn are needed for optimal skin functioning and help keep skin well moisturised. It is also the central ingredient in the enzymes your skin needs to maintain (or restore) youthful radiance. If you are a vegetarian, eat fish. If you don't eat fish, use tofu or make omelettes instead.

COLOUR POWER

My Five Day Facelift Diet is rich in bright coloured low-glycaemic fruits and vegetables. They are just what your skin needs to supply it with optimal levels of vitamins, minerals and phytonutrients in a natural, synergistic balance. They enhance skin metabolism and make it look, feel and behave more youthfully. The antioxidant properties of these plant chemicals counter free radical damage, reduce inflammation, protect DNA, and enhance skin immunity.

IT'S COFFEE FREE

Coffee is a super villain when it comes to skin. Much as we love it (me too!), you need to stop drinking it – at least during your five day facelift. Coffee not only triggers inflammation which shows up on your face as dark circles, puffiness, fine lines, poor colour and highly reactive skin. It also raises blood sugar and disrupts insulin levels. To have great skin, insulin needs to be balanced. In as many as three quarters of people living on a Western diet the insulin/blood sugar balance has become distorted. This makes the body highly susceptible to early ageing – including ageing skin – and degenerative diseases. Remember this: the way insulin behaves in your body is the single most important *internal* determinant as to how rapidly or how slowly your skin ages.

GO GREEN

Rich in polyphenols – as many as 300 to 400mg per cup – green tea is the ideal skin drink. It is well established that these super antioxidant flavonoids it contains help prevent cancer. And, don't forget: what helps prevent cancer also helps prevent skin ageing. By contrast, black tea has been shown to increase the risk of some cancers. Green tea which, after water, is the most widely consumed drink on earth, also contains a small amount of caffeine – just enough to keep you bright but nowhere near as much as in coffee. If you are a coffee drinker, it can help you avoid some of the headachy cleansing reactions that can temporarily occur when you stop drinking coffee. If you are not a coffee drinker and you prefer to take no caffeine drinks, use *decaffeinated* green tea.

'How does one become a butterfly?' she asked pensively. 'You must want to fly so much that you are willing to give up being a caterpillar.'

Trina Paulus, Hope for the Flowers

YOUR FIVE DAY DIET SHOPPING LIST

Here is everything you will need for your Five Day Facelift Diet:

- ❑ Package of *non-instant* porridge oats.
- ❑ 6–8 apples.
- ❑ 2–3 packets of fresh or frozen berries (blueberries, raspberries, loganberries, blackberries).
- ❑ 100–200g shelled walnuts or macadamias (optional).
- ❑ 100–200g almonds (optional).
- ❑ 1 bottle of cold pressed flaxseed oil (must be refrigerated always – never heat this).

- ❏ 1 bottle of extra virgin olive oil.
- ❏ 5 to 7 lemons.
- ❏ A bottle of cider or balsamic vinegar for dressings.
- ❏ Cinnamon.
- ❏ 2 boxes of green tea bags.
- ❏ Fresh vegetables for Powerhouse Salad. Choose from what is in season and looks good. Here's a list for inspiration: broccoli, tomatoes, avocados, courgettes, red, green or yellow peppers, celery, radishes, garlic, cucumber, cauliflower, carrots, mung bean sprouts, broccoli sprouts, mangetout sprouts etc. fennel, beetroot, endive, celeriac, cabbage, mangetout, spring onions, red onions, turnip etc.
- ❏ 1 bulb of fresh garlic.
- ❏ Fresh green vegetables and herbs: Choose from what is in season and looks good i.e. spinach, rocket, endive, escarole, watercress, lambs lettuce, any kind of lettuce, basil, lovage, chicory, silverbeet, dandelion leaves, radicchio, mustard and cress, romaine etc.
- ❏ 500g minimum fresh, frozen or tinned oily fish i.e. mackerel, sardines, wild salmon, tuna, herring etc – *not smoked.*
- ❏ 500g minimum fresh or frozen whitefish or boneless chicken or turkey breasts or organic lamb's liver or a combination of all four.
- ❏ If you are a vegetarian, tuna and free-range eggs instead of meat.
- ❏ 2 pears and/or 2 kiwi fruit.
- ❏ 2 melon (any kind but watermelon).
- ❏ 8 litres (minimum) of spring or purified water.

Big Payoffs

Play it cool and follow the diet for five days. Payoffs will delight you. Not only will you be able to detoxify skin and get rid of a lot of puffiness, it can help calm inflammation, slow ageing, shed fluid retention, and redefine the natural shape of your face. It will also lift your spirits – once you have cleared your system of caffeine, alcohol and other superficial toxins. It can set you on the road to a whole new way of eating and living that may regenerate and rejuvenate your whole body.

If you have excess weight to shed, you might be pleasantly surprised to see the pounds melting away without crash dieting just from cutting out convenience foods riddled with sugar, junk fats and processed carbohydrates. My Five Day Facelift is *not* a slimming diet however. Eat as much as you feel comfortable with. Fat loss occurs naturally in some people simply because it supplies your body with foods which, thanks to your human genetic inheritance, it is programmed to thrive on. (More about exciting discoveries in these areas in Sugar Baby or Lean Machine.)

'The greatest contribution of science is not the discovery of new drugs, but the description of the 'built-in' healing systems possessed by all of us. Modern science shows that these systems are so easy to activate that one wonders how they become stalled in the first place.'

James L. Oschman PhD

EAT YOUR WAY TO BEAUTY

At the centre of *Skin Revolution* you will find two nutritional programmes: one is my Five Day Facelift Diet. It is great for preparing for a big event for which you want to look your best. It is useful in another way too: once you have seen for yourself how effective simple dietary changes can be in firming skin, eliminating puffiness, clearing fine lines and restoring radiance you will have had a taste of just how much transformation can be possible. Then you will be ready to experience mega-regeneration, with my Living Matrix 21 Day Turnaround Programme. It can make you *look* – and *feel* – fifteen years younger.

To kick-start your own skin revolution you need to take a few things on trust to begin with and just give it a go. Soon you will experience it all for yourself. Once you do you may come to look on my Five Day Facelift Diet as a 'secret weapon' – something you can turn to whenever you've been working too hard, eating or drinking too much or if fatigue, life troubles or jet travel has temporarily undermined your good looks and put a damper on your spirits. Experience what it can do for you first. Then you'll be ready to take your own skin transformation to deeper, more longer-lasting levels. Good luck!

BEAUTY WITH POWER

holistic beauty takes off . . . join the revolution

We stand at the brink of a revolution in beauty. Long awaited, its powerful ethos promises not only to transform our skin, it can even change our lives.

Like a phoenix, skin revolution rises from the ashes of fragmented thinking and commercial nonsense which has long dominated the cosmetic industry. The old thinking which it replaces has undermined our confidence and limited our ability to make full use of skin's potential for clarity, radiance and freedom from early ageing. The tools, techniques, lifestyle changes and formulations emerging with the revolution bring power to transform the way you look and feel in ways that have never been possible before.

Off With The Blinkers

For generations we have been looking at skin like blinkered horses. It's the way most dentists still view teeth – as something separate from the rest of the body. We spend endless money on quick fix solutions and yummy smelling creams which promise that some new 'miracle ingredient' will make us beautiful. An ingredient can be terrific, but it needs to come packaged with the synergistic nutrients and energy-enhancers your skin needs to function at its peak. Unless it does and unless it is relatively free of chemical preservatives, artificial fragrances and other chemicals, there is no way it can keep its promises. When our purchase doesn't do the job we are hoping for, we reach out to the next promise of help. More sags and bags appear. We sigh and try to borrow the glow we long for from a large glass of wine.

Now Is The Time

Skin Revolution boldly goes where few have gone before. Based on a deep understanding of the interconnectedness of the whole human being with skin beauty, it makes use of the power of life itself to work its wonders – activating enzymes, triggering energy production and balancing hormones. It protects from damage and initiates your skin's own repair processes. It helps you transform the way your skin looks and behaves in ways which simply cannot happen without addressing the deep processes by which skin manages and renews itself.

'The wrinkle is a serious disease. Do you know of anyone who gets up every morning and worries about illness? But everybody worries regularly about wrinkles . . .'

Albert Kligman MD PhD

Only recently has the science, technology, and biochemistry on which the revolution depends been available. Only in the past decade has science begun to grasp the importance for beautiful skin of supporting skin's *gene expression* on a cellular level. Until recently there was little understanding about how excess glucose in the blood – common because of the kind of foods we eat – triggers the formation of cross-linkage in the skin's architecture, making our skin sag and wrinkle. Even more recently, skin specialists have begun to devise ways by which these and other processes destructive to skin can be stemmed and calmed. We are also learning how to protect skin's DNA from damage. Pioneering dermatologists, molecular biologists and experts in genetics confirm the powerful effect that what we eat exerts on the look and health of our skin. The right combination of foods will not only protect from damage and age-degeneration; it can actually reverse it. These are only a few of the things *Skin Revolution* can help you accomplish for your own beauty.

SKIN REVOLUTION'S MANIFESTO

These are the self-regenerating principles on which *Skin Revolution* is based:
- ❏ Your skin is a dynamic, vital organ with enormous potential for self-repair and self-regeneration provided it gets what it needs to carry out its tasks.
- ❏ Your skin is functionally interconnected with the whole of your body – mechanically, biochemically, energetically – part of the *living matrix* on which health and beauty depend.
- ❏ What you do to your skin you do to the rest of your body.
- ❏ What you do to your body you do to your skin.

'The substrate for systemic interconnectedness is the living matrix, consisting of the connective tissues, cytoskeletons, and nuclear matrices throughout the body.'

James L. Oschman PhD

Biologically Active Skincare

What you will find here is a handbook of tools and techniques for biologically active skincare. It is a unique holistic approach to caring for skin based on a combination of emerging paradigm biochemistry and advanced skin technology. As such, it draws on some of the most important discoveries ever made about how the foods we eat affect the way our skin looks and behaves as well as how slowly or rapidly both it and your body as a whole ages. It shows you how you can deliver skin-enhancing non-toxic compounds as well as life-enhancing energies where they are most needed – to encourage your skin's best biological functions and create radiance no matter what your age.

Make use of the revolution's technologies, its techniques, its awareness of the wholeness of living systems and you can literally transform the way you look and feel. Ignore them at the peril of premature ageing and degeneration which neither expensive creams nor the scalpel of a skilled surgeon can counter. *Skin Revolution* does not exploit. It empowers.

'In every man's heart there is a secret nerve that answers to the vibrations of beauty.'

Christopher Marley

YOUR BEAUTY MATTERS

Anybody who says otherwise must be either blind, politically correct or in denial. Feeling good about yourself coupled with the self-esteem that makes it possible for us to live a free, creative and satisfying life, are all bound up with how we look and how we feel about how we look.

Self Denial Undermines Beauty
We Anglo-Saxons have ambivalent feelings about looking after our face and body. This is probably a legacy from our Ancient Greek cultural inheritance. The unconscious assumptions which come with it infer that the 'soul' is somehow superior to the body. On the one hand, we tend to neglect caring for ourselves, or we disassociate from our body thinking of it as more of a 'thing' than anything else. On the other, we externalise our bodies narcissistically treating them as possessions to be flouted or concealed as the whim takes us.

For some women, the body has become little more than a nuisance – an ungainly, ponderous shell in which they are forced to live. To others it is something to be criticised, prodded, pushed – even bludgeoned – into shape. It can never be good enough or thin enough. It's the wrong form, size, colour, texture. Then, when beaten down by onslaughts of self-immolation, we feel blue, we indulge ourselves with too much alcohol, too many biscuits or behaviour that not only denies our body's value, it even distances us from ourselves.

'No one can make you feel inferior without your consent.'
Eleanor Roosevelt

Sheer Exploitation
Little wonder. Our materialistic, commercially orientated culture makes use of our ambivalence about the body to exploit us. The muscular male with his 'killer abs' and the six foot anorexic blonde running across the pages of the tabloids constantly remind each of us that, whatever shape and size we happen to be, it is just not the right one. They whisper we are supposed to be *different*. We need this eyeshadow, that car, another PhD, three gorgeous new lovers, to fill the 'inadequacy gap'. How are we supposed to make things better? Why, by buying whatever the *purveyors of inadequacies* happen to be selling, of course. Only then are we allowed to feel more handsome, more beautiful, better about being who we are.

Except, of course, it never does. At least not for long. In trying to become something we are not, we lose touch with who we are. Then we are left with not a hope in hell of expressing our own authentic beauty or creating a life for ourselves out of our own values. The human spirit is far too vast, too deep, too rich in its individuality and infinitely too unbridled in its passions to ever conform.

Become Authentic

Being beautiful is about being authentic. It is a process of becoming who you really are. Beauty depends a lot on health, too. The subject of health is not on its own particularly interesting: have you ever noticed how many profoundly unhealthy looking people you can run into wandering the aisles of healthfood stores, desperately worried about how much bran they 'should' be swallowing?

A commitment to real health and beauty is not obsessional, nor is it a means of warding off anxiety through compulsive behaviour. It develops out of an awareness that radiant wellbeing provides the necessary foundation for a rewarding existence. Without it, we do not have the vitality, good looks, clarity of mind and emotional balance each of us needs to live life to the full and to do what we most passionately want to do.

Inside Story

The skin is not a superficial coating to your body – a bag meant to hold you together. Your skin is *alive* with a capacity for magnificently ordered activity. How alive depends on how alive the whole of you happens to be at any moment in time. Your body's largest organ, skin is one of the most reactive too – especially in the way it responds to changes in your metabolic state. It is the living interface between the inner world of your physical body and feelings and the outside world with which you continually interact. The way skin looks and feels reflects both your sense of self and your level of wellbeing. It's the face you show to the world. And, like a magic mirror, the world reflects back to you its sense of who you are.

SKIN TELLS THE TRUTH

When the body is free of toxicity and blood sugar and insulin levels are balanced, your skin glows. Fall in love and it radiates beauty. Plunge into depression; it responds by becoming slack, dull and lifeless. Your skin gives ever-changing, accurate measurement of your overall energy, vitality and emotions.

"'Healing," Papa would tell me, "is not a science but the intuitive art of wooing nature."'

W H Auden

Past Imperfect

For generations our understanding of how to care for skin has been distorted by the dream-sellers. Thankfully things are changing rapidly. You will see evidence of the skin revolution in the emergence of new biologically active non-toxic skincare products, salon-based or medical treatments, some of which use the energy of light itself – a medium by which skin cells communicate to work their magic. In part this is thanks to growing scientific evidence which shows that our exposure to chemicals in the environment, including those which skin continues to absorb from even the most prestigious skincare products, is slowly poisoning us.

The old dream-sellers would have us believe that good looks can be bought in a jar. Not so. A pot of cream is not enough. I don't mean you should throw out all your gorgeous smelling lotions and potions. But it is time to get savvy about what we do and don't choose to smear on our faces, or wash our hair with, and use to care for our bodies.

'Most cosmetic manufacturers will use any kind of slogan to make you disregard their ingredients.'

Aubrey Hampton

Come The Revolution

Much of what is sold in the name of beauty is not good news. It is past time that both the huge cosmetic corporations as well as the so-called 'natural' skincare manufacturers (many of whose products are anything but natural) shed their complacency. They need to invest heavily to clean up their act and clear out unnecessary and potentially dangerous chemicals from their products. In today's atmosphere of expanding pollution, such chemicals can build up and interact with each other, increasing our body's load of toxicity making us vulnerable to cancer, degenerative diseases and wrinkles.

Addressing the vital issue of making *effective* and *safe* cosmetics available demands that we, the public, put pressure on manufacturers urging them to develop new ways of formulating products which deliver *no potentially harmful chemicals at all*. In turn, this depends on our coming to understand the scientific truths which are making the skin revolution possible. We need skincare products formulated using 'organism-friendly' ingredients – substances and compounds which are not 'foreign' to our genetic makeup and which therefore are far less likely to cause harm or to contribute to the toxic overload which makes skin lose its radiance and renders our bodies highly prone to degeneration.

Chemical-Free And Effective

We need creams, lotions and shampoos formulated, preserved and fragranced in *truly* natural ways. Very few cutting-edge companies are doing this, although a growing number are trying to work towards it. Suzanne Hall, founder of the Living Nature range, leads the way. More than a decade ago this skilled, creative and ingenious New Zealand chemist created the world's first effective natural preservative systems, which nobody has so far been able to match. The Living Nature range of products is genuinely *natural*. Hall has been offered a small fortune for her inventions. More interested in creating ever more effective *completely* chemical-free skincare than she is in amassing a fortune, she still refuses.

Such spirit lies at the centre of the skin revolution and is just beginning to permeate every level of the industry. Even some multinational corporations are trying (without ruining their bottom line) to develop ways to get rid of chemicals like the *parabens*, common chemical hormone-disrupters still added to cosmetics and toiletries to preserve them. Parabens can damage DNA. In attempting to find their own solution some manufacturers – still few in number – are also taking part in the exciting transformation happening in skincare.

'I've only ever had one wrinkle – and I'm sitting on it.'
Jeanne Calment (the world's oldest woman,
before she died at the age of 122)

The Pioneers

The work of a growing number of forward-thinking plastic surgeons, dermatologists and scientists, whose research projects and clinical practices are based on holistic skin management, are also part of the revolutionary thrust. They are bringing about major paradigm shifts in the way we view skin problems – from acne to ageing.

Dermatologist Nicholas V. Perricone in the United States, and plastic surgeon Des Fernandez in South Africa, are among them. Perricone was one of the first to recognise the powerful rejuvenative effects which dietary change can have on skin. He advocates the use of natural anti-inflammatory and antioxidant, plant-based ingredients, both as ingredients in skincare products as well as taken in the form of nutritional supplements.

South Africa's Des Fernandez is a surgeon who knows more about how to use topical vitamins in their most effective forms to clear acne, regenerate skin, counter ageing and protect from UV damage than anyone in the world. His pioneering approach to biologically active skin treatment and his fascination with and dedication to skin beauty, is reflected in the products his company – Environ – produces. They make most of the vitamin C 'serums', vitamin E creams and harsh vitamin A analogues used by others look, at best, like the playthings of amateurs and, at worst, like actively destructive formulations capable of doing more long-term damage to skin than good.

Living Matrix Energy

In the early 1990s scientists like D.S. Coffey and K. J. Pienta developed revolutionary new ways of understanding and measuring how an organism functions in health and disease via its 'tissue matrix system' – the *living matrix*. This living matrix is a multi-dimensional, molecular continuum – a dynamic communications network which even has semi-conductor properties. It is a structural, biochemical, energetic, oscillatory informational network which integrates all of the body's parts and activities. The physiological and regulatory processes, on which the health of skin and of the body depend, take place within your living matrix. Support its functioning. It will reward you not only with beautiful skin but radiant vitality. The word matrix means 'womb'. Your living matrix is the womb out of which health and beauty continue to be born.

New England scientist Dr James Oschman, author of the paradigm-breaking book *Energy Medicine . . . The Scientific Basis*, is another of the pioneers whose work is important to the skin revolution. An articulate and exacting researcher, Oschman has evolved scientific explanations and ways of measuring the beneficial effects on the body of such diverse practices as the ancient art of yoga, the Chinese practice of qigong, laying on of hands and Reiki healing. They too influence the living matrix. When your matrix functions with a high degree of energetic order, your body is vital and resistant to degeneration. Your skin thrives.

Light Source – Skin's DNA

Meanwhile Professor Fritz Popp in Germany and Professor Hugo Niggli in Switzerland, together with scientists from Russia, Japan and Australia, have long been busy studying how subtle light energy – biophotons – behave in living tissue and charting their importance to health. Measuring the nature of this ultra weak but super important biophoton energy with the help of high tech equipment, they are able to identify healthy as opposed to diseased tissue. Biophoton measurements verify the vast superiority of fresh organically cultivated foods and the health-giving energy they carry when compared to conventionally grown foods. This complexity of energetic order is imparted to a person eating them.

Niggli worked in the research department of the cosmetic giant Wella for five years. There he created revolutionary models for measuring DNA repair in the skin's fibroblasts – those cells responsible for the production of collagen. He also showed that biophotons are emitted by the DNA of every skin cell.

The findings of these scientists, together with the work of the other pioneers, challenge the traditional view of how we look after our skin. They highlight the inadequacies of most skincare products on the market. Based on the latest 'miracle ingredient' and ignoring the inter-connectedness of skin and overall health, most formulations are far too limited in what they can offer. The pioneering work also points the way to a whole new ethos in skincare. We know now that it is possible to supply skin with a plethora of what it needs to make its *own* transformation happen from within, by activating its own natural regeneration power and that of the living matrix itself. There is no greater power for healing and transforming beauty than the living body's own. All we need to do is call it into action.

Genetic Truths And Falsehood

Are wrinkles inevitable? Are skin disorders the result of our genetic inheritance? Nowhere near to the extent that we have been led to believe. Yes, black skin tends to wrinkle less quickly than white. And yes, you have a greater chance of developing acne in teenage years if your father had it before you. But far more important than the genes you *inherit* is the way your genes are *expressed.* This means whether or not your genetic tendencies are empowered to create the *highest levels* of order by the living matrix. Or are they being expressed poorly as a result of matrix toxicity and energy depletion so you end up with eczema, early ageing, or some other problem.

Your own gene expression is governed by the quality of the fluid your cells are bathed in within your living matrix. This depends on the way you eat, handle stress and use your body, as well as on how great the load of chemical toxicity your body carries. Exposed to high levels of pollutants from water and chemicals in foods and household prod-ucts, and living on the standard modern diet, skin gets in trouble. Follow a *Skin Revolution* way of eating and looking after beauty and you strengthen your whole organism.

Empty Rhetoric

Bold statements abound in the media dismissing almost all skincare treatment products as fraudulent. With tough rhetoric, Anita Roddick, chairman of The Body Shop, decries the belief that skincare products do much of anything for skin. 'Moisturisers do work,' she often says, 'but the rest is pap.' Roddick's attitude is as wrong-minded as that of the dream-sellers who each month launch their latest 'miracle' product based on some exotic sounding ingredient accompanied by sensuous words designed to sell it.

The truth is, there is a lot you can do, both from inside and out, to protect your skin from premature ageing – most of what we call ageing *is* premature – heal skin problems, and even *reverse* degeneration.

'. . . the great increase in knowledge of the physiology of skin has brought the law and biology into conflict. The truth is that all topical substances, whether as simple as water or as complex as multi-ingredient moisturizers, inevitably will affect the structure and function of skin. No topical is completely inert.'

Albert M. Kligman MD PhD

As for the notion that skin products have no effect on skin, as you will learn in the pages that follow, this is utter hogwash. To experience your own skin revolution first hand, you need to throw out the macho rhetoric of the Roddicks of this world and the widespread 'magic bullet' notions used to formulate frothy creams preserved with potentially harmful chemicals. You also need to lose the chemical preservatives, artificial colourings and flavourings in convenience foods and the xenoestrogens in our air, water and foods. For the truth is virtually any chemical that comes into contact with your skin can be absorbed.

Skin Revolution offers an infinitely more powerful approach. It acknowledges the interrelatedness and interactions, not only between your skin and your body as a whole, but between our bodies and the environment in which we live.

Check Out Product Quality

New, more effective procedures for testing the effectiveness and safety of cosmetics are becoming available each year to support the revolution. Flow cytometry is one. It is a laboratory method useful for measuring the effect on functions of living skin cells of a particular compound or formulation – primarily by optical means. Ingredients are fed to live human cells in a laboratory to test whether or not a specific product or substance causes or quells inflammation, enhances or disrupts DNA, increases or decreases cellular energy. It is one of a number of useful technologies when selecting ingredients for new skin products and checking out the effects of formulated products on skin. So far only a handful of manufacturers are making use of it. To do so may challenge the integrity of products already on the market.

Major Alchemy

Thanks to a growing awareness of the positive effect nutrition can exert on skin, the practice of using nutraceuticals to improve its quality is expanding exponentially. Natural anti-ageing substances – from Acetyl-L-Carnitine and Coenzyme Q10 to Alpha Lipoic Acid (ALA) and the sulphur amino acids – are not only being used *internally* to prevent and reverse age degeneration, they are now being incorporated into a growing number of skincare products.

There is a major alchemy involved in creating skin beauty. Most natural compounds for which skin has an affinity travel with relative ease through the skin's surface to improve ageing or ailing skin. They can also support overall health, while enhancing good looks. Hyaluronic acid (HA), an important antioxidant and moisture-enhancer commonly used in skincare products, plays an important role in the functions and structures of the matrix itself. It is even being used as an *internal* supplement as well as in external products. Taken in a highly concentrated, low molecular weight form, it is believed to help lock in vital moisture and promote firmer smoother skin.

'Alchemy: the power or process of transforming something common into something special.'

Webster's Dictionary

Skin Enlightenment

New energy-based skin treatments and non-invasive technologies for professional skin treatments are being developed as you read. Take non-ablative skin rejuvenation – a treatment which does not remove the surface of the skin. It uses intense pulsed light at specific frequencies to restore youthful feel and function to aged or neglected skin. Similar light-based treatments can work other wonders: guided by the melanin (colour) in a person's skin, a few high tech machines are now capable of delivering a charge to hair follicles to disable growing hairs and allow unwanted hair to be shed permanently. This can be a god-send to women with 'moustache' problems and to men who since puberty have kept their shirts on at the beach, embarrassed about excessive hair on shoulders and back.

Then there is the exciting new grow-your-own-cell treatment. Known as Isologen, it may, before long, render injections of bovine collagen and silicon redundant. A person's own skin cells – fibroblasts – are harvested by a surgeon, cultured in a laboratory and later injected into areas of their face to clear lines, redefine smoothness, soften scars, and restore firmness and contours. Like dietary changes and some of the new biologically active skincare products, it is a procedure which aims to activate your body's *own* ability to create good quality collagen.

'What lies behind us and what lies before us are tiny matters compared to what lies within us.'

Ralph Waldo Emerson

The Holistic Revolution Starts Here
'Beauty is truth' Keats wrote. I believe he was right. Beauty is nothing less than the full expression of the unique nature of a man or woman's seedpower in the way he or she looks, feels and lives life from day to day. In my terms, becoming more beautiful is the process by which each of us becomes more who we really are – both at the very deepest levels and in the way we physically appear. In the realm of product development and marketing this 'truth' aspect of beauty becomes even more important. For too long sweeping statements have obscured what is true in the cosmetic industry. This too is changing as the revolution gains momentum.

'Though we travel the world over to find the beautiful, we must carry it with us or we find it not.'

Ralph Waldo Emerson

Why did I choose to write this book? Because I love beauty. I have always been fascinated with it in its every form, from the inner beauty and splendour of each unique human soul, to the fun of playing the makeup game as a way of emphasising individuality, shifting moods, or just making a face shimmer. Having spent thirty years of my life researching skin, health and beauty, writing about it, formulating and marketing internal and external products and playing with the most sensuous treatments and components possible to enhance skin, I think it is time I shared with others who may be as fascinated as I am by lipsticks, powder and paint (as well as what lies beneath), what I have learned and some of the exciting developments happening in beauty right here, right now. Skin is wonderful stuff. Together, let's make it even more wonderful.

ENTER THE MATRIX

get the glow

Beautiful skin vibrates with energy. All twenty-one square feet of it. Skin is not only your largest organ. It is a multi-dimensional interactive system of information, molecules, energy, cells and genetic messages – within your living matrix. Skin is also completely dependent on the matrix for its radiance. Learn about how the living matrix works, what makes it function at a higher level of order, and take action. You may even be able to turn a sow's ear into a silk purse. Many have.

Interface between your inner and outer life, skin both defines the boundaries of your body and interacts with it on every level, as well as with the environment in which you live – molecularly, energetically, chemically. Through the living matrix, your skin responds to the food you eat, the water you drink and the air you breathe, as well as to whatever gets shunted into it from the lotions, potions and cleansing products you use.

'Look deep into nature, and then you will understand everything better.'
Albert Einstein

From the moment you are born until the instant of your death, skin exchanges information. The quality of the chemical, energetic and psychic information it receives determines how it functions. The kind of information it gives out determines its beauty.

'The living matrix is a continuous and dynamic "supramolecular" webwork extending into every nook and cranny of the body: a nuclear matrix, within a cellular matrix, within a connective tissue matrix. In essence, when you touch a human body, you are touching a continuously interconnected system, composed of virtually all of the molecules in the body linked together in an intricate webwork.'
Dr James L Oschman

Outmoded Science

Most of what we think we know about skin is based on last century science. Meanwhile, the majority of skincare products are limited in their effectiveness because most cosmetic chemists don't grasp the necessity of treating skin synergistically. They are still looking for superficial answers – the latest 'miracle ingredient' they can pop into a liposome in the hope that it will do the trick. It doesn't.

Skin products can be 'double handed' too. By this I mean that with one hand a product can bring better moisturisation, while with the other hand it shunts into your skin any number of chemical preservatives, emulsifiers and texture-improvers with a potential to disrupt the biochemical and energetic order of your living matrix by polluting it. There is strong evidence that chemicals commonly used in cosmetics and toiletries build up over years to make the human body toxic, undermine its immunity and encourage early ageing. Chemicals in products can interact with each other too, forming mutagenic and carcinogenic compounds to age skin rapidly and encourage malignancies. All this stuff takes place within the living matrix itself.

'For the first time in the history of the world, every human being is now subjected to contact with dangerous chemicals from the moment of conception to death.'

Rachel Carson, *Silent Spring*

Your skin is also the body's most important sensory organ. Think how yours reacts to lovemaking, to fear, to embarrassment. The way skin reacts to touch is one of the earliest and most formative responses to life we make. It is essential for the physical and emotional growth of any human being. Because skin interacts so intensively, it is your body's most active channel of communication. In a very real way, it *talks* to your environment. Through skin we register affection, dislike, pain, pleasure, comfort and discomfort. Cool water is sensuous, delicious and uplifting. Sandpaper is not. A caress is bliss. A slap is nasty.

Miniature Universes

In some areas, like the eyelids, skin is a mere 0.05mm thick while on the soles of the feet it measures in at a hefty 5mm. Every square inch of this amazing organ contains 78 yards of nerves, 650 sweat glands, 10,000 cells, 1300 nerve endings and tens of thousands of sensory cells and apparatuses – each a miniature universe in itself. What does your skin do for the rest of you? Plenty.

A GOOD FRIEND

Skin does all these things for you:

Protects
- ❏ Its cushiony under layer protects from injury.
- ❏ Its sebum prevents moisture loss.
- ❏ Its melanin protects against UV damage.
- ❏ Its acid mantle wards off bacterial attack.

Keeps You Cool
- ❏ It controls and adjusts your body temperature.

Clears Wastes
- ❏ It excretes toxicity from your body.

Regulates Hormones
- ❏ It helps keep you young.
- ❏ It helps you feel good and look great.

Brings Bliss
- ❏ It carries exquisite sensations of pleasure and pain.
- ❏ It can make sex wonderful – or horrible.

'Commitment is never an act of moderation!'

Kenneth Mills

Sebaceous – oil – glands lubricate its surface and help it retain moisture. Hair follicles embedded within the matrix of nerves shunt sensory impulses to your brain creating exquisite sensitivity, both to touch from without and to emotional change from within. Glands called *eccrine* produce sweat to cool your body while *apocrine* glands, hidden within the skin's deepest layers, secrete compounds which make you more sexually attractive. Ultra responsive sensory nerves known as *Pacinian corpuscles* relay tactile messages to the hypothalamus nestled within your brain from where appetite, temperature, pressure and hormonal secretions are directed. Meanwhile, fine capillaries within the living matrix shuttle nutrients to all the layers of skin and cart away the toxic wastes of its cellular metabolism. They also help dissipate body heat when you feel on the verge of sweltering.

'When the nerve cells are stimulated physical energy is transformed into energy used by the nervous system and passed from the skin to the spinal cord and brain. It's called transduction, and no one knows exactly how it takes place.'
Stanley Bolanowski, Institute for Sensory Research, Syracuse University

BONE UP ON BASICS

The structure of skin used to be divided into three distinct layers: epidermis, dermis and subcutis. The top layer, the epidermis, is highly metabolically active. Yet, until quite recently, the metabolic activity of this layer was hardly recognised. The stratum corneum, the most superficial part, was long believed to be nothing more than a layer of dead cells, devoid of biological activity. Cosmetic chemists and dermatologists once believed it served no greater purpose than to act as a barrier against environmental activity. Now we know that intense metabolic activity takes place. We also know that most of what we smear on our skin or wash our bodies or hair in can be drawn deep into the living matrix.

Deeply Superficial

Knowledge about skin and how most effectively to treat it is increasing exponentially. New discoveries about human physiological processes natural to skin make it clear that the notion of treating the skin as separate from the rest of the body and looking on the epidermis as a 'superficial' shell are not only scientifically inaccurate, they can be actively dangerous. Changes in the skin's deeper layers, shifts in hormones or the effects both of prescription and recreational drugs, all affect *in direct ways* the functioning, appearance and health of the skin's surface. So not only can cosmetics and toiletries alter the health, energy and wellbeing of the matrix, so does what you put *into* your body, in a kind of 'garbage in, garbage out' scenario. Even how you think and feel affects how well your skin looks and functions.

Each layer of skin plays a different part in strengthening it and determining its appearance. Let's take a look at how:

'... the stratum corneum is in active and direct biological interaction with deeper, living layers. No longer do we have strict differentiation between the dead upper layer and the living deeper layers.'

Dr Wilfried Umbach

On The Outside

The outer layer, the epidermis, has at its surface the stratum corneum. The stratum corneum, lubricated by your skin's natural oils, forms a protective acid-mantle barrier essential for healthy, beautiful skin. Chemicals in the environment or from products, electro-magnetic pollution and excessive exfoliations, can breach that barrier making your skin vulnerable to allergy reactions, premature ageing and discomfort. Not only the outer layer of the skin, but all that lies beneath, is highly vulnerable to damage from many sources. The stratum corneum influences many of the enzyme systems on which youthful, beautiful skin depends. Unless it retains its integrity and maintains a controlled moisture content thanks to a good balance of specific lipids, your skin hasn't a hope in hell of realising its potential.

So powerfully do cells in the stratum corneum interact with those of the skin's deeper layers that they directly influence the way the living matrix itself functions, regulating its ability to create new healthy cells. When the lipid composition of the outer layers are altered, or if its natural ability to hold moisture gets disrupted by the use of unsophisticated skincare products or chemicals, coherence of the stratum corneum is undermined. This can be a significant cause in the development of pathological skin conditions from eczema and psoriasis to rapid ageing of skin and acne.

'Never eat at one sitting more than you can lift.'

Miss Piggy

KNOW YOUR ENEMIES

❏ Chemicals common to skincare products can cause inflammation, free radical damage and distortions in acid/alkaline balance.

❏ Excessive exposure to wind, weather and excessive sunlight dries, distorts the skin's functions and ages it.

❏ The wrong diet or prolonged stress depletes the living matrix of energy, nutrients, enzymes and metabolites which it needs to support skin function and looks.

❏ Neglect destroys beauty. Skin needs loving care, day in day out, to thrive.

❏ Exposure to ionising radiation from microwaves, computers, television and mobile phones and mounting electronic pollution in the environment can cause serious (and as yet largely unrecognised) disruption to the health of the matrix and progressive dysfunction in skin.

Relative Truths

Let's look even closer: the epidermis is made up of layers of stratified cells like shingles on a roof. These cells are the first to react to whatever is going on outside your body, whether it is hot or cold, irritating or soothing. They then transmit chemical and energetic signals, which in turn influence functional processes in the skin's deeper regions. All this activity flows through the matrix which encompasses all the layers. The cells at the basal layer – the bottom of the epidermis – are produced by *keratinocytes*. They become the building blocks of the outer skin and are forever displaced by new generations from below. In their journey towards the surface they develop ever more keratin – the protein which helps protect your skin from invasion – shed their nuclei, and finally die to create the skin's horny layer, the stratum corneum, at the surface. Cells right on the skin surface – *corneocytes* – are chock-full of keratin plus lipids to protect the skin beneath from moisture loss. The whole cell turnover process takes about a month. What you do right now to help your skin, whether it be the Five Day Facelift Diet, introducing an effective skin cream, or swallowing an internal product such as fish cartilage or omega-3 fats, will show its benefits progressively so your skin will get better and better as each week passes.

'Beauty without grace is the hook without the bait.'

Ralph Waldo Emerson

Through Thick And Thin

When skin is young and healthy, its epidermis is thick. As you get older, or if you have unwittingly abused your skin through poor skincare or using the wrong kind of product, the epidermis thins leaving the skin much more vulnerable to chemical and physical damage. In the lower epidermis your *Langerhans cells* act as immune watchdogs to guard against invading pathogens, while *melanocytes,* those which produce the pigment melanin, give the skin its natural colour and help protect it from sun damage. Last, but certainly not least, nerve cells called *Merkel* send messages to your brain to register sensation.

Deep Diving

The subcutaneous layer is your skin's most internal realm. It is packed full of fat layers to provide cushions for internal organs and systems, as well as a resilience and a firm yet soft quality and feel. Here in the subcutis, fat cells are interwoven with blood vessels, bundles of nerves and shards of muscle fibre and connective tissue fibres. This deepest layer acts as a protective cushion for what lies above it and draws from the blood stream nutrients and oxygen to feed the whole organ – all the while producing plump, even, smooth contours associated with youth, evident to the eye.

Try this. Gently stroke your fingers over the surface of the opposite hand. Now, do it again but this time exert more pressure. Notice how it has a completely different feeling? When you press firmly, you are stimulating the deeper layers of nerves within your skin. When you stroke lightly, you are triggering nerve endings closer to your skin's surface.

'Most of the over-the-counter products will actually improve your skin for a couple of weeks, but the results aren't very long lasting. What you need is a regimen that will get your skin healthy from the inside out.'

Elizabeth Kinsley, MD, Plastic Surgeon

Structural Support

The dermis, which used to be referred to as the 'living layer' of skin, is nestled safely between the stratum corneum and the subcutis. It attaches to the epidermis through a myriad of 'fingers' which tie the layers together within the living matrix itself. The dermis is filled with tiny capillaries, spiralling all the way through each layer. It is here that you find many of the nerves which make us so sensitive to deep touch.

The dermis, once considered the 'true' skin, is the skin's main supportive area. It is from here that most of its strength, elasticity, smoothness and contour originate. Within a mass of dense connective tissue, cells and extra cellular fibres are immersed in the gel-like basal substance of the matrix. It forms the skin's seedbed of vitality for good looks, feeds all its cells, transfers oxygen throughout and carries the wastes of metabolism away. Collagen is present in several different forms and large quantities in the dermis, to create the skin's architectural structure – an extracellular protein, synthesized by *fibroblasts* – the master cells of connective tissue. Elastin is just what it sounds like: fibres of material designed to let your skin move with each change of expression and then to return to a normal, relaxed state afterwards.

ELEMENTAL SUPPORT

Collagen is high in silicon, the remarkable mineral which has the ability to form lengthy complex molecules by binding with other elements. When it allies itself to magnesium and calcium, it creates firm bones, beautiful hair and nails and helps keep your body free of cellulite. Fibroblasts need optimal quantities of silicon as well as vitamin C, the bioflavonoids, copper from dark green vegetables and shellfish, and zinc to make good quality new collagen. Research going back more than 20 years shows that supporting the body with optimal quantities of these elements helps prevent collagen breakdown and stabilises the skin's structures on which youthful and beautiful skin depend. Elemental support can also undo much of the damage already done from neglect or poor nutrition.

Collagen is the most abundant protein in your body. It configures itself in many forms depending on the job it has to do. Some bundles of collagen are ideal for the twisting and flexing of tendons to join together and bond muscle, others form the lining of arteries and veins.

In beautiful, healthy skin, collagen lies in flat, crisscrossed helical bundles. These fibres are like the warp and weft of fine cloth. So long as they remain smooth and ordered your skin stays young-looking and firm. When fibres in the dermis start to bunch up and harden to cross-link, they become disorganised and all hell breaks loose. Skin begins to sag, wrinkle and age rapidly.

'Nature composes some of her loveliest poems for the microscope and the telescope.'

Theodore Roszak

Toxic Tatters

Back in 1908 Elie Metchnikoff – the scientist who discovered white blood cells – wrote a brilliant book called *The Nature of Man*. It has a lot to teach us about how to create perfect skin and about the cause of early ageing and skin problems, as well as how to *recreate* beautiful skin that needs resurrection. Metchnikoff pointed out that the vast majority of diseases occur because of the build up of toxicity. When this occurs in the living matrix, everything from acne to premature ageing can take hold. Prevent toxicity and you hold back the hand of time. Eliminate it and you rejuvenate skin.

Most drugs are toxic to the body as are most of our manufactured foods. The skin's extracellular matrix – the biological terrain in which its cells live – cannot carry out the tasks the skin is meant to perform when toxicity rises. Unless your skin goes through an *effective* process of detoxification, no amount of expensive face creams or surgical procedures will make a significant difference to it.

'... virtually all disease manifestations are reactions to, and interpretation of, the body's exposure to toxins.'

E. Metchnikoff, The Nature of Man

Terrain Is Everything

Louis Pasteur formulated the 'germ theory of disease' on which our form of drug-oriented orthodox medicine is built. It is based on the notion that disease is caused by exposure to pathogens such as bacteria or viruses. Kill the beasties, and you will fix the problem. Most doctors still believe this. What they don't know is that Pasteur, on his death-bed, completely repudiated his germ theory of disease. Instead he postulated that disease is *not* fundamentally caused by pathogens, but that it is a result of a bacteria or virus being able to get a destructive hold on the body only when the body's internal state becomes depleted, weakened and disordered enough. Pasteur grieved over his mistake, after a lifetime of searching for the truth. Literally breathing his last breath, Pasteur cried out, 'The pathogen is nothing, the terrain is everything.'

These words should be written in stone when it comes to looking after your skin. They also point the way towards your being able to clear skin problems and reverse degeneration. Here's the bottom line: having beautiful skin means creating your own way of living, eating, exercising and handling the demands of stress in your life so all the skin's energetic, chemical and physical activities take place within a vital, unpolluted living matrix. Only then can skin function at its best. Only then will lasting beauty be created. This is true at any age. You can be sixty and have the skin of someone 25 years younger than your chronological age, or 20 and have the skin of someone 15 years older.

'The most effective theory for promoting effective detoxification is a healthy dose of common sense. Avoid putting poisons in your body in the first place. Don't smoke; drink little or no alcohol; don't breathe polluted air; avoid caffeine; drink plenty of water that's been filtered; stay away from harmful chemicals, including solvents and pesticides; use medications only when absolutely necessary.'

Michael Murray ND

Ageless Skin Becomes A Reality
Skin Revolution helps you move progressively towards a way of living, eating and caring for yourself that makes this possible. It can quite literally transform your biochemical, energetic and physical terrain. The bonuses? You won't believe how many there are until you experience them for yourself first hand. Here they are: more energy, a higher level of health, creativity and even greater self esteem. Why? Because skin and brain, immunity, muscles and hormones, psyche and creativity all require the very best possible terrain – the most active, ordered and dynamic living matrix, to live at its peak. It needs to be bathed in a medium largely free of toxicity so the enzymes which guide metabolic processes can work skilfully, and your skin experiences the very highest level of genetic expression.

Gene Power

In recent years, thanks to vast amounts of information and billions of dollars spent mapping human genes through the Human Genome Project which focused on analysing the almost six billion pieces of DNA that make up our human inheritance, we have been bombarded with dazzling claims about genetics. This gene we are told controls this disease. Add an extra gene here or there and you can manipulate life itself. Yet in the midst of all the hullabaloo, the most important truth about genes – especially in relation to skin health and beauty – has been almost completely ignored. Here it is: it is not the genes you *inherit* which are the primary determinant of the health and beauty of skin – indeed of the whole being. It is the way the genes you inherit are *expressed.* Gene expression is a scientific term which is really important to understand to make *Skin Revolution* work its wonders for you. Let me explain.

Yes, the genes we inherit do indeed make us more or less susceptible to various tendencies, strengths and weaknesses. For instance, dark skin is genetically more resistant to wrinkling from exposure to sunlight – a fact that I find particularly infuriating since I inherited that pale Scandinavian skin which is the most susceptible in the world to sun damage, for my ancestors hardly ever saw the sun for generation upon generation. But the genes we have inherited, in truth, do nothing more than define the 'risk' of our getting skin cancer, or sags and bags, excessive dryness or acne. Whether or not these conditions actually develop depends on the biological terrain of the living matrix itself.

> 'The bottom line is very clear: with rare exceptions, only about 30 per cent of physical ageing can be blamed on genes.'
>
> Robert L. Kahn and John W. Rowe

Express Them Right

There are many possible versions of your skin, indeed of the whole of you, tucked within your genes and chromosomes. Which version gets expressed – that is which of your genetic potentials become 'facts' as shown in how your skin looks, feels and functions – depends on how good its biological terrain is kept from month to month, year to year.

Eat convenience foods and drink cheap wine for a couple of weeks, then take a look at yourself in the mirror. That's what poor gene expression looks like. But take heart. Detoxify your skin, strengthen it physiologically and biochemically and your natural, unimpeded life energy released in the process will create a new glowing version of you. Quite simply, there ain't no other way to make it happen. Anything less is like pasting a plaster over a wound, the way sixteenth century women stuck black patches over smallpox scars to conceal them. Get into a *Skin Revolution* way of eating and looking after your skin with skincare products that really work. Make use of some of the new technologies for enhancing the matrix at energetic levels and you will find yourself on a path that revolutionises not only your good looks but your whole life.

PART TWO:

UNLOCKING THE POWER

you've got what it takes . . . so use it

SUGAR BABY OR LEAN MACHINE

AGEs and RAGEs . . . wrinkles and woes

Your skin doesn't age by accident or just because time passes. It loses tone and texture when the order, energy, physiological and biological integrity of the living matrix becomes undermined. Many things can cause this to happen. None is more insidious or more sinister than the chronic high levels of blood sugar and insulin which now threaten the majority of us over thirty. Stop them in your own body. You can not only slow skin ageing, you can reverse its signs.

Sugar destroys skin. And I don't just mean the white stuff that sits in bowls. Most of the foods we eat these days from pastas and breads to packaged cereals and bagels, within a few minutes of entering the body flood the bloodstream with glucose, carrying serious consequences for the skin.

'Youth is the gift of nature, but age is a work of art.'

Garson Kanin

Secrets Of The Dead

The reasons for this are simple and genetic. Yet for almost four generations they have eluded most scientists, nutritionists and doctors. Grain-based foods and sugary foods are a recent invention. For over a million years of evolution the human body never encountered them. Because genetic adaptation is such a slow process – it can take one hundred thousand years for a significant alteration in even one gene to take place – our bodies do not have the ability to deal with them in large quantities for long periods. Yet these grain rich, sugar rich foods, most riddled with junk fats and chemicals as well, make up the largest portion of most people's diets. When our bodies are forced to handle them (and most governments are still trying to sell the idea that a low fat, high carbs diet is *good* for health) our bodies rebel.

What form this insurrection takes depends on our genetic

vulnerabilities. It may show up as adult onset Type II diabetes or obesity, energy swings, raised HDL (bad guy) cholesterol or chronic fatigue, as well as any number of other degenerative conditions. When it comes to skin, the sugar monster fabricates wrinkles, sags, puffy faces, lacklustre complexions and produces a situation where, having learned all this, you wonder if you have the energy to do something about it.

THE WRINKLE MONSTER

Sugar – the wrinkle monster – is two faced. To escape his insidious attacks you need to address both. First there is the all-encompassing glucose-insulin battle you need to win maybe after years of living and eating the way most of us do, in a way which undermines good genetic expression. The second face of the monster focuses on the way excess glucose damages proteins. It attacks skin cells and collagen fibres producing *advanced glycosylation end products*. These nasties, known as AGEs, are like terrorists who wreak havoc within the living matrix causing its collagen fibres to lose their ability to maintain order. AGEs cause collagen proteins to cross-link. This creates wrinkles, sags and bags on your face.

'99.9 per cent of our genes were formed before the development of agriculture.'

Dr S. Boyd Eaton MD

Defeat the first face of the wrinkle monster and the second loses a lot of its power. Your skin will respond by literally rejuvenating itself. So will your whole body, often in medically measurable ways. For more about how this transformation takes place, take a look at my book *Age Power*. It contains the programme which we used in the television documentary To Age or Not To Age when in five weeks we reversed the biomarkers of ageing in men and women between 30 and 60, all the while measuring their remarkable progress using standard, hospital-based medical tests. But right now, let's look at what all this means in relation to skin.

Forgotten Hormone

Insulin is not just of concern to diabetics who don't make enough of it. It is the most important hormone in determining how quickly or slowly your body ages. This is one of the most important discoveries of the past half-century. It began with the work of a brilliant American endocrinologist named Gerald Reaven. In the 1980s, Reaven identified a collection of abnormalities – high blood pressure, distorted cholesterol levels, and others which your doctor commonly worries about – which tend to occur together in people who have them, and have now reached epidemic proportions. These conditions are major factors in the development of degenerative diseases from heart disease and diabetes to obesity – all associated with rapid ageing. Professor Reaven named this collection of abnormalities Syndrome X, or insulin resistance syndrome.

Although its presence often remains hidden to the person who falls prey to it, Syndrome X is a life-threatening, rapidly ageing, perversion of body metabolism which we bring on ourselves by a sedentary lifestyle and – most important of all – by living for decades on a carbohydrate-intensive diet as a good 95 per cent of the population of English-speaking countries still do. How does it happen?

'Syndrome X is a hidden life-threatening perversion of bodily metabolism that is likely to hasten the end of anyone who has it. It is alarmingly common. What's more, evidence is growing that we bring it on ourselves, by the way we eat.'

Gail Vines in *New Scientist*

WORTHY OPPONENTS

In your body, insulin and glucose are antagonists – that is they are meant to balance each other metabolically. Glucose is the particular form of sugar that all carbohydrate foods – from broccoli and lettuce to muffins and chocolate – turn into when you eat them. Insulin has two jobs to perform: first, when glucose from these foods enters the bloodstream, it is supposed to control blood sugar levels. Second, it is responsible for making sure glucose gets turned into the energy form your body needs for metabolism.

When blood sugar is balanced and in control, you have a good supply of ongoing energy. You don't suffer from energy or mood swings during the day or at certain times of the month. It is the pancreas which manages all this. It responds to the level of glucose present in blood at every moment. The more glucose there, the more insulin it secretes to balance it. The less glucose present, the less insulin gets shunted into your blood.

Energy Master

Insulin's second job is equally important. It has to do with getting all this circulating sugar into your body's cells where little energy factories there known as mitochondria can turn it into ATP – the currency your body uses to run all of its metabolic processes, to make hormones, to repair damage to DNA – the lot. The way it does this is interesting. On the surface of each cell there are receptor sites specifically for insulin. They are like locks that only insulin can open so this hormone is able to carry out its second major task – like a key escorting the glucose inside the cell so its mitochondria can get on with their energy producing.

It's a great system. Except that it was never designed to handle the onslaught of glucose we have, for three or four generations, been forcing it to handle by eating so many glucose-producing grains and sugar-based foods. After years of breakfast cereals and toast, sugary sweets and treats, the pancreas is forced to produce so much insulin to control high levels of sugar in the blood that it becomes trigger happy. Day after day, month after month, it secretes so much of the hormone that it continually forces blood sugar to drop too low in which case you get those awful 11 am and 3 pm blues. You then get hungry, eat more carbs in an attempt to get back your energy and wonder why you suffer. The pancreas can also grow weary of the task after a while and literally give out, in which case you end up with Type II diabetes.

'Age ain't nothing but a number.'

Justin Timberlake

But something else happens too – something which not only undermines health and energy but is a major destroyer of beautiful skin and which also encourages cellulite to form and makes us gain weight easily. After years of being flooded with high levels of insulin, the little receptor sites on your cells become jaded. Then, although insulin knocks on their doors in an attempt to escort the glucose through for energy production, your cells have become *insulin resistant* and don't hear the demand to open. Glucose doesn't get through and your body continues to be flooded with unused glucose, you become depleted of energy and your body falls prey to Syndrome X.

When high levels of unused glucose circulate in your body, they seriously disrupt the functions of the living matrix, undermining the beauty of the skin. For when glucose cannot be turned into energy in your body, it poisons it.

HORRORS OF THE SUGAR BABY

Here is what the glucose/insulin scenario looks like:

❑ Habitual eating of high-carbs meals and snacks shunts massive doses of glucose into your bloodstream.
❑ In an effort to maintain balance, the pancreas produces more insulin which keeps insulin levels too high for long periods.
❑ This creates insulin resistance interfering with your body's ability to turn glucose into energy so you feel fatigued, may gain weight easily, become prone to cellulite and can develop the medical abnormalities associated with Syndrome X.
❑ This also stimulates your liver to produce more triglycerides and pour them into your bloodstream.
❑ It can lead to mood swings and hormonal distortions.
❑ As blood fats get converted into HDL – bad guy cholesterol – your risk of heart disease increases.
❑ It also bombards your fat cells with extra calories to tuck away. If you are genetically prone to weight gain you grow fat, but find it more and more difficult to shed it.
❑ This in turn creates yet more insulin resistance and can even start destroying the insulin-secreting cells of the pancreas.
❑ The energy, chemistry and physiology of the living matrix becomes disrupted. Cells no longer receive clear communications in this polluted medium. They become unable to effectively carry out the jobs they are meant to.
❑ Your skin shows the effects of all of this. It loses radiance, thins, sags, wrinkles and ages rapidly. Blotches appear. Spots, too, if you are genetically prone to them. You start to look tired, old beyond your years and, before long, you start to feel as bad as you look.

'I plan on growing old, much later in life, or maybe not at all.'

Patty Carey

Turn Around

Sorry for this long list of bad news. But it is really important that you get a handle on how all this happens. The good news is you can actually reverse it by changing in the way you live – going for a brisk walk every day for half an hour for instance and – most important of all – altering the kinds of foods you eat.

The Living 21 Day Matrix Turnaround can help you do this. Follow it for three weeks. You will experience for yourself your living matrix's transformative power to restore radiance and beauty. Why? Because this way of eating is a modern day equivalent of what the human body throughout its million years has been genetically programmed to require: good quality proteins, the right balance of omega-3 to omega-6 essential fatty acids, masses of fresh, live vegetables and non-sugary fruits rich in phytonutrients, and because it depends on a large part of your foods being eaten raw. This feeds the matrix with not only everything it needs on a biochemical level. It also provides superbly ordered biophoton energy (see Light Up Your Skin) for balance and radiant skin and high levels of vitality. The Living Matrix 21 Day Turnaround programme does something else important too. It eliminates or seriously limits the foods which cause Syndrome X and create AGEs problems, which make skin wrinkle and lose its youthful contours.

Get Into Colours

Our Paleolithic ancestors got an amazing 600 per cent more antioxidant, immune-enhancing phytonutrients present in non-starchy vegetables and fruits than we do today. While the Living Matrix programme may not get you quite that high – depending on how fresh and well grown the foods you choose to eat are – it will take you mighty close.

This is, in no way, a slimming diet, although many people shed excess body fat as a natural part of the metabolic rebalancing it brings about. You eat as much as you like on it – good quality proteins, healthy fats (especially important for skin beauty) and wonderful fresh foods.

Even in the first three weeks it transforms the functions of the living matrix and begins to turn a sugar baby with all her puffs and bumps, sags and cellulite into a lean machine so her skin glows and the body reshapes itself powerfully – from *within.* Six weeks on the programme and it can even rejuvenate your whole body in medically measurable ways. For it helps shift all those parameters of health and biological age measurements which for 50 years have concerned doctors and scientists and which define Syndrome X: high blood pressure, high triglycerides, disturbed cholesterol – the lot. The living matrix does this for us. All we need to do is to supply it with the stuff it requires to carry out the job.

AGEs – The Inside Story

Skin degenerative processes triggered by long term excess glucose circulating in the blood go far beyond the insidious role it plays in insulin resistance and Syndrome X. When glucose levels are too high for too long, because the body is unable to convert it into energy for use, this glucose tends to bind itself to chains of proteins through an abnormal chemical process to form advanced glycosylation end products – AGEs. The binding of glucose to any biomolecule causes whatever it binds to, to alter its nature, so the skin's functions become undermined. This in turn impedes cellular functions, causes inflammation and triggers a high level of free radical production, all of which ages skin fast.

Within the skin, glucose binds to the skin's collagen itself – the living matrix's most important structural protein. Ordered bundles of collagen in a healthy body give skin a firm, well-sculpted look holding back wrinkles and sags. Glucose also binds to nucleic acids in skin cells – DNA and RNA. This produces abnormalities in the way your skin cells function and mutations when they reproduce themselves.

'The bottom line is very clear: with rare exceptions, only about 30 per cent of physical ageing can be blamed on genes.'

Robert L. Kahn and John W. Rowe

THE BEAUTY OF ORDER

Normal, healthy collagen and elastin form a network within the living matrix. It looks a bit like a beautiful hand-woven fabric with collagen forming most of the vertical weave lending skin its structural integrity and density. AGEs cause collagen fibres to stick together and bunch up so they become rigid, losing their flexibility and strength. The first external signs of advanced glycosylation often show up as soft pillows formed around the eyes.

AGEs make your skin look soft and droopy. Cross-linking can become apparent around the mouth, too. It becomes hardened and less flexible. Eventually the cheek area is affected. Cross-linked collagen is a major reason for the deepening of the crease between the edge of the nose and the side of the lips – called the nasal-labial fold. In someone who has advanced AGEs and cross-linking, the skin's surface can actually become a map of lines which form squares to grow deeper by the year, the worse the cross-linking problem becomes.

AGEs And RAGEs

The presence of AGEs in your body accelerate other ageing processes too. They not only physically distort protein tissues, they impair DNA and distort the matrix's fat-based membranes. They alter the chemical functions of cells triggering cascades of destructive events when they attach to cell binding sites and produce 'clinkers' that show up as irregular pigmentation and 'age spots'.

Appropriately the main binding site for AGEs is called RAGEs – receptors for AGEs. The binding of AGEs to RAGEs creates intracellular oxidative stress or free radical damage – another major factor in skin ageing. It also leads to the generation of chemicals which trigger inflammation – the third major force in ageing skin which American dermatologist Nicholas Perricone has spent the last few years trying to make the world aware of.

'Being a sex symbol is an attitude, not looks. Most men think it's looks, most women know otherwise.'

Kathleen Turner

THE FOUR PILLARS OF SKIN AGEING

Here are the four processes at the core of skin ageing which the Living Matrix 21 Day Turnaround Programme helps defeat:
❑ **Non-enzymatic Glycosylation** creates AGEs, cross-links collagen fibres and disrupts cellular metabolism polluting skin in the process.

- ❑ **Oxidation** and free radical damage cause chaos in the living matrix, wreak havoc with cells and deplete the body of the nutrients and metabolites it needs for a high level of order and lasting skin beauty.
- ❑ **Inflammation** compromises immunity and makes your skin highly reactive not only to makeup, the sun, and skincare products but – when severe – even to life itself.
- ❑ **Reduced Methylation** is the process by which a methyl group (a carbon atom plus three hydrogens) is added to a protein or DNA to empower chemical reactions needed to detoxify cells and prevent damage. When methylation is reduced, good gene expression – essential for skin beauty – is undermined. Your body is unable to detoxify itself from excess hormones, toxic chemicals and heavy metals. Skin grows dull and ages rapidly. The more you can support the methylation process the better your skin gets. Foods rich in sulphur like garlic and onions are important in doing this.

More Than Political Activists

These days just about everybody knows about free radicals. Twenty years ago most people figured they were political activists. Following the appearance of Estée Lauder's once-cutting-edge Night Repair, which was designed to counter oxidation damage and assist the DNA repair processes in cells, the rest of the industry jumped onto the free radical scavenger bandwagon and began producing formulas which boasted antioxidant nutrients like vitamins C, E and A.

Eventually cosmetic chemists went looking for plant-based ingredients with similar antioxidant abilities. But few got it right. The secret of creating a high level of protection against oxidation damage for skin lies in understanding the way in which effective antioxidants need to be supplied *together* in *synergy* with other nutrients and substrates the skin needs.

My frustration with 'natural' products which were anything but natural led me to create Origins. Recently, my impatience with the fact that nobody in the entire cosmetic industry seems to understand the principles of holistic skincare has led me to create my new skin spray, Living Matrix Mist™. It supplies skin with everything possible for skin itself to carry out all the metabolic and energetic processes needed to continually regenerate and rejuvenate itself. It eliminates the problems of chemical build up which can lead to toxic overload, pollute the skin and can damage DNA. Living Matrix Mist™ even addresses the skin's need for a high level of biophoton order.

Such products, together with dietary changes and other cutting-edge natural modalities for beauty, are what holistic skincare is all about. Hopefully in the next five years a few leading cosmetic companies will get savvy about what is needed to care for skin at the highest levels and take action, expand their horizons and clean up their act by eliminating chemicals from their products. In an industry still largely blinkered by its search for a miracle ingredient to use as a magic bullet, few grasp this. As a result, despite high-tech complex multi-level emulsions and fancy new delivery systems, most skincare products fall far short of bringing the skin what it needs to resist and reverse age signs, let alone to thrive.

'. . . only a small portion of the genetic information in our cells is expressed. Our diet, lifestyle and environment modify the nature of this information and how it is expressed. We are the products of what and how well our genetic messages are expressed. Healthy ageing is accomplished when our genes continue to express healthy messages throughout our lives.'

Jeffrey Bland PhD

Anti-Inflammation Pioneer

Inflammation is a major concern of skincare and makeup manufacturers. More women complain of highly sensitive and reactive skin. Their tolerance to whatever they put on their faces has become further and further reduced as a result of biological terrain pollution making their skin ever more prone to premature ageing and inflammation. Seldom do they connect this problem with its real causes however: poor diet and exposure to environmental chemicals in air, food, water and products which build up to undermine the integrity and order of the living matrix itself.

BEAUTY EDITOR'S SKIN

Inflammation and high skin reactivity is endemic among beauty writers. My friend Jo Fairley who, like me has a passion for beauty, has struggled with it for years. Beauty writers need to test all sorts of products on their own skin. It may sound great fun to be sent samples of the latest, ultra luxurious creams from Chanel, Dior or Shiseido to try. But using one skincare product after another can wreak havoc with the order and functions of the living matrix, making the skin highly prone to inflammation, so it tends to react to just about everything.

American dermatologist, Nicholas Perricone, is the cosmetic world's great crusader against inflammation. Perricone insists that inflammation is the major cause of skin ageing. In his dynamic American way he has, virtually single-handed, begun the process of making the general population aware of the powerful role diet can play in calming inflammation and making the skin look younger. He puts people on a simple low-carbs diet rich in omega-3 fats from wild salmon and shows them how, in a few days, their skin looks and feels better. An enthusiastic entrepreneur, Perricone a few years ago launched his own range of skincare designed to counter the inflammation he so abhors. It consists of a group of conventionally formulated products – complete with parabens and all the usual chemical ingredients – each of which is based on a different vitamin or nutraceutical like DMAE and alpha lipoic acid (ALA) – one of the most powerful antioxidants yet discovered. And although his products are by no means synergistically formulated, his idea of using nutraceuticals not only internally as supplements but externally in products is an excellent one. This is something the big cosmetic manufacturers should have twigged to and started doing a decade ago. It takes someone like Perricone who was himself forced to learn about ways of enhancing his own health, powerfully and naturally, to lead the way. His skincare business now has a yearly turnover in the tens of millions of dollars. Little wonder, since because each product tends to be based on only one active ingredient, the implication is that you are required to buy and use more than half a dozen of them to reap their benefits. Perricone is a great marketing man. He also firmly believes in what he is doing.

'I made a commitment to completely cut out drinking and anything that might hamper me from getting my mind and body together. And the floodgates of goodness have opened upon me – spiritually and financially.'

Denzel Washington

Winning The War Against Ageing Skin

It is not just one or two anti-ageing battles you need to win to make a significant difference to your skin. Just quelling inflammation or providing more free radical protection from inside and out, or cutting out all the high carbs stuff from your diet to reduce blood sugar and insulin levels and counter the formation of AGEs, or using effective natural methods of enhancing methylation to better detoxify your skin and body as a whole – none of these things on their own will put it off. Yes, of course you need to know how to do all of these things. Then you need to take action. But dealing with one or two of them is only like winning one or two of a great many battles in the war to defeat skin ageing. Each skin improvement process is inexorably woven together with all the others within the living matrix. A true skin revolution doesn't just win a battle or two only to lose the war. It addresses the whole shebang. By altering the way you eat, live and look after your skin externally and internally, this not only makes your skin younger and more beautiful, it brings your whole being access to levels of energy, emotional balance and wellbeing that can turn the dream of living a full and creative life into reality. Such is the promise of the skin revolution. Only this can bring you beauty at the deepest level – genuinely transforming your whole experience of yourself in the process.

FEEDING THE MATRIX

the ultimate wrinkle cure

The ultimate wrinkle cure: feed your living matrix everything it needs for optimal gene expression. The payoff? Younger, firmer, smoother skin, less cellulite and radiant vitality. Here's the how and why of the Living Matrix 21 Day Turnaround. The rewards of this unique way of eating may surprise you: all you can eat of crunchy vegetables, low-sugar fruits and proteins plus (surprise, surprise) plenty of the right kind of fats. What else? Wait for it: hardly a grain in sight.

To understand what kind of diet protects the body from premature ageing and reverses degenerative changes, we need to look back fifteen to forty thousand years. That was long before Syndrome X was even a gleam in some scientist's eye. We need to look forward too – at what emerging paradigm biochemistry and physics can offer to help us protect the integrity of living skin from hormone-disrupters, chemical destroyers and the various electromagnetic pollutions which continue to undermine our skin's integrity and destroy its beauty.

'When we develop reverence for food and the miracle of transformation inherent in it, just the simple act of eating creates a ritual of celebration.'
Deepak Chopra

Exploring all these things and trying to bring what I learned together to make practical use of it all has been a long and fascinating process for me. It has led me to identify what, I believe, will be the food style of the future for anyone wanting to live at the highest possible levels of vitality and get the best protection from degeneration they can. Here are the elements that go into such a diet. For menus and advice on how to put it all into practice to empower your own skin revolution, see Making It Happen (page 199). There you will find what you need to make it all happen for you.

ANCIENT FOOD FANATICS

The biochemistry and physiology of human skin has changed little over the millennia. Our bodies remain genetically adapted to wild foods, not to the refined and processed stuff we now consume. The lives of our hunter-gatherer ancestors who ate this way for more than a million years were not easy. They mostly died young from animal attacks or starved to death when there was no food at all to be found. But, palaeopathologists have discovered from examining the remains of these people, their bodies never experienced the degenerative processes we now do – loss of bone, tooth decay, and infective diseases like tuberculosis. They showed up in the human body a few thousand years ago when, as a result of the agricultural revolution, people began to eat large amounts of cultivated grain-based foods which their bodies had never known before. Palaeopathologists tell us, our ancestors ate so well that today they might be accused of being food fanatics.

'Spiritual growth requires the acknowledgement of one's need to grow.'
M. Scott Peck

Secrets Of The Ancestors

The Palaeolithic era, by the way, began two and a half million years ago in Africa and ended around ten thousand years ago in the Middle East with the beginnings of agriculture. Stone Age man's hunter-gatherer fare gave them far in excess of today's official recommendations for daily intake of vitamins and minerals, essential fatty acids and high quality proteins. They had never seen or heard of grain-based carbohydrates – the French breads and the granolas. Carbohydrate foods made from grains and flours did not exist. They had also never heard of sugar. The odd bit of honey occasionally filched from wild bees was all the sweetness they knew. And they never consumed dairy products – except when nursed as a baby at their mother's breast.

In the words of Dr Loren Cordain, author of *The Paleo Diet*, one of the best books on the subject, 'The blink of an eye. That's how long, in the grand scheme of human history, we have grown food and domesticated livestock . . . yet we have almost completely lost track of the foods our ancient ancestors ate. The so-called new foods that agriculture gave us so completely displaced the old foods that most of us are unaware that these foods were ever new. Many people assume that cereals, dairy products, salted foods, legumes, domesticated meats, and refined sugars have always been part of our diet. Not true! We need to rediscover the foods that brought our Palaeolithic ancestors vibrant health, lean bodies, and freedom from chronic disease. The foods that agreed nicely with their genetic blueprints are the same foods that agree nicely with our genetic blueprints.'

Examining the stomach contents of early man's remains, scientists have been able to determine that they ate more than two hundred different kinds of plants regularly. Today we are lucky if we get eighteen or twenty. Eating a wide variety of non-starchy vegetables and herbs provides the human body with nutritional diversity. Our Palaeolithic cousins got their proteins – quite a bit more than we do today – from fish and shellfish, grubs, insects, large and small animals – all of which were rich in anti-inflammatory omega-3 essential fatty acids. Their foods were eaten fresh since they had no way of storing them. Most were eaten raw. This enabled their living matrix to suck a high degree of biochemical and energetic order from what they ate. And, although Palaeolithic man died young as a result of the hard life he led, generally he died healthy. He was tall and strong. He ate in a manner that provided his cells and living matrix with all they needed to engender first rate genetic expression.

GENES GO SLOW

Genetic adaptation is an excruciatingly slow process. It takes a hundred thousand years for the body to make even one significant gene change – helping our bodies, say, to adapt to a significant change of diet. Refined sugar, concentrated carbohydrates like breads and cereals, junk fats and convenience foods showed up on our tables less than a hundred years ago. They only became widely used in the last fifty or so. Our bodies continue to be overwhelmed by the onslaught of such novelties. Not only do our bodies not have the enzymes to adequately digest and assimilate them, eating them long-term depletes us of the essential minerals, trace elements and vitamins needed to cope with them.

'Eating a meal with full awareness can be a powerful, enlightening and healing experience.'

David Simon

Programmed For Health

What happens to us? We experience degenerative diseases – from diabetes and obesity to heart disease and chronic ill health. So much for the bad news. The good news is great for skin. Your body has phenomenal powers for self-healing, regeneration and rejuvenation. Begin to eat in a way that provides it with what it does require for good gene expression, in the form of foods it handles well. Clear out the unfamiliar, hard to deal with foods which it has been silently trying to struggle with. One minor miracle after another begins to happen. This is what feeding the matrix is all about. Here are some of the elements that make up The Living Matrix 21 Day Turnaround Diet and a description of why it works so well.

'The belly rules the mind.'

Latin Proverb

Genes, Antioxidants And Immune Support

The sweetness in vegetables and fruits is an indication that they are ripe – that they hold optimal complements of vitamins, minerals and trace elements. In the case of fresh organic foods this can be very high indeed. When we eat plant-based carbohydrates – whether in the form of apples, broccoli or muffins – our digestive system extracts the nutrients we need from them. But the difference between how our bodies handle the carbohydrate in a slice of French bread and the carbohydrate in a fresh apple or a spinach salad is like night and day. Until recently in our evolutionary history, our bodies have never had to process carbohydrates from grain sources like wheat or corn. The carbs to which we are genetically well adapted come from low-starch vegetables and herbs – green leafy vegetables and simple non-sugary fruits (the high glycaemic banana did not exist in the form that we know it until very recently), as well as masses of herbs. These foods not only provide energy for us, they are brimming with vitamins, minerals, beneficial phytohormones and phytonutrients offering first rate antioxidant support to protect skin from age damage. They are also rich in immune-enhancing plant factors, bringing yet another string to the bow for skin regeneration and rejuvenation.

FROM PLANT SUGAR TO ATP

Within their leaves, all plants make carbohydrates – starches and sugars. The process of photosynthesis absorbs the sun's light energy and thanks to a mysterious alchemy – which chemistry can chart but still nobody really understands – turns it into nourishment. The main sugar plants use for energy is fructose just as the main sugar we use is glucose. Our bodies have the ability to turn fructose and plant starches into glucose so we can convert them to create ATP.

'All food is the gift of the gods and something of the miraculous, the egg no less than the truffle.'

Sybille Bedford

Grain and flour-based foods – the cereals and breads as well as the sugary stuff made from them – are different. When you eat them, they quickly shunt vast quantities of glucose into your bloodstream with all of the potentially devastating consequences to skin and the body outlined in the last chapter including rapid skin-ageing and cellulite. There are other important reasons too why a low-grain or grain-free diet works best for good skin.

Good, Bad And Ugly

Grain-based foods come in two varieties. The worst for skin – and thankfully more people are finally becoming aware of this – are the refined carbs – breakfast cereals, sweets, pasta, white breads and rolls. Whole grain foods, so popular in the seventies and eighties, are little better. Whole grain foods supply the body with vitamins E, B complex and important minerals essential to life. But these are all lost in the refining process. Even most of the fibre – important to digestion and the elimination of wastes and toxins from the body – gets thrown out. Food manufacturers add back only a handful of the vitamins lost in refining, and then in their chemical form – through a process ironically known as fortification. There is even evidence that some of the chemical vitamins used may be dangerous to the body. The safety of bromating and bleaching agents used in the refining processes is also highly questionable. So the first thing to do for the sake of your skin is open your cupboards and throw all this stuff out.

'Let thy food be thy medicine and thy medicine be thy food.'

Hippocrates

Good For Some

Whole grains are different. They can be useful for some people in small quantities. These people are the fast-burners – the men and women who, no matter what they eat, seem never to gain weight. Sadly, they are much in the minority. The rest of us tend to be better off without whole grains – provided of course that we can break through established habit patterns and give up outdated notions about how 'essential' bread is to the 'good life'. Not only can your body function better without them, your skin becomes far more beautiful.

There is another important caveat with regard to eating whole grains, too. The phosphorous they contain – essential for healthy skin and bones – is bound up and unavailable to the body when we eat them because grains contain a substance called *phytic acid.* Phytic acid combines with the zinc, copper, iron, magnesium and calcium in our own intestinal tract when we eat these foods, blocking our ability to digest and absorb these nutrients well.

Although our ancestors did not know the science behind all this, in traditional societies intuitively they either soaked or fermented their grains before eating them. The Japanese are masters at this. They still produce an enormous variety of delicious, naturally fermented foods. Both processes neutralise phytates as well as enzyme inhibitors also present in grains, in effect partly digesting them before we eat them.

Soaking a seed or grain does this too. Even better is sprouting them for a day or two in a bowl on your kitchen counter. Sprouting a seed not only breaks down complex starches making them easy to digest, the sprouting process increases the vitamin content of these foods dramatically. All this makes sprouts powerful sources of nutrition parallel to the live foods our hunter-gatherer ancestors harvested as they wandered through the woods gathering leaves and herbs, berries and roots.

'I was raised almost entirely on turnips and potatoes, but I think that the turnips had more to do with the effect than the potatoes.'

Marlene Dietrich

Most grains and legumes in your local supermarket have been treated innumerable times with pesticides and herbicides – to inhibit the growth of moulds and to kill insects. If you are going to eat grains at all, choose the unrefined varieties and if at all possible, go organic to help protect your skin and body from accumulating high levels of chemicals.

Watching It Happen

Most people find when they leave aside grains, sugar and refined foods, their skin not only loses its puffiness, lines on the face begin to disappear and skin's natural firmness rapidly returns. Once the body has made the adjustment to a new way of eating, they report that energy levels have soared. Colleagues who volunteered to be guinea pigs during my research for *Skin Revolution* and while I was formulating my Living Matrix spray, reported this again and again. One friend, an actress, was especially resistant to the idea of giving up grains for three weeks to find out what the Living Matrix 21 Day Turnaround diet might do for her skin. She said she couldn't imagine living without bread. 'It's the very staff of life,' she insisted. One week into the programme she rang me. 'My God,' she said. 'I have never had more energy in my life.' 'Good,' I replied, 'But what about your skin?' 'My skin looks great.' 'Wait another couple of weeks,' I told her. 'It should only get better and better as your body gets used to this new way of eating.' It did.

'What you eat is not the goal. What you are is the goal.'

Osho

Living Carbs – Beauty's Powerhouse

The living matrix way of eating is *by no means* a low carbohydrate diet. You eat as much carbohydrate as you like – masses of the best kind – from bright coloured peppers and apples to fresh herbs, rocket, avocados and tomatoes, berries, melons and sprouted seeds and legumes. These foods promote your skin's highest genetic expression. They bring your body optimal levels of vitamins, minerals, trace elements and natural sugars in superb balance. And they carry none of the negative influences on your skin and health which can come from eating significant quantities of flour-based carbs and convenience foods. Here are some of the ways matrix eating sets your skin up for rejuvenation, and how:

'Food should be prepared with butter and love.'

Swedish Proverb

❑ PHYTONUTRIENTS COLOUR YOU BEAUTIFUL: non-starchy vegetables and low-sugar fruits boast high levels of phytochemicals – microscopic natural antioxidants to help your body resist degeneration. They support immunity, stabilise vitamins in skin tissues, protect from illness and halt premature ageing. It is these recently discovered but now much studied plant factors which give vegetables and fruits their bright colours. They work in synergy with vitamins, bringing more nutritional clout. Some clear our cells of toxic substances like herbicides and pesticides. Others act as free radical scavengers against oxidation damage.

There are now over 20,000 phytochemicals identified in fresh fruits and vegetables. They offer synergistic power to smooth and firm your skin, improve eyesight, counter infection, degeneration and cancer, and can calm allergic reactions. They have names like *catichins, quercetin, hesperidin, sulphoraphane, carotenoids, flavonoids and licopene.* Many act in the body as they do in the cells of the plants from which they come – creating a cellular screen against photoageing from overexposure to UV radiation or chemicals in the environment. The wider a variety of phytonutrient-rich plant foods you eat the better your skin can become.

'I consider the discovery of a dish which sustains our appetite and prolongs our pleasures as a far more interesting event than the discovery of a star.'
Henrion De Pensey

❑ LIVING SPROUTS BRING ENERGY AND ORDER TO SKIN: the Chinese invented them centuries ago. They carried mung beans on their ships, sprouting these seeds to provide vitamin C and prevent scurvy in sailors. In their dormant state, chickpeas, mung beans and lentils are filled with enzyme inhibitors. This makes them hard to digest even when cooked and is one of the reasons why eating beans and lentils creates so many digestive troubles. Our bodies are not very well designed to handle them in this form.

Enzyme inhibitors interfere with our ability to absorb minerals present in a food. But, when you sprout a seed, all this changes. Its content of B vitamins and vitamin C soars. Enzyme inhibitors get neutralised. Meanwhile, enzymes themselves present in these embryonic plants improve the way your own body's enzymes function. Sprouted seeds of mung, chickpeas, unshelled sesame seeds, lentils, adzuki and buckwheat are delicious in salads, as snacks, or used to create live muesli for breakfast. You can buy them from a shop already growing or sprout them yourself in bowls on the kitchen counter. Because they are young plants and because they are eaten raw they also convey the highest levels of *biophoton order* to your living matrix. Ironically, the only sprouted seeds you should avoid are the most widely available: alfalfa sprouts. Research shows that alfalfa embryos may inhibit some of our immune functions. In some people they may also contribute to inflammatory conditions like lupus or arthritis. This is because alfalfa contains an unusual amino acid – *canavanine* – which can actually be toxic to humans when we eat large quantities of them. As the alfalfa plant grows to maturity this amino acid is metabolised so it is no longer present in the mature grass.

'Good food is a celebration of life.'

Sophia Loren

❏ LOW-SUGAR ENDS WRINKLES, SAGS AND BAGS: Living Matrix Turnaround eating draws on low-to-medium glycaemic fruits and vegetables. This is important. The glycaemic index (GI) is a measure of how much a specific food will raise your blood glucose level – and how fast. Eating high GI foods on a regular basis, like bananas or bread, sugar, crisps or cereals, can lead to the skin-degenerated changes described in the last chapter. Lower glycaemic foods protect your body from blood sugar disorders and insulin resistance syndrome – Syndrome X. They also prevent high levels of untransformed glucose from circulating in the body and stop skin from producing a lot of advanced glycosylation end products – AGEs – which make it wrinkle, sag and age. Low glycaemic carbohydrate foods can even reverse age signs – fading wrinkles, firming your face, restoring contours, clearing deposits of cellulite and – a special bonus if you have trouble shedding fat from your body – encourage natural weight loss. They restore metabolic balance to your body.

❏ RAW POWER FOR BEAUTY: as many as possible of your living matrix foods are eaten raw. Not only is a food's biophoton energy depleted or destroyed when we cook it, even the biochemical structure of the nutrients it contains can be altered by heat. Fibre in raw plant foods is broken down and turned into a soft, passive substance when foods are cooked. This makes fibre lose its natural magnetic cleansing effects on the intestines. Not only are vitamins and minerals depleted by cooking, amino acids in protein foods can be denatured by it and cross-link in much the same way AGEs make this happen to the collagen in your skin. The water content of foods is also decreased when they are cooked. The quality of water healthy fruits and vegetables contain is the best in the world. It is 'living' water – complete with life energy and important trace elements. Foods carry within them the enzymes that help our body digest and assimilate them. The enzymes present in raw foods become destroyed when they are heated to 40 degrees C or above. This loss puts extra strain on our own enzyme systems in order to digest and assimilate them. It can use up essential supplies of our own co-factor vitamins and minerals which we need for other purposes like protecting us from age degeneration. Raw foods lend a high support to your body's immune system. This is important to counter premature ageing. These are only a few of the reasons why living matrix eating relies heavily on raw vegetable foods. While the odd phytonutrient can be absorbed more easily when a food is heated – licopene in tomatoes for instance – this is not true of the vast majority of plant nutrients. When foods are eaten raw they are delivered to the body in a superbly ordered chemical and energetic synergy. Our skin thrives on it.

'An onion with a friend is roast lamb.'

Egyptian Proverb

☐ GOOD FATS FOR GREAT SKIN AND SMOOTH THIGHS: fat matters for ageless skin. If you doubt this take a look at any thirty-five year old woman who, struggling to keep her weight down, has been on and off low fat diets. Her skin grows thin and lined, pasty and haggard, because she has not supplied it with enough of the *right kind* of fats. The right kind of fats won't make you fat either. In fact they can actually help you grow leaner. It is not *fat* that is dangerous to life and health, it is *junk fat* which undermines both. What *is* the wrong kind? Trans fatty acids in convenience foods. Margarines. Highly processed golden polyunsaturated oils like corn and safflower, groundnut and sunflower which line our supermarket shelves. These fats are destructive to the body. It's they, together with sugar, that promote heart disease. They undermine hormone balance, disrupt the integrity of cell walls making skin lose its capacity to maintain moisture balance and to nourish its cells so it can keep its firmness. What your skin *does* need is three kinds of fat:

○ **A GOOD BALANCE OF ESSENTIAL FATTY ACIDS** – the **Omega-6** group, found in avocados, nuts and seeds, and the **Omega-3** group, in good supply from eating wild fish, game, flax seeds, flaxseed oil, and walnuts. The ideal ratio of one group to the other is 2 parts omega-6 to one part omega-3. This is what our palaeolithic ancestors got. Most of us these days get 22 parts omega-6 to 1 part omega-3. This is a long way from what we need for the best possible gene expression for beautiful skin. In short supply in most people's diet, the omega-3 oils are vitally important to skin beauty and body health. They increase the body's metabolic rate – great for fat burning. They have powerful anti-inflammatory properties – great for skin. They heighten your ability to deal with stress and increase your insulin sensitivity helping to protect you from Syndrome X.

○ **Omega-9** fats are found in good supply in extra virgin olive oil. Olive oil is rich in oleic acid, a monounsaturate which is resistant to the damaging effects of heat and light – far more than any polyunsaturated oil. Great for salads, olive oil can also be gently heated without turning into a trans fat.

○ **Coconut Oil**. What? 'But isn't this a saturated fat?' It is indeed. So is butter which you can eat on the matrix diet too. The fats in coconut oil are something special, however. Far from contributing to heart disease and other degenerative processes, medium-chain triglycerides (MCTs) found in coconut can actually help *lower* cholesterol. In Sri Lanka, where coconut oil is the main source of dietary fat, you will find the lowest death rate from heart disease. They also encourage your body to shed its fat stores and offer great help to sugar babies wanting to become lean machines. Years ago farmers figured a good way to fatten cattle for market would be to feed them coconut oil. After all it was cheap, widely available and high in calories. Their experiments failed dismally. The animals only grew leaner and more muscular. Over 50 per cent of the fat in a coconut consists of MCTs. Great for skin and your whole body, they also fill you up and provide energy when you need it, while helping to eliminate cravings for sugar and muffins.

'Exciting food should exercise the senses and stretch the palate.'

Alan Wong

❑ PROTEIN POWER FOR GREAT SKIN ARCHITECTURE: your skin assembles and uses almost fifty thousand different proteins to carry out its work – creating collagen, nerves, muscles, enzymes, hormones and antibodies on which beauty depends. It needs the highest quality protein to pull it off – to build good cell walls and manufacture glycosaminoglycans – the gel-like substance in which your skin's cells are immersed. For the sake of your skin you need protein. Certainly when you are over thirty. The best quality proteins come from animal sources – eggs, fish, game, meat – preferably organic, and, to a much smaller degree, dairy products. All proteins are built from a combination of only 22 amino acids, eight to ten of which are considered 'essential' since your body is capable of making the others from them. However if just *one* essential amino acid is low or not available then the body is unable to synthesise the proteins it needs even when your overall intake of protein foods is high. It is possible to be a vegetarian and build beautiful skin but it is a lot harder: animal proteins are our only source of *complete* protein. Vegetable foods contain only *incomplete* protein. The two best kinds of food for vegetable proteins are grains and pulses. Legumes, like beans, lentils and cashews, are high in the amino acid lysine yet low in methionine. Grains have an opposite protein profile. So when you eat the two together, as many traditional cultures do, usually with a little animal protein added in, you get a more complete protein. However, it is important to remember that most people's bodies are not equipped to handle large quantities of grains and pulses. Such foods tend to raise glucose levels, disturb insulin balance, and make many people fat.

Mexicans mix corn with red beans. In the Middle East they combine chick peas with wheat. The Japanese mix rice and soya. But studies of our primitive ancestors show that they were most certainly *not* vegetarians. They lived on a diet of animal protein and fat, with herbs, vegetables, seeds and fruits. They had strong dense muscles, excellent bone formation and perfect teeth. Once the agricultural revolution set in and they added grains and legumes to their diet – even though they were far healthier than we are today living on refined and processed foods we find evidence that they had abscesses, dental caries, bone loss and infections. All the long lived peoples of the world like the Vilcabamba Indians in Ecuador and the Georgians in Russia ate good quantities of vegetables and fats and also consumed flesh and animal-based foods including milk and pork. This is one of the major reasons why animal proteins form an important part of the Living Matrix 21 Day Turnaround. If you are a vegetarian and want to follow it, make use of microfiltered whey – the most highly bioavailable protein anywhere – eggs, organic tofu and even fish if you can. In addition to supplying a high level of top quality complete proteins, fatty fish is a great source of the omega-3 essential fats.

'Anyone who doesn't believe in miracles is not a realist.'
David Ben-Gurion

These are the major players in *Skin Revolution* eating. Together they work to detoxify and rebuild the living matrix, enhance cell functions, eliminate puffiness, clear pockets of cellulite and regenerate skin. You may well find, as all my volunteers who tested the programme reported, that once you get a taste of eating this way and once you experience for yourself what it does for your skin, as well as how it reshapes your body – making it leaner and firmer – builds strength and balances moods, that you want to eat this way permanently. I do. It's a great foundation on which to build a lifetime of beautiful skin and vitality – at every age.

MAGNUM FORCE

search and destroy ammunition you can't
afford to miss

Living matrix eating is the all-encompassing transformative
power behind your own skin revolution. That said, there is
wonderful natural support on offer when you feel the skin
needs extra help: the powerhouse nutraceuticals. Check out
what they can do, choose the best for you and forget the rest,
at least until you need them.

At last the cosmetic world has discovered nutraceuticals. Also called
functional foods, phytonutrients and phytochemicals, these natural
substances are currently being added to skincare products at a rate of
knots. Most manufacturers remain naïve about how to combine them
to get the best effect. We are going to see a lot more of these: unique
forms of vitamins with the ability to repair DNA damage, extracts from
plants to enhance immunity and protect from ageing, each bringing
specific benefits for skin. Learning how to use them can give you yet
another tool for your Skin Revolution tool-kit.

'Natural forces within us are the healers of disease.'

Hippocrates

Meet The Big Three

There are three little-known nutraceuticals which are musts when the
skin needs extra help. Together they create a magnum force against
ageing, wrinkles and skin problems. They form the core of a wide-
based anti-ageing, anti-inflammatory, antioxidant army, and work to
protect the integrity of the living matrix. The big three work wonderfully together. They also work well when taken with the more common
antioxidants from alpha-lipoic acid, grape seed extract and Co-enzyme
Q10 to vitamin C and zinc. Let's explore these three biggies first. I use
them myself all the time. Then we can look at others which, like foot
soldiers, make up a whole anti-ageing army.

Universal Sulphur For Perfect Skin

Sulphur is the third largest elemental component in your body. The hottest item in offices of savvy plastic surgeons these days is a unique form of this element: MSM – methyl-sulphonyl-methane. It is at the top of the list for extra support. MSM, also known as 'physiological sulphur', is a superb free radical scavenger. It neutralises free radical molecules that damage skin. Found in every tissue of your body, MSM concentrations diminish with age. They need to be supported by the right kind of diet and supplements after the age of 25. MSM is also found in rain water, the sea, and all living organisms. It exists in especially high concentrations in raw vegetables, fruits and sea foods. Even the cocoa plant from which chocolate is made is a good source. But, unless your diet is composed primarily of raw foods like the living matrix programme is, it is highly unlikely that you are getting enough MSM for optimal health and beautiful skin.

'MSM, an odourless, essentially tasteless, white crystalline chemical, demonstrates usefulness as a dietary supplement in man and lower animals. Our research suggests that a minimum concentration in the body may be critical to both normal function and structure. Limited studies suggest that the systemic concentration of MSM drops in mammals with increasing age. This may be due to dietary habits where one ingests foods with lower MSM potential with maturity, or possibly there is a change in the renal threshold.'

Dr Stanley Jacob

The crème de la crème source of sulphur for the human body, MSM slows down the loss of collagen, stabilises connective tissues, and is important for clearing toxic build up both on a cellular level and in the body as a whole. It even helps regulate the way insulin behaves in the body. MSM is light years ahead of other forms of sulphur. It is completely safe as well as highly effective. Even people who are 'allergic' to sulphur-drugs and sulphite-based food additives thrive on it.

Great Nails And Hair

Sulphur is the most beautifying of all the elements. Even the curliness of hair depends on it. It regulates the sodium/potassium balance bringing in nutrients and oxygen to cells and neutralising wastes. Every time your body clears out destructive chemicals it uses sulphur to remove them. MSM provides elasticity and healing repair to skin tissues. It may even alter cross-linkages, smoothing out scars. It is not only useful as an internal supplement, it is essential for beauty all round. As a prime free radical scavenger, physiological sulphur helps rid the body of allergies. It even protects the lining of the digestive tract from parasites and pathogens. This is important for skin since when leaky gut or dysbiosis occurs in the digestive tract, skin suffers. If you have a tendency to acne you can break out. If your skin tends to be dry, this can make it drier and give the face a colourless, lifeless look. Sulphur is essential for cartilage strength and to build keratin – the fibrous protein out of which hair and nails are made – as well as to virtually every function of the skin. With extra MSM your nails grow faster and stronger. Your hair gets thicker and shinier. A good dose of MSM is 2000 milligrammes (2 grammes) for each 60 kilos of weight a day. Start with 500 mg per 60 kilos of weight and work up. Use together with half that amount of vitamin C, preferably in the form of calcium or magnesium ascorbate (so if you take 2 grammes of MSM take 1 gramme of vitamin C).

'We must remove the word "impossible" from our vocabulary.'

Bernie S. Siege

Carnosine – Master Of Paradox

The second master nutraceutical for skin is carnosine. Carnosine is not to be confused with the amino acid L-carnitine which transports fatty acids into the mitochondria of cells so they can be turned into ATP. Carnosine is a dipeptide – a two-part protein – made out of the amino acids beta-alanine and L-histadine. Like MSM, it is a natural metabolite in your body as well as a powerful antioxidant. It occurs in particularly high concentration in long-lived cells like nerves and muscles. Carnosine levels decline as our body ages. In muscles its concentration falls by more than 60 per cent between the ages of 10 and 70.

'Many antioxidants are aimed at preventing free radicals from entering tissues, but have no effect after this first line of defense is broken. Carnosine is not only effective in prevention, but it is also active after free radicals react to form other dangerous compounds. So it protects the tissues from these damaging "second-wave" chemicals.'

Marios Kyriazis MD

Carnosine addresses the great paradox of life – the fact that the elements which support life – glucose, lipids, oxygen proteins and trace elements – also destroy it. This nutraceutical binds toxic metals so your body can eliminate them safely. Carnosine both supports life and protects from its destruction. It guards cells and protein tissues from oxidation damage. It prevents glycosylation – the process that produces AGEs to build up leading to collagen cross-linking, wrinkles and sags. Carnosine both rejuvenates old cells and extends the functional life of skin's building blocks – DNA – as well as its lipids and proteins. As such it is identified as an 'agent of longevity'. This amazing dipeptide also clears toxicity. When chromosomes are exposed to high levels of oxygen, carnosine is the only antioxidant known to protect them from oxidative damage. It rejuvenates connective tissue and speeds wound healing. Carnosine may yet prove to be an important key to dissolving AGEs and destructive cross-linking of collagen after it has occurred, but it is too soon to tell for sure.

In 1999 researchers in Australia confirmed that carnosine increases the longevity of fibroblasts – the skin cells responsible for producing collagen. It also extends the *Hayflick limit* – the maximum number of times a cell can divide before dying – by a remarkable 20 per cent. Because of its ability to repair protein tissue, Russians use carnosine, with great success, in a special form called N-alpha acetylcarnosine or NAC in eye drops to eradicate cataracts. Carnosine improves overall skin condition and can treat tough leathery skin as well as preventing many age signs on the face. Used as an oral nutraceutical the recommended dose is 50 to 200mg of carnosine a day taken on an empty stomach. In the case of carnosine *more* is most certainly not *better*. Doses above this amount can actually be *less* effective.

'Be yourself, no matter what they say.'

Sting

Nicotinamide – Golden Thread Of Youth
The last place you might expect to find a golden thread in the tapestry of living skin is in the form of a special form of vitamin B3 – nicotinamide or niacinamide. This form of the vitamin behaves quite differently than the well known nicotinic acid which causes hot flushes when swallowed. As far back as 1968 Nobel Laureate Linus Pauling published research reporting success in the treatment of psychiatric patients using moderate

doses of this vitamin together with ascorbic acid. Nicotinamide has long been used both topically and orally for its anti-inflammatory abilities. It has a quite stunning ability to reverse many aspects of skin ageing when used internally and even externally in skincare products:

- ❑ As a precursor to electron carrier substances in living cells – NAD and NADP – nicotinamide enhances energy production within the living matrix. It takes part in many metabolic pathways including turning glucose into ATP making fatty acids important for skin beauty, and metabolising proteins.
- ❑ It increases collagen synthesis by stimulating the activity of fibroblast cells, prolonging their life, and protecting them from senescence.
- ❑ It decreases skin inflammation by inhibiting the release of histadine and its ability to trigger the production of anti-inflammatory mediators.
- ❑ It enhances the synthesis of lipids important for good cell walls and overall skin health and beauty.
- ❑ It diminishes wrinkling.
- ❑ It repairs DNA after skin has been exposed to too much UV light, electromagnetic or chemical pollution.
- ❑ It increases the biosyntheses of ceramides and other important moisture-holding gels in which skin cells are suspended.
- ❑ It fades age spots and helps prevent the formation of new ones.
- ❑ It plays a central role in blocking genetic messages which can result in skin cell ageing and delays cellular strangulation leading to apoptosis – cell death.

In the past five years, much research has been carried out into the external use of this nutrient in skincare products. Proctor and Gamble long experimented with nicotinamide and concluded that, together with vitamin E in the form of tocopheryl acetate and panthenol – a pro-vitamin form of B5 – it could form the basis of a new range of anti-ageing products – Olay Total Effects. Studies are now in progress at various universities to explore its possible use in protecting the body from cancer. Others indicate that nicotinamide may help prevent diabetes. The usual dose for improving skin is between 500mg and 1000mg a day. It is best taken with a good multiple B vitamin.

'*Clinically, niacinamide has been shown to significantly improve type I sensitive skin (associated with abnormal barrier function) by decreasing sensitivity and stinging. Improvement of the skin barrier may account for the increased skin smoothness and improved skin texture reported by patients using niacinamide containing products.*'

Dr Leslie D. Baumann

Broad Spectrum Works Best

'Antioxidants' and 'free radicals' have become buzz words. Go into any pharmacy or healthfood store and half of the products on the shelf have them written all over their labels. Yet most people are not clear about what they mean. Simply put, a free radical is a highly reactive oxygen molecule which can destroy tissues – particularly cell membranes and genetic materials. Electrons in molecules usually come in pairs. When oxygen is burnt in the body – a process absolutely necessary for life – one member of an electron pair can get stripped away turning the molecule into a free radical and making it highly unstable. So it rushes about frantically looking for another electron to mate with. It desperately grabs on to any electron available, often destroying the molecule it has stolen it from, creating a chain reaction. These beastie molecules can tear through cell membranes and mitochondrial membranes, shredding them, screwing up a cell's functions and even threatening its life.

Free radicals attack skin cells from all directions – when we come in contact with chemicals in products or the environment, when we lie out too long in the sun, when we inhale passive cigarette smoke – even when we exercise long and hard. They are formed in great number when we are exposed to environmental contaminates. We also generate them in our body when we are exposed to radiation like x-rays or cosmic rays flying in aeroplanes. Free radicals even occur during normal metabolic processes. Because they can disrupt and destroy cells, excessive free radical activity is not only one of the critical reasons why the skin ages, it is also a major factor in the development of degenerative diseases – from heart disease to cancer. Your body has a number of skilful methods for quenching these troublemakers: the problem is that too often, given the kinds of foods we eat and the kind of pollution we are subjected to, our bodies are bombarded with more free radicals than our natural internal antioxidant enzymes can disperse. That is when we can benefit from a lot of extra help from antioxidants in our foods and as supplements.

'There's a great woman behind every idiot.'

John Lennon

From Pigments to Vitamins

Antioxidants are substances and compounds – from vitamin C and selenium to licopene in tomatoes – which carry the ability to deactivate free radicals, rendering them harmless. Over the past thirty years masses of population studies, trials and laboratory experiments have shown that antioxidants are *good* for us. Antioxidants from vitamins C and E, Co-enzyme Q10 to pinebark extract and nicotinamide appear more frequently as ingredients in skincare products. They help protect skin from age damage. But the benefits of free radical scavengers don't stop there. Some can calm inflammation, enhance the skin's moisture holding ability and improve its immune functions as well. Vitamin C's overall talents as a vitamin, for instance, are quite distinct from its antioxidant properties. Some antioxidants such as the bright coloured carotenoids in vegetables and tocopherols – forms of vitamin E – are also involved in cellular signalling. Others can play a role in gene expression or in guiding and regulating the actions of enzymes. Antioxidants antidote skin's toxins. By counteracting them, they help create better skin health, prevent damage and slow down skin ageing.

'Take a day to heal the lies you've told yourself and the ones that have been told to you.'

Maya Angelou

Pure Synergy

Many different antioxidants occur together in nature. The leaves or the flesh of a plant or a mushroom can contain many different antioxidant immune-enhancing phytochemicals, each of which has something different to offer skin. Antioxidants work together. They empower each other.

To get the highest level of antioxidant support for skin, there is nothing as good as a diet high in fresh organic fruits, vegetables, sprouted seeds and herbs, plus first rate protein foods and plenty of essential fats. It supplies an almost perfect balance of essential antioxidant vitamins: A, C and E and the antioxidant minerals zinc and selenium, all of which bring significant anti-ageing help. This way of eating also provides skin with a high complement of potent plant-based antioxidants which have proven to be of value. If you want to use phytonutrient supplements, it is best to buy a wide spectrum, plant-based antioxidant formula which includes most of the best phytonutrients since they work in synergy. You can also find formulas which include antioxidant vitamins and minerals. When it comes to combining nutraceuticals, the whole is far greater than the sum of its parts:

- **Carotenoids** give vibrant fruits and vegetables their colour. More than 600 varieties have been identified. Fat soluble, they seek out the lipids in cell membranes where they protect from free radical damage, look after the integrity of DNA, improve cell communication necessary for growth and reproduction and support immune functions.
- **Licopene**, a red carotenoid found in tomatoes, pink grapefruit and watermelon, is the most efficient quencher of singlet oxygen free radicals. It protects against degeneration and cancer.
- **Flavonoids** and other **Phenolics** belong to a large group of organic plant molecules produced by plants to protect themselves from attack by disease and insects and protect them from damage by intense UV light. Some, such as the anthocyanins found in wine are deep red, some purple, others bright blue. They often have an astringent or slightly bitter taste. Green tea is rich in these flavinoid antioxidants which is one of the reasons it is an excellent drink for skin. You will find them in onions, apples and citrus fruits. They mop up free radicals, help fight off viruses, calm inflammation and help protect from allergies.
- **Sulphur Compounds** in vegetables like onions and garlic, broccoli and watercress bring protection from cancer and age degeneration.

'Carnosine's ability to rejuvenate connective tissue cells may explain its beneficial effects on wound healing. In addition, skin ageing is bound up with protein modification. Damaged proteins accumulate and cross-link in the skin, causing wrinkles and loss of elasticity. In the lens of the eye, protein cross-linking is part of cataract formation. Carnosine eye drops have been shown to delay vision senescence in humans, being effective in 100% of cases of primary senile cataract and 80% of cases of mature senile cataract.'
Karen Granstrom Jordan MD

Master Protector

If, in addition to the three master nutraceuticals – MSM, nicotinamide and carnosine – you want to take only one more nutraceutical with first-rate antioxidant properties, you can't do better than thiotic acid – also known as alpha-lipoic acid – ALA. The 'universal antioxidant' this sulphur-based vitamin-like substance is an important co-factor in the production of cellular energy. When it is not in sufficient supply, muscle mass shrinks and the skin's energy is diminished. ALA protects your DNA and mitochondrial membranes, inhibits inflammation and remodels collagen. It also inhibits the formation of AGEs, improves insulin sensitivity and helps clear excess glucose from the bloodstream.

'Healing is embracing what is most feared; healing is opening what has been closed, softening what has hardened into obstruction, healing is learning to trust life.'

Jeanne Achterberg

Thiotic acid is used as a drug in Germany because of its ability to enhance sugar metabolism. A unique free radical scavenger, thiotic acid is both fat and water soluble. This means it travels easily across cell membranes to quench free radicals, both inside and out. A very small molecule, ALA works together with other antioxidants to recycle them. When vitamin E quenches lipid peroxidation, a new free radical is formed. Thiotic acid *reduces* that new radical, turning it back into vitamin E so it is ready to fight the battle for yet another day. It does the same with vitamin C. Dermatologist Nicholas Perricone has popularised the use of ALA in skincare. Like a number of other cosmetic manufacturers, he bases some of his products on it. The usual internal dose of ALA is 100 mg taken twice a day with meals. ALA is an excellent nutraceutical. I use it especially when I am travelling or under a lot of pressure from work. But it doesn't hold a candle to the magnum force the 'big three' – MSM, nicotinamide and carnosine – have to offer when used together. If you are going to explore the power of nutraceuticals for skin, I suggest you begin with this combination, then work your way down the list adding ALA and others if you need them.

PUMP UP THE HORMONES

how to grow your own and steal the rest

Your skin ebbs and flows on a tide of hormones. The agony of adolescent acne, the glow of pregnancy, the wrinkling and thinning of menopause, all have one thing in common: hormones. When your body's symphony of hormones is well played, skin is radiant. When hormonal harmony turns into cacophony and youth-supporting hormones dry up, there is a lot you can do to put things right.

All the metabolic processes on which beautiful skin relies cannot happen without hormones. The word itself comes from a Greek word, *hormao*, which means 'I excite'. This is exactly what the hormones do. They are messengers made in minute quantities in the brain, endocrine glands like the thyroid, adrenals, pancreas, testes and ovaries, then transported throughout the body. Even the skin itself makes hormones. So much hormonal activity takes place in there that some authorities look upon our skin as an endocrine gland in its own right.

'Be like the flower, turn your faces to the sun.'

Kahlil Gibran

Intracrine Synthesiser – Par Excellence
When an organ – like the skin – can produce specific hormones for its own use (rather than only using those made elsewhere in the body) this is called *intracrine biosynthesis*. Give your skin access to all the nutrients, energy, essential fatty acids, and proteins it needs, and it becomes a master synthesiser.

Hormone activity in the skin goes on all the time. Some hormones are continually being destroyed – metabolised and used up. Others are created as the skin's need for one or another develops. In a body whose living matrix is ordered and vital, this takes place in much the way a theme or cadence in a piece of music will give way to another melody – part of the coherent symphony. So rapidly can hormonal shifts take place and so closely interwoven is your endocrine system with thoughts, feelings, and external events, that measuring the levels of a certain hormone – say oestrogen or progesterone, testosterone, DHEA, or melatonin – in blood can give you or your doctor only a vague idea of what your hormone levels are really like. Measurements he takes at 10 am will have changed by noon.

'My problem lies in reconciling my gross habits with my net income.'
Errol Flynn

GO FOR BALANCE

Whenever hormonal levels in the living matrix become unbalanced, or depleted or both, the skin shows it. And if skin beauty has become undermined by hormonal disorder or depletion, there are three possible steps you can take to restore order.

1. Detoxify your body and rebuild it. Use the Five Day Facelift Diet and then go onto the Living Matrix 21 Day Turnaround Programme. The right diet, exercise and life changes alone restore hormonal balance in most people. And they do it better than drug-based therapy with *none* of its risks.
2. Use herbal hormone supporters to help the body restore its own hormonal balance.
3. Supplement your own supply with nature-identical hormones as supplements or in creams. These are *not* artificial drugs but the exact same molecules as those found within your own body.

Hormones at Work

Each hormone is designed to affect the cell it targets in specific ways. Cells have receptor sites on their surface to which a hormone molecule attaches. The more receptor sites available in a particular tissue, the more sensitive that tissue will be to a specific hormone. A hormone is only able to direct the functions of a cell or tissue if it can bond to its receptor sites. Regardless of how high your hormone level may be, when it cannot bond, it will exert no effect.

'. . . it's sort of bloom on a woman. If you have it you don't need to have anything else; and if you don't have it, it doesn't much matter what else you have.'

James Matthew Barrie

Skin cells boast receptors for many hormones, each of which plays an important part in beauty. Provided your body has not been polluted with cigarettes, drugs or oestrogen-mimicking petro-chemically-derived herbicides and pesticides, your skin-regulating hormones are likely to be well-balanced. Through the passage of time, more often as a result of a lifestyle that does not support hormones in an optimal way, hormone levels decline, including the sex hormones testosterone and oestrogen, and skin deteriorates.

Cycles Glories and Miseries
The skin's hormone flow both directs and follows life cycles. Puberty, PMS, pregnancy, menopause, all bring about hormonal changes in the skin. At puberty, levels of oestrogen soar, the skin softens and becomes more vulnerable to damage, oestrogen triggers the maturation of the female reproductive organs, spurring the development of secondary sex characteristics like breasts and pubic hair. There are three different forms of oestrogen. Together they redirect the distribution of fat giving a female body broader hips, breasts and a slender waist, as well as far softer skin than a man's.

'There is nothing mysterious about ageing. Ageing is simply an inherited hormonal, neuroendocrine program . . . that can be modified, delayed or even reversed.'

Walter Pierpaoli MD

Not For Men Only
Testosterone is an important hormone for skin too. This male repro-ductive hormone, found naturally in women's bodies as well, not only gives you a healthy sex drive, it also makes for strong skin. Adequate levels of testosterone promote a rich head of hair in women, too. Too

much testosterone can produce unwanted hair on the face and other parts of a woman's body. It is all a question of balance. In a healthy female body, most testosterone is converted into oestrogen.

Help For Skin At Period Time

Menstruation is a time when the level of the female reproductive hormone progesterone falls dramatically as certain prostaglandins – hormone-like compounds made in the lining of the womb – increase. This makes it a breakout time – especially for women whose skin tends to be oily. Water-based foundations can help. Mineral-based foundations are even better (see More Than Makeup). A period is not the best time of the month to have a facial. Facials involve massage and only make matters worse by rupturing whiteheads beneath the skin surface. During menstruation, a woman's skin is excessively sensitive as well. So stay away from tweezing and waxing. PMS is largely a disorder of hormonal imbalance. What you do to help your skin also helps clear premenstrual tension.

PMS SKIN

The common causes of PMS are the common causes of skin trouble at menstruation:

❑ Too much oestrogen.
❑ Too little progesterone.
❑ Hypothyroidism – low levels of thyroid hormones.
❑ Stress and adrenal dysfunctions which cause too much cortisol – your body's stress hormone – to be secreted.
❑ A diet high in sugar, carbohydrate of grain origin, and junk fats – all of which destroy insulin sensitivity and screw up blood sugar.
❑ A deficiency of vitamins, minerals, and trace elements – especially B6, zinc and magnesium.

'The career of flowers differs from ours only in audibleness.'

Emily Dickinson

HERBAL HELP FOR PMS SKIN

Here is some of the most effective help for PMS skin:

CHASTEBERRY

Chasteberry is my favourite plant helper to alleviate PMS and to clear the skin troubles it brings. Both are related to a lack of progesterone and/or an excess of prolactin. In studies more than 50 per cent of women using a chasteberry extract reported significant improvement in both areas. Look for a chasteberry extract standardized to contain 0.5 per cent *agnusides* – the most hormonally active ingredient in the plant. You will find it in tablet or capsule form. The usual dose is 200 to 250 milligrammes a day. 2ml a day is the equivalent dose of liquid extract. Use chasteberry from day 14 of a menstrual cycle until menstruation stops.

LICORICE ROOT

Licorice root is a great hormonal balancer for PMS, pill-caused hormonal disturbances and any number of other hormone-related skin disorders. It's particularly good for puffy skin caused by excess water retention and the build up of pollution in skin. Licorice root taken daily, two to three months at a stretch, helps lower oestrogens and raise progesterone. This plant blocks the enzyme which breaks progesterone down, so more remains in your tissues. You can make a delicious licorice tea from the powdered root or you can swallow it in capsule form – one to two grammes at a time – two to three times a day. You can also take a fluid extract three times a day, or use a dry extract of the herb (choose one with 5 per cent *glycyrrhtinic* acid content) from 250 to 500 milligrammes three times a day.

DONG QUAI

Dong Quai (Chinese angelica) is another good-guy herb for skin troubles at period time. The best way to use it is three times a day starting on day 14 of the cycle and stopping at the onset of menstruation. Menopausal and postmenopausal women can take it all the time. (See below.)

'Time is nature's way of keeping everything from happening at once.'
Woody Allen

STEER CLEAR OF THE PILL

There was a time when doctors believed that taking birth control pills was good for the skin. Happily that notion is fading. Birth control's artificial hormones deplete your body of nutrients like vitamin B-6 and zinc, both of which are essential for good skin. If you're going to take the Pill, you need supplements of these nutrients to counteract the negative effects of the artificial hormones it contains.

Bitter Pill For Skin

Oestrogens, even in a low dose, make blood vessels dilate. This can produce broken capillaries on the face as well as spider veins and varicose veins in the leg. Drug based oestrogens also increase melatonin production but only in certain spots. So when the sun hits your skin these spots get darker. The Pill can also trigger acne and pimples as well as lowering your sex drive. Libido itself is entirely governed by the flow of hormones. When sex hormones are not in balance and libido falls, the skin's glow diminishes. Think of how glorious your skin looks in the throes of passion.

When a woman has been taking drug-based birth control for a long time and then stops, her prolactin levels rise. The primary purpose of *this* hormone is to regulate the development of glands in the breast involved with milk secretion during and after pregnancy. High levels of prolactin is the main reason why many women cannot get pregnant so long as they are breast-feeding. When prolactin levels are high in women who are not breast-feeding this can cause disturbances in the menstrual cycle and sex drive, as well as oily, highly reactive skin, acne, ovarian cysts and PMS. A high potency multiple vitamin and mineral supplement, plenty of fatty fish and flaxseed oil – both rich in omega-3 essential fatty acids – together with chasteberry extract help counter this.

'We are indeed much more than we eat, but what we eat can nevertheless help us to be much more than what we are.'

Adelle Davis

Pregnancy Changes Everything

When pregnant, your progesterone levels soar. High progesterone during pregnancy is, in no small part, responsible for the wonderful glow pregnant women can have. For some women, pregnancy is the best time of their lives and their skin shows it. For others pregnancy wreaks its own havoc. If you're pregnant and prone to acne, steer clear of antibiotics and under no circumstances touch Accutane – the vitamin A derivatives prescribed to treat it. It can cause birth defects. It's a no-no while you are breast feeding as well. Accutane is something I would not touch at any time. It profoundly disrupts hormonal balance and may create depression.

Levels of oestrogens also rise during pregnancy. This can make skin prone to eruptions and irregular pigmentation. You can also end up with melasma – dark splotches on cheeks, forehead, or upper lip. Between 50 and 75 per cent of pregnant women do. More common amongst dark complexioned women, melasma is made worse by exposure to ultraviolet light. More than any other time, during pregnancy it's important to use a good mineral-based sun block. (You don't want chemical sunscreens absorbed into your body.)

Whatever colour skin you were born with, it will tend to darken while you're pregnant. Nipples get darker. These changes, too, are hormonal. So is dry itchy skin in the later stages of pregnancy. Make sure you get plenty of essential fatty acids all through pregnancy, particularly the omega-3 fats from oily fish. They can help a lot to alleviate itchy dry skin not only during pregnancy but anytime.

'The tragedy of life is not that it ends so soon, but that we wait so long to begin it.'

Anonymous

Skin's Passage To Power

Menopause brings its own hormonal challenges. Even before periods stop, falling levels of oestrogens and progesterone create skin changes. Excessive dryness is one. Moisturise, moisturise, moisturise. Also increase your level of omega-3 fats: eat mackerel, herring, sardines, wild salmon. Use cold-pressed flaxseed oil on your salads. Explore what natural hormones – progesterone, tri-oestrogens, even testosterone – in cream form can do to improve skin texture and firmness. They supply low doses, not of drug-based hormones used for HRT, but of exactly the same molecules your body itself produces.

EXTRA HELP

If you have not already done so, peri-menopause is the time to pay close attention to the kind of skincare and makeup products you're using. Look for ranges genuinely free of preservatives, chemicals, alcohol (see Resources) and other chemicals which can cause reactions. Low doses of a natural progesterone cream rubbed all over your body helps to restore youthful thickness to skin that has lost it.

Herbs Can Help

Plant remedies can be used alone or in combination since hormone-regulating herbs work well in synergy. Apart from their being generally safe in almost all circumstances, the great bonus with herbs is that they have the wisdom to do the balancing of hormones for you. The same herb that increases a hormone in a woman's body who needs more can reduce it in another woman who needs less.

'It is never too late to be what you might have been.'

George Eliot

Here are my favourites for skin:

BALANCED SKIN AT MENOPAUSE

DONG QUAI – MASTER BALANCER

The most valued of all Oriental plants in the treatment of women's hormonal problems, Chinese angelica has the ability to energise the skin and support its functioning. It helps de-age it, improves circulation, and adds a youthful radiance to the face, smoothing out fine lines and thickening skin. It can also help thicken the walls of the vagina and bladder and relieve rheumatic aches and pains associated with hormonal shifts. 15 to 30 drops of the fresh root tincture three times a day is the recommended dose.

BLACK COHOSH – SNAKE MEDICINE

Called Sheng Ma in Chinese medicine, and also known as black snakeroot, this plant is a favourite of Native Americans. It has been used for hundreds of years to treat disorders of the womb, to restore healthy menstruation, to soothe irritation and congestion, and improve the look of skin during menopause. Black cohosh is rich in phyto-oestrogens and in the adaptogens – plant chemicals – which enhance the body's ability to handle stress by countering high levels of cortisol. Make an infusion of black cohosh using one teaspoon of the dried root to a cup of boiling water. Let it steep for 12 minutes then take a dessertspoonful every few hours. You can also use Sheng Ma in the form of a tincture made from the fresh root. Caution: black cohosh is never used during pregnancy or when there is menstrual flooding.

'The system of nature, of which man is a part, tends to be self-balancing, self-adjusting, self-cleansing. Not so with technology.'

E. F. Schumacher

EXTRACTS OF RED CLOVER – SILKY SOFTENER
Rich in plant oestrogens, red clover is the best herbal skin softener I know. It sleeks and soothes skin, while increasing its ability to retain moisture. Like the fruit pomegranate, this plant can be especially useful to overcome dry skin in mid-life. It also clears a build up of wastes and toxins that happens over time and refines skin's texture. Use it as a tissane – simply pick up the red flowers from a fresh clover plant, toss them into a cup and steep for 10 minutes. You can also take it as an extract – a few drops in a glass of water three times a day.

'Nature does nothing uselessly.'

Aristotle

WILD YAM – SKIN STRENGTHENER
A chemical called *diosgenin* extracted from wild yam was long used to manufacture steroid drugs, including oral contraceptives, testosterone, oestrogens, and corticosteroids through a series of chemical steps. But there is a lot of confusion surrounding the use of wild yam and wild yam cream, so beware: ignorant or unscrupulous companies, knowing that there is a high demand for natural progesterone cream and that natural progesterone can be made from this

chemical taken from the wild yam, sometimes sell wild yam creams letting their customers believe that wild yam itself contains natural progesterone. It does *not*. Wild yam creams are pretty useless. The progesterone cream that my close friend John Lee has made the world aware of is *not* a wild yam cream or a progesterone cream. It is a cream which contains a natural hormone chemically identical to your body's own progesterone.

An infusion of the dried root – ½ to 1 teaspoon in water, once or twice a day – or 10 to 30 drops of a tincture – can not only improve the quality of ageing skin, it helps ease joint and muscle pains and headaches, as well as moistens a vagina which has lost its lubrication because of hormone disruptions. Used from day 14 to 28 of a menstrual cycle, wild yam can help many women still menstruating clear their PMS.

Steroids And Your Skin

Now let's look at the third option for rebalancing hormones and clearing related skin problems: nature-identical hormone support. The reproductive hormones progesterone, testosterone, and oestrogen, as well as DHEA and pregnenolone, belong to a group known as the steroids. They have a characteristic molecular structure which looks a lot like the cholesterol in your own body. This is not surprising since they are all made out of it. Cholesterol is the vital fatty substance which has had such a bad press for years. It is absolutely essential to the health and the beauty of skin. Women who go on and off high-carbohydrate low-fat crash diets ruin their skin and look drawn and haggard. They do not get enough essential fatty acids from their food to be able to produce the cholesterol their body needs to manufacture the steroid hormones skin needs to stay beautiful, so it ages rapidly. So does the rest of them.

Out of each steroid hormone your body manufactures from cholesterol, yet another and another can be made from it in a rich hormonal cascade. Pregnenolone is the steroid manufactured directly from cholesterol, for instance. It is a precursor to progesterone, as well as to many other hormones, including those made from progesterone further down the cascade.

'Increasingly women ask their physicians for guidance, but most physicians don't have the answers or the experience with natural hormones. The prescriptions that physicians have written for years are largely patented, chemicalised hormonal substitutes. These products are not exact replicas of what you have in your body and you will not be able to achieve optimum individual balance with them.'

Uzzi Reiass MD

Progesterone:

A derivative of pregnenolone – mother of all sex hormones – progesterone is a precursor to the oestrogens, testosterone, and even cortisol – the stress hormone. It is progesterone which gives skin a high resistance to stress. It helps keep it firm and thick and it increases the strength of its blood vessels and capillaries. Progesterone used as a cream can reverse many of the signs of ageing in the skin of a woman whose levels have decreased and also promote healthy bone growth. When progesterone levels fall too low, skin loses its tone and thins badly.

'A good face is the best letter of recommendation.'

Queen Elizabeth I

Oestrogens:

There are three major kinds of oestrogens found in human skin: oestrone (E1), oestrodiol (E2), and oestriol (E3). E1, commonly used in artificial form in conventional hormone replacement therapy, has quite rightly come under attack as a major risk factor in breast cancer. Like E2, it is considered an 'aggressive' oestrogen. At high levels, both of these forms of the hormone are associated with increased risk of both uterine cancer and breast cancer. E3 – oestriol – is more benign. All three of these hormones in their natural state and in balance work together in a woman's body to create soft sleek skin. In their drug forms, I personally would never use them. Oestrogens in skin increase the rate of cell turnover at the basal layer, slow the rate of hair growth, reduce the activity and size of sebaceous glands, and increases the production of hyaluronic acid – one of the skin's most important metabolists which helps it stay moist and plump. Hyaluronic acid also helps skin retain its ability to stretch. When there is an excess of oestrogens in the body – this is common living in the sea of artificial chemicals which are oestrogen mimics, or when women are on the Pill or HRT – this can thin the skin far too much.

Testosterone:

Found at far higher levels in a man's body than in a woman's, testosterone is a major reason why a man's skin ages less rapidly than a woman's. Testosterone increases the rate of cell turnover in the basal layer, enhances collagen production by stimulating fibroblast activity, and increases the size and activity of sebaceous glands. Because testosterone increases collagen production, like progesterone, it helps thicken skin. This can be important as the skin ages. Some women find that small quantities of testosterone applied to the skin in cream form can help restore tone and firmness. The down side of using natural testosterone on skin is that, when high levels of this hormone circulate in the blood, some women become highly prone to acne. An excess of testosterone can promote the growth of body and facial hair in some women, while this does not happen to others.

BEST NATURAL FEMALE HORMONES FOR SKIN

It is best to work with a doctor informed about the use of natural hormone therapy who can guide their use, for hormones are highly individual in their effects on the body. These come in cream form, and are not chemically-made drugs, but based on nature-identical molecules – the same as those you have in your body.

Tri-Est or Triple Oestrogen
A balanced combination of three forms of oestrogen in cream form: oestrone, oestradiol and oestriol.

Micronised Natural Progesterone
Micronised means that a hormone has been reduced to very small particles so it absorbs rapidly.

You use natural hormone creams everywhere on the body, not just on the face. Most doctors who work with natural hormone creams follow this protocol: if you menstruate regularly, use Tri Est from day 1 to day 14 of your cycle. Use progesterone from day 15 to day 28. If you are post menopausal, both creams can be used simultaneously on an ongoing basis.

'From the time she first enters puberty until the end of her last menstrual period, every woman is keenly aware of the constant hormonal changes going on inside her body. Except during the months of pregnancy, she will experience the complex interplay of the oestrogens, progesterone and other hormones, ebbing and flowing on a usually regular 26 to 28 day cycle, until she reaches her late 40s or early 50s.'

Jonathan K. Wright MD and John Morgenhaler

Beware The Death Hormone

Not all of our hormones decline with age. Cortisol, a stress hormone secreted by the adrenal glands, increases. It can be one of the most destructive, pro-inflammatory, ageing forces on skin of any age. No wonder cortisol is sometimes called the 'death hormone' because, when circulating in high levels, it is capable of undermining the immune system, shrinking the brain and skin, forcing blood sugar up, undermining insulin sensitivity and triggering the release of inflammatory prostaglandins. It even encourages the body to lay down excess fat and predisposes us to hypertension.

Necessary to enable us to meet the challenges of stress, cortisol keeps blood sugar levels at constant highs by triggering the formation of glucose from fats and proteins. In a young healthy body the level of blood cortisol rises in the morning and goes down at night. When you are under constant stress, cortisol is continually secreted into the bloodstream. Real problems arise when the body makes too much cortisol for too long, either as the result of using steroid drugs such as cortisone or from living under stress for long periods.

When we are young it is reasonably easy to move back and forth from the dynamic stressed stage to a deeply relaxed restorative one. As we get older, our body can lose this ability and we often produce excess quantities of the death hormone. A six-year-old has far higher levels of cortisol than a 21–year-old.

'The question that really must be asked is whether the pharmaceutical hormones routinely prescribed for women are safe. These are hormone formulations often extracted from horses or concocted in test tubes. Can they possibly be safer than natural hormones that are exact replicas of what a woman's own body makes? I don't think so. Research, in fact, shows that pharmaceutical hormones can have very disturbing side effects.'

Jesse Lynn Hanley MD

CUT THE COFFEE

As little as a cup or two of coffee a day can dramatically increase levels of cortisol in your body. This can undermine the immune system on which the beauty of the skin depends, distort blood sugar and insulin balance making you prone to the formation of AGEs, collagen cross-linking, sags, bags and wrinkles. Coffee drinking also triggers weight gain in many people. A number of studies show that when we reduce coffee intake – better still cut out coffee altogether – our skin improves dramatically within a few days, body fat levels go down, water retention decreases while skin becomes more hydrated and loses puffiness.

'To be truly motivated, one must make personal commitments.'

William G. Dyer

Check Your Stress Index

Long term stress not only raises cortisol levels, it depresses DHEA – another important steroid hormone for skin. Elevated cortisol and low DHEA are associated with rapid skin ageing as well as depression, fatigue, osteoporosis, heart disease and poor memory. So closely related as antagonists are DHEA and cortisol that a person's adrenal stress index can be measured by comparing the levels of DHEA and cortisol in saliva.

One of the most important things you can do to lower cortisol levels and counter the negative effects stress has on skin is to change your diet. The Living Matrix 21 Day Turnaround is a high-raw diet rich in fresh vegetables and low glycaemic fruits complete with good quality protein. This way of eating not only detoxifies the skin and rebalances hormones, it increases levels of potassium. People who live on convenience foods or who eat a lot of cooked carbohydrates – cereals, pastas, bread and sugar – tend to have a severely disturbed sodium-potassium ratio. For beautiful skin and a healthy body we need five times as much potassium in our diet as we do sodium. Most people today get less than a tenth of the potassium they need. By the time they are 35 or 40, their skin is puffy, sallow, and lines easily. The average diet of convenience foods also makes the body highly prone to degeneration on all levels, quite literally putting it under severe stress and encouraging the production of cortisol and a lowering of DHEA.

CALM STRESS

When it comes to hormones, the single most important thing you can do is protect your body from high levels of cortisol. In addition to changing your diet and getting plenty of exercise, consider taking a good multiple vitamin rich in nutrients which are especially useful in supporting adrenal function: pantothenic acid, vitamin B-6, vitamin C, zinc and magnesium. If you want good skin at any age, be sure you get enough of them. Eat more organic liver. Take good supplements.

Youth Hormones

The anti-stress hormone DHEA and the body clock regulating hormone melatonin are both found in human skin. Each in its own way affects skin tissues and has important tasks to perform. Your body can turn DHEA into oestrogen and testosterone. The exact roles of DHEA and melatonin in human skin are still being closely scrutinised. The levels of both decrease as we get older. Many experts believe both these hormones taken as nutritional supplements can slow age-related changes.

Melatonin decreases the cortisol level in the body and promotes deep sleep. It is also useful in re-establishing normal body rhythms after jet travel. DHEA helps alleviate menopausal symptoms in some women, enhances libido and produces a feeling of wellbeing when natural levels of anti-stress hormones have dropped. Creams containing the natural sex hormones – tri-oestrogens, progesterone, and testosterone are available through compounding pharmacies under a doctor's prescription. If, after making changes in the way you eat, you find that the hormonally related herbal remedies don't do enough, natural hormone creams or supplements of DHEA and melatonin can be worth investigating.

Chill Out

Another useful way to balance hormones and improve your skin is to practice daily deep relaxation, meditation, autogenics, or yoga breathing. Each helps your autonomic nervous system learn, at will, to move from the dynamic state of stress and excitement to a deeply restorative one in which the cells of your skin, indeed the whole of your body, repair themselves. I like Dr Herbert Benson's relaxation response techniques. Like many forms of meditation, it works by concentrating on a particular word or sound that is pleasing to you. The word can be anything – for instance 'flower', 'peace', or 'love'. Benson likes the word 'one' as it is simple and has a connotation of unity about it.

CONTROL STRESS HORMONES

This is a particularly useful hormone-balancing stress-protective technique, once you have practiced it a few times because you can do it in so many different places, such as in a waiting room or on a commuter train or bus. I know people who've made this a part of their daily trek to and from work, with tremendous benefits not only for their skin but for their whole lives.

1. Find a quiet place where you won't be disturbed for 15 to 20 minutes and sit in a comfortable chair that supports your back.
2. Close your eyes. Give yourself a moment to settle in and you are ready to begin.
3. Simply sit there, feet on the floor and eyes closed, quietly repeat your word over and over to yourself: "one . . . one . . . one . . ."
4. When your mind wanders – and it will – or you are disturbed by a sound or thoughts, simply turn your attention gently back to repeating the word again.
5. That's all there is to it. After 15 to 20 minutes, stop repeating the mantra and get ready to come back to your normal state of consciousness refreshed.
6. Open your eyes, stretch, and go about your everyday activities.

The Teacher Krishnamurti once remarked that any word would be better than the fruitless and often destructive thoughts that normally run through our minds. He then wryly suggested using Coca-Cola.

PART THREE:

MAPPING THE MINEFIELDS

enter the cosmetic labyrinth . . . get savvy

TOXIC OVERLOAD

don't let chemical conspirators get under your skin

The United Nations Environmental Programme calculates that 70,000 chemicals are now in common use across the world. Another 1,000 new chemicals are introduced each year polluting the planet and our bodies. Legal loopholes in every country still allow beauty products to be sold which contain potentially deadly toxins which can disrupt the order of your living matrix, undermine skin beauty and encourage degeneration. Continually threatened with *toxic overload*, to clear it our bodies need help.

A recent headline in the Sunday Times shouts 'Top Perfumes Linked to Cancer Scare Chemicals'. The article goes on to report that when a Swedish government-accredited laboratory analysed 34 common products, researchers found that well known perfumes like Chanel No. 5, Dior's Poison, Calvin Klein's Eternity and Tommy Girl all contained diethylhexyl phthalate (DEHP) or similar chemicals. Phthalates are commonly are used as 'plasticisers'. And phthalates are dangerous.

'The growing list of synthetic ingredients manufacturers add to their products are turning the most innocent-looking shampoos and moisturisers into cocktails of toxins that could cause cancer over years of sustained use.'
Amelia Hill, *The Observer*, April 17, 2002

This is hardly big news. Phthalates have long been known to be both carcinogenic and mutagenic. They can adversely affect sperm in men and disrupt reproductive processes in women. Nonetheless they have continued to be used in our cosmetics and toiletries. Phthalates have been found present in other common products as well – body sprays, compacts, and a great number of hair mousses. Now, largely in response to the Swedish study, the EU is proposing to ban their use based on the fear that they may be responsible for genital abnormalities recorded in 4 per cent of male babies. But – *this is important* – phthalates are merely a pale echo of the problem – a minute concern

– in a much more threatening and complex multi-dimensional and pervasive chemical toxicity which pervades our lives.

'Chemicals that affect animal and human health in this way should not be in cosmetics at all. Many people are exposed to multiple doses every day from the range of cosmetics they use, while workers in the cosmetics and beauty industry face greater exposure.'
Helen Lynn, Health Co-ordinator, Women's Environmental Network

Sickening Sea

In the 21st century, in the industrialised world, we now live in a sea of petrochemically derived chemicals dangerous to skin, health and life. Our bodies take in massive cocktails of *xenoestrogens*. They behave like female hormones once they get inside us. We absorb them through herbicides and pesticides in the foods we eat and from the air we breathe. We swallow them along with other insidious compounds in the drugs we take. We even absorb them from the plastic cups from which we drink our tea. The last thing we need is even more hormone disrupters or other metabolic poisons absorbed through our skin from the products we slather on our faces and bodies.

Chemical hormone mimics not only carry dangers for male health, being largely responsible for the fall in male sperm count by almost 50 per cent since 1940. They are also major culprits behind the exponential growth of reproductive disorders in women – from PMS, endometriosis and fibroid tumours, to infertility, osteoporosis and menopausal miseries.

The phthalate scare is but a tip of a chemical iceberg: it has developed out of ignorance sometimes because cosmetic manufacturers have been more concerned about corporate bottom lines than the wellbeing of their customers. Much of the skincare and toiletry world still remains ignorant of all this. Either that or they are choosing to turn a blind eye to it.

FAST TRACK TO RAPID AGEING

Common cosmetic ingredients can age skin. Take the preservatives EDTA and disodium EDTA. They have been shown to accelerate the formation of hydroxy radicals which damage cell

membranes and trigger degenerative changes in the cells.
Meanwhile, sorbic acid, used as a preservative in many skincare
products and over the counter medications, can trigger the
formation of AGEs, cross-linking collagen and elastin and
making skin sag and wrinkle.

*'There is unequivocal evidence that a number of man-made chemicals have
caused serious damage to the health of wildlife and humans all over the globe.
However, the full extent of the threat they pose is unclear since only a handful
of the tens of thousands of chemicals in everyday industrial and domestic use
have been adequately tested.'*

World Wide Fund For Nature

The EU's concern about banning DEHP and other phthalates is
commendable. Immediately it had Boots denying the presence of phthalates in their hair products. Soon after they promised, as the newspaper
reported, 'We are investigating this reported presence, and if confirmed
we will take all necessary steps to remove it.' But to worry only about
the way a specific individual chemical can be dangerous to health and
life side-steps the real issue of chemical toxicity which the skin revolution addresses head on.

Dangerous Reactions
There are now over 7000 ingredients commonly found in cosmetics
and toiletries. These include a few thousand aromatic compounds
frequently used to perfume products. More than 1000 of these have
been individually shown to produce toxic effects on living systems. But,
here's the rub: far more important than the potential harm any single
chemical can do, is the dangerous way in which these chemicals can
interact to produce far more toxic compounds within our bodies.

So far behind the times are methods used to check out the 'safety'
of chemical ingredients, that it may be decades before the depths of
the chemical danger to which we are now being exposed become
common knowledge. The outdated analytical methods still used to identify carcinogenic chemicals examine the effect of only *one* chemical on
living tissue. It is at least a hundred and fifty years behind what it
should be – based on nineteenth century toxicology. As such, it takes no
account of the dangers of mega-toxic compounds created by chemical

interactions with one another as well as with the pollutants in our foods, water and air. All these chemicals, and others formed by reactions between them, contribute to mounting toxicity. This, in turn, undermines immunity and makes our bodies highly susceptible to degenerative disease and makes our skin age more rapidly.

'We live in a toxic world . . . every toxic substance can damage the body, of course, and usually the damage is worse with the greater the extent of exposure and the idea of total toxic load grew out of physicians' observations that small exposures to more than one toxic substance often resulted in large damaging effects on the body . . . exposures to more than one toxin in small amounts can be as bad as exposure to a large amount of one toxin.'

Parris M. Kidd PhD

Get Savvy About Toxic Overload

Apart from inadequate nutrition and all the fatigue, cell damage and degeneration which accompany it, the build up of waste products and foreign chemicals polluting the living matrix interferes with skin health more than anything else. Toxicity in the body builds up from a multitude of sources. Some – the *xenobiotics* – come to us from outside. The word 'xenos' means foreigner in Greek while 'bios' means life. Chemicals in the environment and from products are foreign to life. They are not familiar to our metabolism, which is why they can cause problems. Others – the endogenous toxins – are formed in our own bodies as by-products of metabolism. They often accumulate as a result of over eating, or from prolonged stress, excessive exertion or long-term fatigue. The exogenous and the endogenous toxins come together within our living matrix to establish what a body's 'toxic load' is – in other words, just how poisoned it has become as a result of the build up of stuff it would be better off without. Nowadays, your body's toxic load can be measured in a medical laboratory. Doctors trained in functional medicine use toxic load measurements to guide sophisticated natural detoxification treatments when healing chronic illness.

How Toxic Are You ?

The extent of a body's toxic load matters. A continuous interchange is supposed to take place between your body's trillions of cells and the surrounding interstitial fluids. This is how nutrients and oxygen enter the cells of the skin and cellular wastes are cleared from them. Wastes are then carried through lymph vessels to be eliminated from the system on the breath, and through urine, the bowels and the skin itself. The exchange of nutrients and oxygen in cells and the elimination of waste is an exchange regulated by subtle electrochemical energies. A build up of toxicity in the living matrix results in poor circulation and electro-chemical stagnation so cellular metabolism, the transmission of information, and the regulation of hormones can break down.

When cells thrive and skin is radiant you have a high level of protection from ageing. This happens when plenty of nutrients and oxygen get into its cells and toxic wastes can be efficiently removed from them. And, although the living matrix has elegant ways of clearing wastes including its own antioxidant enzyme system and detoxification processes through the liver and kidneys, chemical and electromagnetic pollution becomes ubiquitous when we eat foods which supply neither the essential nutrients nor the energetic order which the living matrix needs. The toxic overload replaces them.

FOREIGN DANGERS

Man-made chemicals are foreign to living systems. As such they are potentially dangerous to them, including our own body. Why? Because in a million years of evolution, our bodies have never come into contact with them. Our genes are not adapted to handle them. We do not have the enzyme systems needed to clear them from our bodies. Included in the group of potentially destructive chemicals are hundreds, perhaps thousands, of common cosmetic ingredients – from artificial preservatives to fragrances.

From Nature But Unnatural

Some common ingredients in cosmetics that contribute to toxic build up have originally been derived from a natural source. Take sodium laurel sulphate and sodium laureth sulphate, surfactants found in the majority of shampoos, bubble baths, toothpastes and shower gels. These foamers are derived from coconut oil and palm oil through a series of chemical reactions in the lab. Technicians take the original molecule and change it out of all recognition into something that the body recognises so that our bodies respond to these chemicals too as 'foreigners'.

It is the 'foreign' character of these manipulated molecules which causes problems for living systems.

SLSs easily penetrate human skin. They can build up in the body. They have been shown to cause eye irritation, skin rashes, hair loss, flaking skin and mouth ulceration. They too are capable of combining with other chemicals used in the formulas of products to form *nitrosamines* which are carcinogenic.

Cleaning Up Your Act

Your body needs a constant supply of energy and supportive nutrients to quench free radicals and clear wastes before they can undermine health, create fatigue and destroy the beauty of your skin. Toxic overload, which happens from a combination of causes, makes normal functioning impossible. Sure signs of it include many skin conditions from premature ageing to acne, psoriasis, cellulite and dehydration. Toxic overload is also a major cause behind all degenerative diseases associated with ageing.

'Compared to the toxins found in our air, soil and waterways, cosmetics seem a trivial pursuit to many environmental health and consumer advocacy groups. But many of the same poisons that pollute our environment, from dioxins to petrochemicals, can be found in the jars and bottles that line our bathroom shelves.'

Kim Erickson, *Drop Dead Gorgeous*

BETTER OFF WITHOUT THEM

Here are some of the most widespread chemicals commonly used in makeup, skincare and toiletries. A cosmetic manufacturer of integrity should, by now, be working diligently to eliminate them from the products they sell.

❑ **Parabens:** made from toluene, a petrochemical derivative, these are the most common synthetic preservatives. They are still used in 99 per cent of all products. They show up on labels with names like *butyl paraben, methyl paraben,* and *propyl paraben.* Naïve cosmetic manufacturers claim parabens are 'safe' since they don't directly cause inflammatory reactions to skin. But these enzyme inhibitors *do* damage the DNA of skin cells – something easy to verify by feeding placebos to live cells in a laboratory and then recording what happens to the cells via flow cytometry. Research carried out in Japan, Germany and Britain also implicates parabens – which we absorb in significant quantity day in day out – as a causative factor in male fertility problems and breast tumours in women.

❑ **DEA** diethanolamine, **MEA** monoethanolamine, and **TEA** triethanolamine: hormone disrupting chemicals which can form carcinogenic nitrates and nitrosamines, these are widespread in the United States and other countries. They are in the process of being restricted in the UK.

❑ **Isopropyl Alcohol** SD-40: a drying and irritating solvent which disrupts your skin's immune protective barrier making it more vulnerable to invasion by microbes and to penetration by other destructive chemicals. SD-40 promotes the formation of irregular pigmentation and age spots as well.

❑ **DMDM** Hydantoin and **Urea** – Imidazolidinyl: a couple of the many preservatives commonly found in products, these can release formaldehyde into the body, triggering skin reactions, allergies, joint pain, dizziness and lowering of immunity. Formaldehyde undermines the life processes of the living matrix. This is why morticians use it to embalm dead bodies.

❑ **Coal Tar Dyes** FD&C Colour Pigments: these are common synthetic colours made from coal tar. They can contain heavy metals to pollute the body and deplete it of oxygen. They can also be carcinogenic. Coal tar dyes are major culprits in skin reactions. They engender skin sensitivity.

❑ **Fragrances:** many chemicals used to make artificial fragrances are known to be both toxic and carcinogenic. Specifically they can affect the central nervous system, even triggering emotional disturbances and behavioural problems in some people. This is a wide group, the majority of which are dangerous – in no small part because of the solvents used to disperse their molecules and to suspend these complex organic chemicals in solution.

'There is no question that people are being damaged by their cosmetics. How can they not be? So many things are put into cosmetics now that are carcinogenic and it is allowed because cosmetics are not considered to be as serious as drugs or foods.'

Dr Jean Munro

Make Choices

Does this mean you should never again sleek on that yummy lip gloss or that you need to toss the light-as-air cream you just bought into the bin? Not necessarily. What it does mean it that it is time to become aware of the dangers of toxic overload to your own system and take action both to minimise it happening to you, and to spring clean your body of any toxic build up already present. You might, for instance, choose to use the lipstick or a favourite mascara but look for a shampoo with a natural saponifier like kumerhou or soap wort and to forget the foaming bath lotions. It is important not to take on trust cosmetic and skincare manufacturer's assurances that everything they put in their products is perfectly safe. It simply is not.

A growing number of conscientious companies are striving to formulate products without potentially dangerous ingredients. Some of them are excellent. Others, although they may have been conceived out of a genuine wish to produce good safe skincare and makeup, fall short on effectiveness and aesthetic feel. Organic wines can be wonderful. But just because a wine is organic does not make it beautiful to drink. Delicious organic wines rely both on chemical-free vineyards and on the sophisticated skills of the winemaker who creates them. So it is with cosmetics.

Living Matrix Detoxified

Make some changes in the products you use, not only for skin and hair care but for cleaning in your home. Then try the Five Day Facelift Diet. It is a great way to begin the process of detoxification and reducing your body's toxic load and in the process clearing fine lines and puffy skin. Follow this with the Living Matrix 21 Day Turnaround. It is an effective way not only to reduce your body's toxic load, enhancing the look and functions of your skin, but to raise your vitality and bring you a high level of protection from premature ageing all round.

DECREASE TOXIC LOAD FOR LIFE-LONG BEAUTIFUL SKIN

Here is a checklist for preventing toxic overload and decreasing the toxic build up in your body in an on-going way. Make use of it. Your skin can only get better and better.

❑ Decrease your exposure to harmful chemicals by choosing your skincare and makeup products carefully.

❑ Clear your cupboards of chemical cleaners, sprays and solvents. You don't need them.

❑ Eat organic foods free of hormone disrupting pesticides and herbicides.

❑ Get plenty of exercise – walking for 30 minutes a day is a great way.

❑ Stay away from cigarette smoke, both active and passive.

❑ Eat masses of fresh, raw, non-starchy vegetables and clean protein foods like fish, game, organic meat and eggs.

❑ Limit your alcohol intake to a glass or two of wine a day – at the most.

❑ Improve kidney function for better elimination: drink purified, spring or ultra clean water – at least eight 200ml glasses of it a day, more if you can manage it, or have a cup or two of green tea too.

❑ Take a sauna often – preferably infrared (see page 192) to induce sweating, remove toxins and activate your skin's eliminating processes.

❑ Stay away from sugar and avoid artificial sweeteners.

❑ Limit your coffee intake to a cup a day – none if you can.

❑ Open your windows for an hour a day – even when it is cold, to air out your home.

❑ Improve your liver function – your body's main organ for detoxification – and your body's ability to cleanse itself by eating sulphur-rich garlic, onions and broccoli often.

❑ Take extra antioxidants and immune enhancers (see page 70) to neutralise free radicals.

'Nothing in the world is more dangerous than sincere ignorance and conscientious stupidity'.

Martin Luther King

You might get to know a few of the good, natural skincare and cosmetic ranges too. See if you can find alternatives to what you use on your skin now. But beware, not all that glitters with the word 'natural' is worth its weight in gold.

WINNIE THE POOH – TAKE TWO

optically active molecules make a difference

'Pooh looked at his two paws. He knew that one of them was right, and he knew that when you have decided which one of them was the right, then the other one was the left, but he could never remember how to begin.' *A.A. Milne*

Pooh is not the only one confused about left and right. With a few notable exceptions, our multi-billion dollar cosmetic industry is not even at Pooh's level yet when it comes to understanding the tremendous significance of using *chirally correct* ingredients – either 'left-handed' or 'right-handed' molecules – when formulating skincare products. If you want to produce biologically active, effective formulas which do more good than harm to the skin's living matrix, chirality matters. As yet, either few cosmetic chemists have awakened to this fact or few companies are willing to address the challenge of chirally correcting their products. For the sake of your skin, you should know about chirality and why it matters. Let me explain.

Mirror Image Twins
The word *chiral* (pronounced KI-RUL) comes from the Greek *kheir* meaning *hand*. It is the word chemists use to describe pairs of molecules which are identical twins *chemically* yet mirror images of each other *physically*. Like your right and left palm. There is a lot of attention paid to chirality when it comes to cutting-edge nutritional supplements nowadays. For instance, the left-handed form of a certain amino acid, L-carnitine, builds muscle while DL-carnitine, which is much cheaper and more common, is toxic to the body.

'A chiral molecule is one that is not superimposable on its mirror image; it has the property of rotating the plane of polarisation of plane-polarised monochromatic light that has passed through it. This phenomenon is called optical activity.'

Dr Rod Beavon

Check It Out

Right now, hold your hands in front of your face, palms facing *towards* your body. You will notice they are *identical* – except that at the same time, they are opposite. The thumb on your right-hand faces to the right while the thumb on your left-hand faces left. Organic molecules – those containing a carbon atom, found in living things – are just like your hands. They too exist in mirror image form. Such molecules are known as *chiral* twins. One is *dextro* – that is *right turning* (D-) and the other *laevulo* – *left-turning* (L-). If you try to superimpose them, like your palms, you can't since each 'thumb' of the molecules would go in the opposite direction.

Scientists measure chirality by directing polarised light at a chiral molecule and watching whether the molecule rotates to the right, which makes it a D molecule – or to the left, in which case it is an a L molecule. To make things even more complicated, when both left and right forms occur in equal amounts, the compound is called *racemic.* A racemic molecule such as DL-carnitine always has 'DL' in front of its name.

Less Damaging Drugs

So what? So plenty. In the past twenty years giant pharmaceutical companies from Pfizer in New York to Zeneca in Europe have been busy chirally correcting drugs they sell as a result of scientific studies and the realisation that the effect of a particular compound can vary dramatically depending on its chiral or optical orientation.

The pharmaceutical market for 'chirals' or optically active compounds is now well over $100 billion a year and growing rapidly. There is increasing evidence that the optically pure form of a drug not only has better therapeutic actions, its side effects can be dramatically minimised. More than fifty per cent of the top 100 drugs are now chirally resolved. So are more than seventy-five per cent of the applications for new drugs. Not long ago the FDA issued, with Europe running close behind, a mandate that any new drugs be chirally correct. Do a search on www.google.com and you will get back around 369,000 hits for 'chiral'. Even the Nobel prize for chemistry in 2001 went to scientists working with chirality.

CHIRAL FACTS

❏ An organic molecule containing four different groups can exist in two mirror image forms. These are called *enantiomers*, from the Greek word for opposite. They are like your right and left palms.

❏ When a molecule causes a ray of polarised light to rotate to the right, it is a dextro – or 'D' molecule.

❏ When a molecule causes a ray of polarised light to rotate to the left it is a laevulo – or 'L' molecule.

❏ When D form molecules and L form molecules occur in equal amounts in a mixture – a DL molecule – this is called *racemic*.

❏ In drugs and to a large extent in nutritional supplements and cosmetics only one form of a molecule is active, safe or beneficial.

'Consider the curl of a pig's tail or the spiral on a seashell. Does it turn left or right? Many of us would not notice these natural manifestations of chirality. But stereochemists such as Christopher J. Welch, a process research fellow at Merck Research Laboratories, do. Stereochemist's eyes get trained in seeing shape and chirality, he says. And chirality pops up all over the place.'

A. Maureen Rouhi, *Chemical & Engineering News*

The beauty and health of your skin, like that of your whole body, demands that the ingredients which you put on it and introduce into it have the right molecular shape. Sometimes using the wrong chiral molecule can be disastrous in its effect.

Courting Disaster

The drug Thalidomide is an excellent example of what can happen when the wrong enantiomer is used. Back in the 1950s doctors prescribed it to pregnant women to calm nausea. Not long after, scientists discovered that thalidomide produced gross deformities in the babies of women who had used it. Many were born with stubs instead of arms and legs. The drug was a racemic mixture of both D and L molecules.

It took researchers until 1979 to discover that while the D, the L, and the racemic DL form of thalidomide exhibited equal sedative activity, only the L form of the drug caused foetal deformities.

Choose Supplements Carefully

When it comes to using amino acids and nutritional supplements it can be important to pay attention to the chirality of anything you decide to take too. Take free-form aminos. Amino acids are the building blocks out of which your body makes hormones, enzymes, glands, nails, hair, collagen and muscles. For beautiful skin you need an adequate supply of the right combination of amino acids day by day, year by year. Most amino acids – excluding glycine – come in two forms, either D- or L-. The L- series of free-form amino acids are in the same natural form as amino acids found in living plant or animal tissue. As such they are far more compatible with human biochemistry. Those that make up a long-chain protein molecule are all of L- chirality, except *phenylalanine* which can also appear in its racemic form DL-phenylalanine.

FREE-FORM AMINO FOR BEAUTY

As free-form nutritional supplements, certain single amino acids can be helpful for enhancing beauty as ingredients in products and also from inside out. *Arginine*, for instance, helps increase muscle mass, detoxify the skin and body as a whole, and encourages the release of youth-making human growth hormone. *Carnitine* is useful in weight loss, and contributes to firmer, smoother skin. *Glutathione* is a powerful antioxidant which inhibits the formation of free radicals and protects skin from rapid ageing as a result of oxidation damage which undermines the order of the skin's living matrix and contributes to wrinkles and sagging. But it is vitally important to make sure you are taking these things in the proper chirality, and ideally the skincare products you use should only contain chirally correct ingredients.

'According to the market research firm Freedonia Group, demand for chiral raw materials and active ingredients will grow by 9.4 per cent annually between 2000 and 2005.'

A. Maureen Rouhi, *Chemical & Engineering News*

Fat Shifting Amino

Take carnitine, a good weight loss helper, for instance. Your body fat is held in adipose cells. It is only burnt in the tiny energy factories called mitochondria. Carnitine is the means of transport by which fat molecules can travel into the mitochondria to turn into energy. The higher the level of carnitine in your muscles, the more stored body fat is likely to be transported and burnt. Two to four grammes of L-carnitine taken on an empty stomach before exercising can be useful to help with weight loss. But make sure you only use L-carnitine. The racemic DL-carnitine is widely available too. It is a lot cheaper. But it is also toxic and interferes with L-carnitine metabolism in your body. Using the wrong form may even *increase* your body fat.

The Right Vitamin

Vitamin E is another one to watch. Natural forms of the vitamin are D- forms as in d-alpha-tocopherol. Synthetic forms are DL- as in DL-alpha-tocopherol. Only the D- form of this vitamin is properly recognised by the human body. The racemic mixture of the vitamin – which you can find on shelves of pharmacies and healthfood stores everywhere – does indeed exhibit antioxidant activity. But, because it also contains some of the L- form, taking it can actually inhibit the D- form of the vitamin from passing through your body's cell membrane. Natural vitamin E which boasts a mixture of tocopherols is the best choice (alpha, beta, gamma etc) all in their D- form. They work together synergistically. When buying vitamin E avoid the DL- synthetics.

IT'S A CHIRAL WORLD

❑ Smell is our most chirally aware sense. We can actually perceive the 'shape' of a molecule depending on the handedness of it through its fragrance. Left-handed carvone for instance smells like green mint. The right-handed molecule of the same chemical smells like caraway. A major reason why poorly formulated cheap perfumes make people feel sick is that many of their ingredients are not chirally correct. They both offend the nose and send the wrong chemical messages to the brain.

- ❑ In tobacco, nicotine is found in its L form. The D form is far less addictive and less toxic. If cigarettes were chirally corrected they would be less likely to wreak so much havoc with people's bodies.
- ❑ Sugars, such as glucose which our bodies manufacture from carbohydrate foods we eat, are also chiral. Humans metabolise only right-handed glucose. Left-handed glucose – which can be produced in small amounts and is expensive to make – tastes sweet but it travels though the digestive system without being absorbed.
- ❑ Right-handed pheromones – the chemicals by which animals send sexual signals to each other through scent – can be hundreds of times more potent in their effects than their left-handed cousins.

'What could be more similar to my hand or my ear, and more equal to it in every respect, than its mirror image? And yet I cannot substitute the hand as seen in the mirror for its original; for if it is the right-hand, the other in the mirror is a left-hand, and the image of the right ear is a left ear, which cannot take the place of the other either.'

Emmanuel Kant, 1783

An awareness of the importance of chirality in drugs is already high. In the realm of nutritional supplements, it has been slower to come although all of the leading researchers in biochemical nutrition now write about it. With a few exceptions, the cosmetic industry still lags far behind.

Chiral Hydroxies – Protect Your Skin

Since the early nineties skincare products and salon treatments have contained a lot of alpha hydroxy acids. The most widely used is glycolic acid, a caustic chemical related to the amino acid glycine, used for peels and to dissolve the dead cells on the surface of the skin. The problem with glycolic acid, which exhibits no optical activity, is that it has a highly corrosive nature. It is well-known to cause serious irritation and it can precipitate a free radical cascade initiating the skin's immune responses.

A gentler and more effective AHA is lactic acid in its correct enantiomer L-lactic acid. This is the same chemical that gives athletes muscle ache after a workout. Unlike glycolic acid, lactic acid *does* have optical activity. It comes in three forms, D-lactic acid, DL-lactic acid and L-lactic acid. The first two are most commonly used by skincare manufacturers since they are inexpensive and easy to come by. Neither the D- nor the DL- form is natural to the body. This does not mean that they will not do the job of sloughing off dead cells, but the chirally correct L-lactic acid, can not only refine the skins surface, it can improve the way it functions.

L-lactic acid does not behave like a foreign invader. It has its own ability to calm skin metabolism. It is a natural anti-inflammatory, which both softens skin and reduces the chance of scarring when used for peels. L-lactic acid also encourages the skin to manufacture more glycoproteins, glycolipids and glycosaminoglycans, which form the gel-like medium of the skin's matrix. It also supports the skin's plasma membranes and basement membranes – rich in strengthening and moisturising compounds. D-lactic acid and DL-lactic acid cannot do this. L-lactic acid offers effective skin refining and resurfacing yet it carries a minimum risk.

'Everyone who is seriously involved in the pursuit of science becomes convinced that a Spirit is manifest in the laws of the Universe.'

Albert Einstein

Double The Benefits
Some of the most potent and effective skin products these days are made from natural ingredients. Ideally the active ingredients used to compound natural cosmetics should be chirally correct as well. The *alkaloids, terpenes* and *sesquiterpenes* for instance, which give a plant its taste and fragrance, live side by side in a plant cell. One can be an L- *isomer* while the other may be a D- isomer or come in the racemic DL- form. Take limonene found in more than 300 known plants in both the D- and the L- form. The difference between the right-handed and left-handed form of this phytochemical is tremendous.

TWO FACES OF LIMONENE

Left-handed L-limonene	Right-handed D-limonene
- promotes hair growth.	- industrial degreaser.
- inhibits tumour growth in animals.	- solvent used to dissolve and recycle old tyres.
- enhances production of antioxidant enzyme *glutathion peroxidase* which protects from age-related free radical damage.	- potent allergen. - inhibitor of hair growth. - teratrogenic – can cause birth defects in foetuses. - triggers free radical damage.

Which would you rather have a manufacturer put in a skin cream you smear on your own skin?

Hooray For Pioneers

In the autumn of 1996 a forward thinking British marketing expert with a scientific bent, Nigel Allan, became fascinated with chirality. Allan recognised that a great deal of the potential skincare products have for transforming the health and beauty of the body is being wasted in the hodgepodge way in which most – even some of the world's most expensive and successful products – are being formulated. They are making no use of the power of chirality. Allan got together with a brilliant chemist, Mike Bollman in Canada. Together they created the world's first chirally correct cosmetic line.

'Women who live for the next miracle cream do not realise that beauty comes from a secret happiness and equilibrium within themselves.'

Sophia Loren

Allan knew that when you use synthetic lactic acid – which is still used in most lactic acid containing products, you are using the racemic DL-form. It can have harmful effects on the skin. He was also aware that a racemic mixture, at the very least, could cancel the good effects of its chirally correct form, at worst it can be seriously damaging.

Many expensive and widely used products are. A well known vitamin

C serum often prescribed by doctors for the vitamin's antioxidant, anti-ageing properties is an excellent example. The form of the vitamin used, causes serious inflammation and can destroy skin tissue. People using it report that it 'erases' fine lines, yet this phenomenon occurs only temporarily as skin becomes 'engorged' by the product's inflammatory properties making it look smoother. Meanwhile, deep within the skin, the form of the vitamin in the product spurs age degeneration.

Bollman and Allan together got off to a good beginning, creating an effective salon-based range of cosmeceuticals using only chirally corrected active ingredients. Later, these products were manufactured by a private label company in Arizona, then shipped in one form or another to distributors who sell them under their own brand name labels. Some of these companies show what can only be called *excessive* imagination in their sales materials. Some claim, for instance, that their own Dr So-and-So conceived of the 'unique' range they sell or that their products contain no chemical preservatives. Having examined most of the chirally correct ranges on the market, I am virtually certain such claims are not true. Even so, despite the nonsense, most chirally correct skincare lines are far in advance of run of the mill products, including most top of the market ranges.

When it comes to cosmetics, Nigel Allan knows more about the importance of chirality than anyone in the English-speaking world: he has returned to Britain where he continues to advise upmarket French skincare companies. Hopefully a few of his clients are waking up to the importance of what he and Bollman have created and are beginning to make use of his knowledge, incorporating chirality into their own formulas. It is easier for a small or medium sized company to do this than one of the multi-nationals. For it means only having to reformulate a few products compared to the volume of creams and lotions that will need to be redone once the big guys wake up to the power of chirality.

Nature Weds Science

Pioneering chemist Suzanne Hall, whose Living Nature range is genuinely *without* chemicals of any kind, was one of the first to realise the importance of chirality and make use of it. When an existing product in her original range needs updating, she checks out each ingredient in the formula. Where one or another turns out not to be in the best chiral form, she replaces it – with its correct chiral twin. In formulating Living Nature's new Professional Range – the best collection of natural face and body products I have found anywhere – she went to great trouble to ensure that chirally correct ingredients went into it. Not to do so, she felt, would be to undermine a product's potential to bring maximum benefits. Hall's work spearheads a new wave of effective, safe, natural formulas, making much so-called natural skincare look fifty years behind the times. She is always searching for inventive ways in which science can be used in the service of nature to bring the very highest support to skin and body.

'In recent years, many dermatologists and skin aestheticians have been using laser and infrared technology to affect the skin on a cellular level – either via "resurfacing" or by stimulating cellular activity. With optically active compounds, we can achieve these same effects, not on a cellular level, but on a molecular level, deep within the structure of the skin – without the need for lasers.'

Nigel Allan

As the skin revolution gathers momentum, you are going to hear a lot more about chirally correct products. Meanwhile, try some. I think you will be pleasantly surprised by the results. Ask questions about the chirality of the ingredients in any range you are thinking of buying as well. Unless the company who manufactures and sells it is pretty savvy, chances are they will not even know how important chirality is to biologically effective skincare. The short list of references to this chapter at the back of the book (page 342) is a great place for them to begin to learn. The sooner they do, the better all of our skin will fare.

PERMA YOUTH

authentic beauty comes of age

Self-obsession . . . narcissism? That's past history. Authentic beauty is tough, ageless, and all-encompassing. It comes out of a demand for self-actualisation, not self-obsession. Discernment, self-respect, ecological savvy and aesthetic awareness – these are its watchwords. Beauty now is not just holistic. It's *holographic* and powerfully transforming to the lives of those who pursue it. Such is the shape of skin to come.

The coming revolution calls for products that not only de-age skin but shift moods, dissolve stress, enhance health and transform the way we feel about ourselves. New 'ageless consumers', driving revolutionary change, are turning away from 'magic bullet' formulations. They want more power, more synergy, more effectiveness. They are demanding skincare which can make significant changes to the way their skin looks, feels and functions. Some of the new cutting-edge formulations are beginning to keep that promise.

'When you really listen to yourself, you can heal yourself.'
Ceanne Derohan

The people who buy these products are far removed from our parents' generation. They purchased dream creams and hoped for the best. We have become tough-minded. We are not easily fooled by products that don't keep their promises. And, according to Mintel consumer polls, 'keeping young looking' is top of our list of priorities.

THE PERMA YOUTH CULTURE

Even youth ain't what it used to be. The Future Laboratory in London – a brilliant group of futurists, involved in brand profiling, data mining and cultural brailing, coined the phrase 'rainbow youth' to describe the richest and largest growing segment of the beauty-concerned, cosmetic-buying population: this is a new breed of men and women – often 50-plus – healthier, wealthier and more clued into what is real and what is hype than any 25 year old. Skin revolution consumers are *ageless*. Martin Raymond, Future's Director sums it up beautifully, 'Forty-two is the new twenty-two'.

'There's a few things that we know about this generation, which I think are gonna create a huge consumer demand, which is going to fuse with this enormous new medical scientific capability to create dozens of amazing new products and trillions of dollars being spent.'

Ken Dychtwald

Perma youth consumers are ageless revolutionaries. Many grew up in the sixties. Others have taken on a post-modern sixties fascination with change and hope that existed before the cynicism of the seventies and the nihilism of Generation X set in. They wear stylish clothes – Calvin Klein, Gant, Ralph Lauren, Patagonia, Armani and Paul Smith. They use Botox and pulsed light therapy. They find the best plastic surgeons in a desire to undo the ravages of time. Yet they are far from focused only on the *appearances* of beauty. They demand more and have the energy, money to spend, and determination to get what they want. The over 50s buy 80 per cent of all top-of-the-range cars and 50 per cent of all skincare products. Even the average Harley Davidson cruiser is now 52. Rainbow Youthers own 80 per cent of the EU's disposable income. They want real quality of life. They want to be more creative and to have a lot of fun. As far as growing old gracefully is concerned – forget it. The holy grail of life expectancy is fast approaching 100 for men 110 for women. Thirty or sixty, 'Perma Youth' is in for the long haul.

Politically aware and demanding, the new breed of ageless consumers care more about how a cream *performs* and what Power Yoga may do to strengthen their bodies than they do about *brand names*. Computer literate and open to new ideas, they are the prime movers behind the skin revolution. Ironically, it is now the lost generation of sugar coated, coke-sniffing, makeup-buying 20 year olds who make up the 'old guard'. Trans-generational revolutionaries are on to something bigger and better. Forty something? Fine. Fifty something? OK. Want to revolutionise your life? Go for it.

'...miracles don't come from cold intellect. They come from finding your authentic self and following what you feel is your true course in life.'

Bernie S. Siegel

SKIN REVOLUTIONARIES WANT IT ALL

Skincare products and self-care treatments for the trans-generational revolutionaries need to fit with the kind of clothes they buy, and the high-tech devices they use – from ipods to portable ionisers – with the organic foods they like to eat and the rowing machines they work up a sweat over. Few of the giant skincare manufacturers are switched on to their needs.

- **Authentic Beauty:** natural, potent, chemical-free products which make us look and feel younger, more vital and more who we uniquely *are* – not like some photo in a magazine.
- **More Dynamism:** vitality is the essence of the new authentic beauty. Skin revolutionaries find it in low-grain no-sugar eating. They swallow the best nutraceuticals they can lay their hands on. They rejuvenate skin and body in *medically measurable ways*. The exercise they choose has to be fun, or they won't do it at all. They are determined to live the life they want – not the one they are *supposed* to live.
- **Bioactive Chemical-Free:** Perma Youthers demand safe *and* potent products – free of harsh surfactants, artificial fragrances and colorants. They not only need to smell good and feel good, they have to *work* – reversing age damage and not producing inflammation in the process.
- **High Synergy Skincare:** they go for natural treatments formulated from a cutting-edge, holistic perspective where health and beauty merge to make skin function so well that it helps us look as ageless as we want to feel.

> ❑ **Holographic Beauty:** the new authentic beauty doesn't stop at the edges of the body either. It encompasses sensuous products and practices to lift moods, counter stress, induce sleep, and heighten energy. Each product or process – from an aura spray based on the energy of top grade essential oils, to ionisers, air and water purifiers, music, and scented candles – needs to be *holographic.* It needs to enhance the *whole* of us: our capacity for joy, vitality, good looks, and excitement about being alive.

'Beautiful young people are accidents of nature. But beautiful old people are works of art.'

Marjorie Barstow Breenbie

To Rise In Flame Like The Phoenix

The drive for greater authenticity, which lies at the core of deep, authentic beauty, is intrinsic in all of us. Perma Youth revolutionaries are well equipped to make quantum leaps. These people are capable of changing their lives in any way they choose. Rise in flame like the phoenix? Right. Let's do it. My friend Kathy Phillips, Beauty Director for British Vogue, is a good example. She has not only practiced yoga for 30 years, she literally wrote the book about it: *The Spirit of Yoga.* Kathy knows about nutraceuticals, biochemistry and orthodox medicine, yet she is equally comfortable with energy medicine, aromatherapy and natural healing. When she finds herself in the midst of major life change she feels afraid – just like the rest of us. Then she does it anyway. Kathy makes use of whatever is appropriate from day to day to care for her skin, feed her body and nurture her soul. And in true revolutionary fashion, she shares what she knows with the rest of us.

'Healing may not be so much about getting better, as about letting go of everything that isn't you – all of the expectations, all of the beliefs – and becoming who you are.'

Rachel Naomi Remen

HOLOGRAPHIC BEAUTY

A life-changing shift from whole body treatment to whole being treatment is happening everywhere. Authentic beauty is holographic: it encompasses the energetic and biochemical interconnectedness of the living matrix with psyche and spirit – the matrix of consciousness. It recognises that what takes place within each of our skin cells is connected with our thoughts and feelings, with the choices we make and values we live by. Like a hologram, each minute part of our life holds within it the 'whole picture.'

We now want products, techniques and treatments to clear cellulite, protect our skin from ageing and reverse degeneration. But we also want new ways to alter our consciousness, without alcohol or drugs. We want to feel better, avoid the ravages of stress, to turn our homes and workplaces into environments that can satisfy the soul and feed our senses. We want sexy food, mood beauty, makeup that makes us look like who we really are, yet even better. We use aromatherapy, chromatherapy, phytotherapy as well as electronic energy, to protect us from the ravages of urban life.

'Deep down, I'm pretty superficial.'

Ava Gardner

Ions For Holographic Beauties
Computer monitors wreak havoc with skin, make eyes sore and leave operators looking and feeling drained. The electrostatic charge on the screen and the resultant field created between the screen and user is good neither for health nor beauty. Here's why: charged particles enter this field and are deflected either towards you or towards the VDU. Negatively charged particles – the 'good guy' ions – go towards the screen and are neutralised. Positively charged 'bad guys' flood the face and body, impingeing where they abrade delicate surfaces. Sore eyes in computer operators are not caused by flicker or glare – they only produce headaches – but by these charged particles.

A similar situation exists on aircrafts. Jets become highly positively charged as a result of air friction combined with near-zero humidity – not to mention exposure to cosmic radiation when cruising at 35,000 feet. The net result is that positively charged particles remain airborne almost indefinitely, wreck skin and mucous membranes. In such an atmosphere, super bugs and other micro organisms inimical to human health thrive – a major reason why we become prone to infection after long haul flights.

Back in the seventies, ionisers were considered little more than electronic pep-pills. Now reborn in highly effective, scientifically validated forms, they have become part of the skin revolution. Although some on the market are pretty useless, the new generation like Ion Air Technologies Air-Care Portable are based on significant advances in technology. Portable, powerful and uplifting to the spirit, using one can not only benefit your skin, it can raise your energy and promote a sense of wellbeing all around – holographic beauty goes electromagnetic.

Old Guard And New Bullets

New 'miracle' ingredients continue to appear. Take *kinetin* – one of the latest skincare buzzwords. This plant growth hormone is the main player in Almay's Kinetin Skincare, in ICN Pharmaceutical's Kinerase Cream and in Osmotics' Kinetin Cellular Renewal. Other magic bullet ingredients include the amino peptides used in L'Oreal's Age Perfect range. Meanwhile, dimethyl amino ethanol and tyrosine – used to stimulate collagen production – form the core of Evian's joint venture with Johnson and Johnson's skincare products for menopausal women. Some of these magic bullet ingredients will join the liturgy of skin treatment, hopefully to become part of more synergistic formulations in the future. Others will go the way of Gary Glitter platform shoes and 1970s false eyelashes.

'Sacred cows make the tastiest hamburgers.'

Abbie Hoffman

As for the Botox frenzy, it is still on course. But furrowed brows who hate needles can now buy do-it-yourself lotions instead of suffering. Jennifer Flavin-Stallone, wife of Sly, promotes a product known as A-Tox. Other companies sing the praises of similar formulations like Botoc and Wrinkox. I couldn't resist trying them. I was not surprised to find, at least for me, they had more to do with wishful thinking than erasing wrinkles.

The biggest, richest, cosmetic company in the world – L'Oreal – followed closely by Estée Lauder and Proctor and Gamble, are busily involved in makeovers of global proportions – expanding core brands, planning new product launches, looking for more profitable offshore markets. So are next level corporations like Shiseido, Yves Rocher and Boots. After all, this is the name of the cosmetic game. Meanwhile, unbeknown to most of them, newer, younger, more inventive companies, have been listening closely to the demands of the perma youthers, and responding to them with ever more revolutionary offerings – products which not only feed corporate bottom lines, but enrich our lives in the bargain.

'To me, old age is always ten years older than I am.'

John Burroughs

Vitamins Reborn

Vitamins have long been important ingredients in skincare. They will continue to be. Vitamins do penetrate the skin and do good: *tocotrienols* – the new age form of vitamin E – vitamin A and its analogues, nicoti-namide, pantothenic acid and of course the ubiquitous vitamin C. Vitamin C is essential in the biochemical transformation in your skin cells which takes the amino acid *proline* and incorporates it into new collagen and elastin. This vitamin also helps maintain good capillaries and converts burnt out vitamin E back into a usable form so it can fight another free radical battle. The problem is that, in the wrong form, vitamins – especially vitamin C – can do skin a lot of damage too. Even the majority of companies who sell C-based products appear to be ignorant of this fact.

Some of the most well known vitamin C-based products are formu-lated with the *wrong* forms of the vitamin. While using them can, as manufacturers claim, 'smooth out lines' they do this by creating inflammation so that skin looks 'plumped up' while causing age-damage at its deeper layers.

American dermatologist Nicholas Perricone insists that vitamin C *ester* is the answer – a combo of plain vitamin C and palm oil. Esters are more stable; they react differently than ascorbic acid with other ingre-dients in a formulation. South African plastic surgeon Des Fernandes is also into esters. He approves of combining vitamin C with a mineral such as magnesium to form *magnesium ascorbyl palmitate*. Better still, he likes the *ascorbyl tetra-isopalmitate* form where *four* molecules of

135

palmitic acid are attached to each molecule of vitamin C. 'With only a tiny amount of vitamin C, this fat soluble form passes easily through the horny layer,' says Fernandes, 'and enters the cell wall with great ease and you can get up to ten times more active vitamin C into the cell itself.' Fernandes knows more than anybody else in the world about how to create effective vitamin-based skincare products. His Environ range bears witness to this.

Meanwhile, a whole new generation of natural antioxidants, like a new extract from the Ambla plant, may solve the vitamin C dilemma altogether by simply replacing it. An ayurvedic remedy from exotic fruits, ambla has a long life and contains low molecular weight tannic acids. Like other newer natural antioxidants, it has an ability to combine with iron and copper ions, preventing the formation of hydroxy radicals and AGEs which can be a problem with the 'bad guy' forms of vitamin C.

'The way living systems return to balance is by continually expanding to encompass more of the whole.'

Joel and Michelle Levey

Innovative Instrument

The forward-thinking Fernandes is not content to formulate products. He recently designed a simple but brilliant device for increasing the penetration of vitamins and other active ingredients through the skin's surface. Known as the Roll-Cit, it consists of a small roller impregnated with minute needles. Roll it gently over the surface of your skin and it makes micro channels in the stratum corneum – the epidermal barrier to the skin's deeper layers – allowing active ingredients to reach skin depths perhaps thousands of times more effectively than when you only apply a product to the skin's surface. You apply a product, say the right kind of vitamin C or A, repeating the process several times a week. The tiny holes created in the horny layer seal themselves naturally within 24 hours. But here's the rub: you want to be very careful about what you choose to apply. It will also increase the penetration of chemicals, fragrances and preservatives which you most certainly *don't* want to get inside.

When penetration of vitamins is increased, skin manufactures more collagen, it becomes thicker, firmer and tighter. Fine lines soften. The Roll-Cit may not be a tool for the faint-hearted but it works a treat for some. The Roll-Cit is an excellent example of skin revolution ingenuity at its best. There is also a medical version of the Roll-Cit which probes far deeper allowing a dermatologist or surgeon to increase keratinocyte and fibroblast activity in a patient's skin to soften lines, tighten and firm, restore elasticity, and reduce pigmentation – even improving the appearance of dilated blood vessels. It can be used on all areas of the face and body for skin rejuvenation.

'Red meat is not bad for you. Now blue-green meat, that's bad for you!'
Tommy Smothers

SO HOW *DO* YOU SPELL NATURAL

The new trans-generational revolutionaries love *natural* products. They are into organics in a big way. The market for naturals is growing at a rate of between 10 and 20 per cent a year. But, far from naïve, perma youthers are sick to death of hype surrounding words like 'natural' and 'organic'. They have been misused for the past twenty years – at best carelessly, at worst dishonestly – so much so that most of us don't even know what they mean. Most skincare manufacturers have only just begun to meet the demands of trans-generational revolutionaries. But exciting things are happening elsewhere.

Wild And Wonderful
American Kate Rossetto's Take Me There sprays are another example of never before seen revolutionary beauty products – this time with a spiritual twist. They can help insomniacs sleep, they counter the stress of urban life, they can even make you feel more confident. More about these in a moment. Effective ionisers, sprays to counter the negative effects of VDUs and the damaging effects of jet travel, home spa products and consciousness-altering CDs for meditation, all with scientific clout are also part of the revolution.

Riding The Waves Of Revolution
In no small part the ingenuity of people like Des Fernandes, the passion of Nick Perricone, the wisdom of Rossetto, the vision of

research scientist James Oschman, inspired me to develop my own contribution to the skin revolution: Living Matrix Mist™. To my knowledge it is the first and only holographic skin complex. You spray it on your skin each morning and evening – when you brush your teeth – and as often as you like throughout the day whenever your skin or your spirits need brightening (especially when you are exposed to computers, stress or air-conditioning). Living Matrix Mist™ supplies in pure, natural, biologically active form, the nutrients, energy and biochemical triggers your own living matrix requires to create beautiful skin at any age. It is also energetically charged so it lifts the spirit as it nourishes the skin. Free of all chemicals, artificial fragrances, parabens and other substances foreign to living tissue, Living Matrix Mist™ has been synergistically formulated to give the skin what it needs to carry out all the processes necessary for ongoing regeneration and rejuvenation:

- Cellular energy production.
- Optimal gene expression.
- DNA protection.
- Strengthening of cell membranes.
- Cellular nourishment and elimination of waste.
- DNA repair.
- Production of new collagen and elastin.
- Protection from AGEs and cross-linking of collagen.
- Evening out pigmentation.
- Increasing skin vitality.

Far from the magic bullet approach, Living Matrix Mist™ is pure synergy, and in keeping with all the principles of natural health: it provides the wherewithal. The skin's own metabolic wisdom makes the magic. That is what skin revolution is all about for me.

Let's Go Shopping

When it comes to skincare, the 'good stuff' out there falls roughly into four categories. This is what I call them:

1. THE ETHICAL-NATURAL-POTENTS: these products have muscle, perform and contain no artificial chemicals or unnatural preservatives.
2. THE NATURALS: these really *are* natural, but nowhere near as sophisticated as the pioneering ethical-natural-potents.

3. THE BIOLOGICAL ACTIVES: these are based mostly on vita- mins and nutraceuticals. Sometimes called 'cosmeceuticals', the name is actually more a marketing term and has no legal meaning. These products tend to be conventionally formulated, chemically preserved and fragranced. The best are good. The rest are hype.

4. THE FEEL GOODS: these products are delicious to use, mass market or up market formulations, they make up the bulk of what's on the market.

What follows is by no means an exclusive list. There are many good ranges available but there is also a lot of junk out there, so beware.

'Beauty is not in the face; beauty is a light in the heart.'

Kahlil Gibran

1. **THE NATURAL-ETHICAL-POTENTS:** the smallest group but growing fast, they work well and are a superb marriage of nature and science in service of revolutionary skincare.

○ *Living Nature* lead the field in ethical, completely natural, chem- ical-free skincare. Their products contain no synthetics and no genetically modified plants. Created by Suzanne Hall, all Living Nature ingredients are of plant origin, including unusual gums and clays as well as Manuka Honey – from its native New Zealand. They are preserved using a complex system of natural plant frac- tions which varies from product to product depending on what is needed to do the job. SOME OF THE BEST: Rose and Herb Radiance Oil and Manuka Honey Hand and Body Lotion.

○ *Living Nature Professional* is more advanced, next generation, cutting-edge revolutionary stuff. Therapeutic spa and clinic prod- ucts, as well as face creams and body lotions for home use, Living Nature Professional is made from organic, wild-crafted (gathered in the wild) and chirally correct ingredients, with its motto – much in keeping with the ethos of the new holographic beauty – 'As you nourish your skin, you can nurture your spirit.' New Zealand's Kumerahou, reishi mushrooms, towai, rewarewa, and algaes coupled with advanced natural antioxidants and immune enhancers come together here in real synergy. Products come packed in biophoton- enhancing violet jars and bottles. SOME OF THE BEST: Creamy Cleanser, the smell of which is a work of art in itself, Honey

Exfoliant, Firming Serum for Night, and Body Polish – a remarkable green stuff you spread on skin before slipping into the shower to make skin smooth as silk.

O **Barefoot Botanicals** is a fine British entry in the natural ethical potents. A simple but effective collection, it was created by an eccentric and gifted European chemist under the direction of British homeopaths Jonathan Stallick and Hilery Dorrian. The products are chemical-free and preserved with a paraben-free form of grapefruit seed extract plus other plant derivatives. The products are full of antioxidants, phytonutrients, vitamins and specific essential oils. SOME OF THE BEST; Rosa Fina Cream and Body Lotion and SOS Cream for eczema or psoriasis.

O **Scents of Balance** originates in the high planes desert of Montana. Its creator Kate Rossetto grows a lot of what she uses in her products herself. A passionate woman, Kate not only formulates pure, natural skincare and therapeutic spa products *by hand*, she is a master at working with focused intention and prayer, which she uses to good effect in preparing them. Some are designed to regulate moods, make shifts of consciousness and enhance self-esteem. Her Take Me There Mists are high frequency emotional sprays. Water-based with the tiniest bit of alcohol to hold the frequency of the pure essential oil complexes she creates, you can keep these sprays on a desk or at the side of a bed or carry them in a pocket. They come in six different varieties including one called Freedom to help shed addictions, and another, Power and Grace, to increase confidence, courage and determination. Kate also packages her products in special dark violet glass to preserve them. SOME OF THE BEST: Rose Silk Face Cream – one of the lightest and most delicious on the market, Take Me There mists, chakra oils, and Breast Toning Oil.

O **Green People:** some of the best in this category are the organic ranges. Green People heads the list. Few skincare products and toiletries carry the Soil Association's organic guarantee symbol. Many of these products do. Green People creator, Charlotte Vohtz, worked long and hard to get organic certification for her products. A woman with great determination, integrity and a firm belief in holistic beauty and health, Vohtz single-handedly put organic skincare and toiletries on the market. The company is absolutely straight about what is in every formula. Vohtz got into cosmetics and homecare products while in search of a solution to her daughter's skin problems. The Green People range encompasses toothpastes, hair care, body products and herbal tonics as well as non-toxic baby products. SOME OF THE BEST: Body Butter, Rosemary and Pink Clay Shower Gel, Baby Salve, and Dry Zone.

'Believe in yourself and what you feel. Your power will come from that.'
Melissa Etheridge

2. **THE NATURALS:** the most rapidly growing category in skincare, these products often contain parabens or other chemical preservatives but they are produced by companies seriously committed to natural ingredients of good quality.

○ *AD Skin Synergy:* a new British company making top quality natural products whose philosophy is to provide the products which make a real difference using the finest blend of natural ingredients available in the world. Their first entry into the market, Nourishing Night Treatment, is an ultra-fine blend of top quality essential oils and other lipids. Many of their products are organic or wild-crafted including rose hip seed oil rich in GLA with powerful natural antioxidant power. Their products are free from petrochemicals, artificial fragrances and animal ingredients.

○ *Kyra:* most chirally correct skincare ranges fall into the natural category. Kyra is the best. It was put together by Canadian Taylor Sinclaire. Simple to understand and a pleasure to use, formulas are derived from those originally created by chiral experts Nigel Allan and Michael Bollman. Sinclaire has a complex website full of both cutting-edge science and fascinating speculation. The company is committed to caring for people and the earth. SOME OF THE BEST: Mellow Yellow Daily Defence Cream, Ice Shower Body Wash and Mint Mantra Anti Aging Cleanse

○ *Weleda* and *Dr Hauschka* also belong to the natural category. So do *Aveda, Decleor, Just Pure, Neways, Ren, Juelique, Liz Earle, Annemarie Borland, Aubrey Organics* and *Clarins.* Each boasts some particularly delicious products.

○ *Origins* also fits into this category although they use a lot of man-made ingredients as well as plant-based substances. Origins does not use animal-based ingredients; neither do most of the other manufacturers of the naturals. When Origins discovered that the glucosamine they had been using was not made in a laboratory but had come from shellfish, they published 'a profound apology' to customers and began using something else. SOME OF THE BEST: no Puffery, Night-A-Mins, and Pure Cream.

'If a woman hasn't got a tiny streak of harlot in her, she is a dry stick as a rule.'

D.H. Lawrence

3. **THE BIOLOGICAL ACTIVES**: conventionally formulated, but better than 'magic bullet' products, each of these ranges is based on vitamins or other nutraceuticals like ALA, Co Enzyme Q10, bearberry and other plant extracts.

○ **Advanced Skin Therapy:** this British range of products, formulated by Californian chemist Sam Dhatt under the steely eye of Nuala Briggs, is one of the best in this category. An expert in cutting-edge high-tech resurfacing and laser treatments, Briggs has shrewd judgement, and is well informed about advances in cosmetic ingredients. She seems to know what's coming before almost anybody else. The range is big, and not without its drawbacks. But Briggs is completely open about what and how much goes into each of her products, and her formulations are often far in advance of others. SOME OF THE BEST: Q10 Cream, Advanced B5 Serum, and Skin Vitalight W/MDI Complex.

○ **N.V. Perricone:** American dermatologist Nicholas Perricone is a major pioneer in the skin revolution. He is also the world's most vocal promoter of neutraceutical based skincare. His books have helped to break through outdated blinkered attitudes towards skincare and have awakened people to the powerful effect dietary change can exert on skin. He is into wild salmon the way kids are into sweets: he wants people to eat it twice a day. Believing passionately in the rejuvenative power of ALA, ascorbyl palmitate and tocotrienols, he insists that skin ageing, like degenerative diseases, is the result of inflammation triggered by sun, pollution, cigarette smoke, alcohol, stress – you name it. His product range is huge. He also claims that *dimethylaminoethanol* – DMAE – an antioxidant found in abundance in fish, tightens muscle tone thanks to its ability to release neurochemicals like acetylcholine at neuromuscular junctions. Topically applied DMAE is supposed to firm the face and make it look younger. Having reviewed the clinical experiments he carried out to validate this and examined before and after photographs of his subjects, I remain unconvinced. SOME OF THE BEST: Alpha Lipoic Acid Face Firming Activator, Spider Vein Face, and Lip Plumper.

O ***Environ:*** brainchild of Dr Des Fernandes, this unique range may not be the most aesthetically pleasing to use, but it certainly is one of the most effective anywhere. Fernandes' vitamin C products are excellent, as are his vitamin A offerings. They come in different strengths. You begin with the lower concentrations and work up as skin strengthens. Environ products are favourites of dermatologists and plastic surgeons. I became a convert when faced with skin like leather not only on my face, but all over my body after a bout with measles. I used everything I could think of on my face for three days before my skin began to soften and return to something approaching passable. But the dry leathery skin on my body refused to yield. I was sent a bottle of Environ's Derma-Lac Lotion. I applied it four times. Within 24 hours my leathery body skin turned back into soft, smooth flesh. SOME OF THE BEST: Rich Night, C-Boost, and Colostrum Gel.

'I've been through it all, baby. I'm Mother Courage.'

Elizabeth Taylor

4. THE FEEL GOODS: Mmmm . . . delicious frothy moisturisers from ***Lancome***, gorgeous cellulite products from ***Dior***, light reflecting lotions from ***Estée Lauder*** and creams from ***Prescriptives***, new pro-endorphin products from ***Guerlain*** . . . ***Yves St Laurent, Lancaster, Shiseido***. Mass market offerings from ***L'Oreal, Olay*** and ***Neutragena***, they all belong to the group. We buy them, love them and find them impossible to resist. Quite right. An important part of beauty is the luxury of texture, smell, feel and all the glamour that comes with the images used to sell it.

A few of the most expensive cosmetics in the world, and the most luxurious, are also among the best. But, to my knowledge, not one of the giant corporations has yet been able to create their own natural preservative system as Suzanne Hall managed to do single-handed, or come up with mood-altering and consciousness shifting products as Kate Rossetto has done, or demonstrated the ingenuity of Des Fernandes with his Cit-Roller or combined neutraceuticals taken internally with external skincare products based on them, or ever bothered to investigate the way dietary change can rejuvenate skin as Nick Perricone has done. The Feel Good manufacturers, powerful though they are, can learn from these people whose knowledge is cutting-edge, who are tuned into the perma youthers culture, understand the nature of the new holographic beauty and are willing to make quantum leaps to explore new territories.

Move Up To Age Power

More skin revolutionaries have objections to GM and Bio-tech procedures in the natural world. They want environmental, human and ethical audits – that corporations get into triple bottom line accountability. Books appear every year revealing cosmetic dangers, toxic substances, cancers caused by a shampoo ingredient or bone marrow being undermined by hair colourings. Cosmetics riddled with dubious ingredients from coal tar dyes and benzene to phenylenediamine and formaldehyde are no longer acceptable to perma youthers. Meanwhile, the cosmetic industry continues to be attacked by genuinely concerned customers, health and animal welfare lobbyists, and issue-driven organisations who want it to clean up its act fast. The Future Laboratory pointed out in a presentation at the In Cosmetics Exhibition 2003, '360 degree reporting means all are now targets: shareholders, CEOs, workers, researchers, R&D labs, non-compliant consumers. Alternatives are needed.' Right on.

'Forty is the old age of youth, fifty is the youth of old age.'

Hosea Ballou

With an increasingly sophisticated and demanding market for holographic beauty and ever more vocal consumers hungry for products they can trust, we need companies which tell us the truth and listen to our needs. The beauty care industry is a wonderful industry – blessed with the ability to bring more happiness to its customers than any other I know of. If only they can make the leap into revolutionary enthusiasm, who knows how life-changing what they produce can become.

MORE THAN MAKEUP

make magic with minerals . . . next generation makeup

When it comes to makeup marketing hype no word is more tossed around than *revolutionary.* 'It shimmers, it gleams, it refracts light, it de-ages . . .' Then you open the bottle and what do you get? Another liquid riddled with film formers, thickeners and surfactants plus the inevitable chemical preservatives and colorants. For my money, only one form of makeup is truly worthy of the title. It's so unique that you need lessons in how to apply it.

Natural mineral-based cosmetics represent a whole new technology. The developers have used pure micronised minerals to create foundations which are makeup, concealer, and sun block all in one. Based on non-reactive elements like titanium dioxide and zinc oxide, these foundations create weightless coverage and instant broad-spectrum (dealing with UVA, UVB and UVC rays) chemical-free protection from the elements. Used properly they can disguise virtually any skin discolouration while looking so natural (provided you know how to apply them) that even a spotty teenage boy can get away with using them to cover his blemishes. Unlike conventional liquid, cream or pressed foundations, they contain no chemical dyes. So calming are the mineral foundations to skin, they can even be used after a skin peel. Little wonder cosmetic surgeons and dermatologists throughout the world rave about them.

'Even I don't wake up looking like Cindy Crawford.'
Cindy Crawford

Mineral makeup products – sold primarily in salons – come in all sizes and shapes out of companies with names like Youngblood and ColourStrokes Cosmetics – contract manufacturers in New York who make them for own-brand label medical practices and marketing companies throughout the world. The most extensive and best collection of this new breed of makeup is Jane Iredale's.

Secrets Of The Screen Trade

Jane began her career as a casting director for television commercials working a lot with models. Later she moved onto television and films. She formed her own production company in the United States and produced over 50 programmes for PBS and HBO, won an Emmy for a film series which she wrote, and later moved from film to theatre where her work was nominated for a Tony award.

Working with actors who wear a lot of makeup for long periods under harsh studio lights and continually struggle with skin sensitivities and reactions, Jane felt inspired to create a range that would give better results as well as protect skin from harm. She was looking for a makeup technology that was non-reactive, lasted all day, looked natural and could be used by all skin types – even the most sensitive – without causing problems. She found it in minerals.

'If the practice of beauty were a religion, New York would be its Vatican.'
Sharon Krum

Mineral Alchemy

The list of ingredients used to formulate Iredale's foundation reads like the labels in an alchemist's laboratory – mica, iron oxides, manganese violet, titanium dioxide, bismuth oxychloride – all in micro fragments. Each element brings its own non-reactive properties to the formula. Mica gives slip and slide and minimises shine, titanium extracted from the minerals rutile and ilmenite provide covering and tinting power. Titanium is described by the American FDA as one of the purest and most effective active ingredients available for sun protection. Zinc oxide, taken from limestone, has long been used to encourage the healing of skin disorders. Jane's formulas contain no talc, no perfumes or sensitisers such as chemical colorants. The coverage they give doesn't fade, crease or smear and carries an SPF somewhere between 17 and 20. One light brushing of foundation provides a sun block which is both water and perspiration resistant and lasts.

Mineral makeup is rich in concentrated pigment which gives complete coverage yet looks natural. Iredale's Amazing Base, which looks like loose powder, and its easy-to-carry form PurePressed Base, is non drying. They adhere to the skin better than any makeup I have ever used, providing a day long sheer, natural finish to skin. I recently used PurePressed base when photographing a young man who had highly sensitive acne skin that reacts to just about everything. He wore the foundation all day, even after the photography was finished. No one even noticed he was wearing makeup. Not only did it cause no reaction, it actually calmed his skin. The Iredale formulas come in many different shades, each one can act as a concealer, foundation and sun protection all in one.

'As a physician who treats patients with environmental illness and multiple chemical sensitivities, I was delighted to find a line of makeup that is truly non-toxic, hypo-allergenic and attractive that I can enthusiastically recommend to my patients.'

Erica Elliot MD

Too Good To Be True
Does this sound too good to be true? I thought so when I first opened a compact of what looks like nothing but another pressed powder. I took hold of the applicator which came with it and began to spread it on my face: I was *not* impressed. Why? Because the downside of mineral makeup is this: to create a perfect, natural finish which lasts, you have to know how to apply it. Mineral makeup is very different than the foundations we have grown up with.

HOW TO MAKE MINERAL MAGIC

❑ Give yourself an hour or two to play and practice with mineral-based products. They are highly concentrated and can be applied in many different ways depending on the kind of skin you have and the finish you want – light as a feather or strong coverage.
❑ Apply whatever moisturiser you like to use over clean skin.
❑ Using a special blunt-ended fat brush (this is important) brush the pressed base or loose powder base – I preferred the pressed one – in a light layer over the face.
❑ Go easy. Mineral makeup is richly pigmented so it needs to be applied in thin layers until you get the depth of coverage you are looking for.
❑ If you are covering blemishes, you can use a special 'flocked sponge' instead.

- ☐ If you prefer a liquid makeup base to one applied 'dry', simply mix the loose powder form of the foundation in your hand with a little of your moisturiser and apply as you would a normal liquid or cream foundation.
- ☐ If you like a dewy surface, mist on mineral water afterwards.

'I use Jane Iredale on and off stage and my complexion is smoother and healthier than it's been for years. And, incredibly, my makeup doesn't run even during the most strenuous performance.'

Marina Kvitka, Bolshoi Ballerina

Although it takes some practice to get the hang of perfect mineral makeup application, half an hour or so experimenting brings great results. Try it all sorts of ways until you find which works best for you. If you can, get some advice from an expert makeup artist who loves the stuff as much as I do and uses it all the time. Once I discovered for myself what terrific benefits minerals brought my skin in terms of look, feel and health, I rang my friend – and favourite makeup artist in Europe – Valentine Gotti and asked Valentine to show me how to work some of her magic.

The Touch Of The Master

Like all the great makeup artists, Valentine is just that – an artist. She could easily have been a fine designer or painter had she not fallen in love with working on the human face. Her list of clients range from Catherine Deneuve, Sigourney Weaver and Juliette Binoche to top women in business and the media. She has the rare ability to create both fascinating highly eccentric faces for the covers of magazines and to take any woman's face and make it an even more beautiful expression of who she really is. Except when you are using makeup just for fun and games, this is what good makeup artistry is all about.

'Exuberance is beauty.'

William Blake

Valentine sees every woman's face as a canvas. She loves Jane Iredale foundation but is as eclectic as I am about using products from conventional ranges for mascaras, lipsticks and light reflecting creams. She tells women never to be afraid of their face but to look at it dispassionately and learn its proportions. She generally prefers to blend colours on the back of her hand and then applies them with her fingertips. She insists that the natural oils on the hand help in the blending and application processes. Applying makeup, she insists, should be a mind-stilling ritual. Here's what she taught me:

SET THE STAGE: face the daylight if at all possible in front of a window with your brushes and applicators and a magnifying mirror. Make sure you have all the tools you need before you begin including a flat brush – which Jane Iredale calls the Handi – for applying mineral foundation.

PREPARE THE CANVAS: regardless of the age of the face Valentine is working on, she uses an optical reflector cream like Prescriptive Vibrant before applying foundation – especially around the eye area. To erase dark shadows around eyes and in the nasal labial fold or to cover broken veins, she applies YSL's Touche Éclat – another of my own 'must haves'.

UNIFY THE FACE: Valentine applies mineral foundation either with a brush or, if you want a high level of coverage, with the special flocked sponge, blending carefully. Do one area at a time starting at the forehead, down each side, then chin, beneath the jaw and finally the nose. Blend lightly under the jawbone. You can use a darker foundation or bronzer around the outside of the face to frame the 'canvas'.

DEFINE THE BROWS: then using your index finger placed just above an eyebrow pull the flesh gently upwards to reveal your brow's true arch. With a slanted eyebrow brush like MAC's 266 and brow colour use light quick strokes to create and define the arch then fix it with transparent mascara.

PALE WASH YOUR EYES: sweep a fine layer of gossamer-fine pale eye shadow on the upper lid and around the socket. Then apply whatever other shadows you want to use.

MAKE A FISH FACE: squeeze in your cheeks as though you were pretending to be a fish. Your natural cheek bones will show themselves so you can sweep a mineral blusher upwards in a half moon shape up to the temples. For a diaphanous look, you can touch on a bit of compact powder over this.

PRIME THE LIPS: use a lip primer to protect against 'bleeding' and make lipstick last longer, then apply a neutral toned lip liner on the whole mouth to redefine its shape. This also makes a good base for either gloss or lipstick. Once they have set, touch a bit of shimmer in the centre of the mouth.

CURL AND DEFINE: give your lashes a firm curl from Shu Umera's eyelash curler (my own favourite) to open them up. Apply mascara from the base of the lashes to the tips. Curl them again.

GO FOR GOSSAMER FINISH: if you want a truly well-blended diaphanous look, you can mix all your mineral-based blushers or eye colours with a tiny bit of translucent pressed powder so they slide perfectly onto the face eliminating blotches of colour.

'No woman should ever be quite accurate about her age. It looks so calculating.'

Oscar Wilde

Unique Beauty

Valentine thinks her mission as a makeup artist is to teach women how to see their faces the way they really are – a unique collection of planes and forms which good makeup can make even more interesting and attractive. She believes the kind of carping self-criticism most of us indulge in – about a nose that's too big or black circles under our eyes – is actively destructive to a woman's self-esteem. Without self-esteem, real beauty can never shine through. Valentine researches the tools of her trade, pigments and products with a passion only those of us cursed by a similar obsession with colour, beauty, form and texture, understand. She loves using optical creams and pigments beneath her colours. Valentine is catholic in her choice of ranges. She insists that, although some of the best products in the world are expensive, there are good alternatives available to anyone on a limited budget.

LESLIE'S SECRET MINERAL MAGIC

My skin tends to be a little dry. I usually apply mineral makeup in pressed form using a blunt brush. But I love to experiment. I discovered that a very fine oil is a wonderful medium to work the loose powder pigments into when I want to create a liquid foundation instead of applying it dry. My favourite oil is AD Skin Synergy Nourishing Night Treatment. Forget the 'night' part. It is one of the finest blends I have ever found anywhere. I place four or five drops of it on the palm of my hand, add a pinch of the powdered mineral makeup colour I use and blend with my fingertip for a few seconds. It goes on like silk for a long-lasting smooth-as-satin finish which delights me.

Crystalline Scales

All Jane Iredale Cosmetics are ultra low risk when it comes to allergy, since they come free of sensitisers. Because the pigments used in them are concentrated yet come in the form of tiny fragments of minerals, they offer complete coverage. You can use them to advantage to camouflage large or small blemishes or irregular pigmentation. And because the minerals are inert – in effect inorganic – they don't support bacteria. This is one of the reasons mineral-based products are so benign even on troubled skin, provided whatever you use to apply them is scrupulously clean. Mineral products are non drying and adhere better than anything else to the skin. Like fine artists' pigment, well applied, they can seem to take on the qualities of living skin itself.

'Beauty is how you feel inside, and it reflects in your eyes. It is not something physical.'

Sophia Loren

Other cosmetics contain fillers used to stretch small quantities of pigment so they go a long way. Fillers can be drying. They also tend to fall into minute cracks on the skin's surface, accentuating lines. Not so these cosmetics. Under a microscope the minerals out of which they are made look like miniscule, overlapping crystalline fish scales which create a filter allowing a free exchange of oxygen and preventing damage by ultraviolet light. Minerals in such tiny particles have a superb surface-area-to-volume ratio so they hold firmly and don't run, crease or smear. You can even go swimming in them. Later they come off easily with a cleanser.

Jane Iredale pressed blushers and shadows are similar to the bases. You can use them wet or dry. Her lip colours and glosses have been created without any chemical dyes, preservatives or animal products – not a bad trick when you consider that a woman wearing lipstick every day ends up devouring 2 tubes of whatever she uses each year of her life. Most lipsticks contain cold tar dyes and synthetic preservatives. You won't find any in the Iredale range.

Fickle By Nature

Two years ago I fell in love with mineral makeup. I have tried most of the mineral-based ranges on the market in their various incarnations – from foundation to blusher, lipstick, mascara and eye shadow. Do I prefer mineral-based products in all makeup categories? No, I do not. I love the mineral blushers, foundations and pressed powder as well as some of the peripheral products such as the eyebrow fixatives and flocked sponges. But so far, nobody has come up with a mineral-based lipstick or mascara that turns me on.

'I have a woman inside my soul.'

Yoko Ono

I go out of the way to protect my skin and body from the build up of chemical colorants, preservatives, and sequestering agents which are ubiquitous in makeup, toiletries and most skincare products, and which can pollute our bodies daily. But I never make a 'religion' out of anything I do. If I fall in love with a product – a lipstick, a mascara, or cream which *works* for me even though it contains something I would rather it didn't – I will use it until I find something else that does equally as well and is also a more pure product. Jane Iredale mineral makeup very much belongs in the pure category. Maybe before long the mineral technology will get so good that I will be tempted by a mineral-based lipstick or mascara too. Not yet.

PART FOUR:

TAPPING
THE
ELEMENTS

fire power . . . skin's soul support

LIGHT UP YOUR SKIN

cell communication, DNA and biophotons . . .
hooray!

Your skin feeds on light. Light keeps youth hormones flowing, regulates sleep-wake cycles so stress doesn't make you haggard, fuels DNA repair, feeds cells, carries messages, keeps your spirits high and makes your face glow. Light even enhances the strength of the musculature on which firm, well-contoured skin depends. It is no accident the ancient Romans trained their gladiators naked in full sunlight.

This does not mean we are being given license to spend hours lying in the sun or that we need not protect our face from over exposure. But make use of light in all its incarnations – from the sun's rays to the light-enhancing biophotons in living foods – to expand the health and beauty of your skin and you are more than one step ahead in the how-to-look-beautiful game.

More Than A Little Light Magic

Some light magic you may already know about. The way light entering your eyes affects the skin's rhythms and supports hormonal balance, for instance. Other ways in which light enhances health and beauty are based on scientific discoveries so far in advance of consensus physics that they challenge the very basis of scientific assumptions about the nature of reality. Did you know that light continuously pours forth from the 60 billion cells of your body? That the nucleic acids of DNA trap light in the same way your eyes do, to trigger chemical changes in your skin? That new forms of light therapy can be used to rejuvenate skin in ways which, even five years ago, seemed impossible? Let's look at some of the good things light does for skin. Then we can delve into the politics and practices of good sun/skin management so you can make use of the very best sunlight has to offer and suffer none of the negative consequences to skin that over exposure to UV radiation can bring.

Great Flaring Forth

It is little wonder that light is so important to the body. All light came into being fifteen billion light years ago at the great flaring forth – the Big Bang – which gave birth to the universe. Light in the form of photons flared forth from the void, then hydrogen atoms, helium atoms, and eventually matter itself. In a very real sense our bodies are made of light. The food we eat comes to us thanks to photon energy absorbed by plants which convert it into the chemical nutrients we take in when we eat them. In addition, healthy living plants hold a great deal of biophon light energy which gets transmitted to our own bodies when we eat them fresh and raw. Light is enigmatic. It comes in many different forms and wavelengths, each of which affects living systems in a myriad of ways. The more we understand about them, the more power for beauty we can extract from this mysterious form of energy.

'For the rest of my life, I will reflect on what light is.'

Albert Einstein

LIGHT BEGINNINGS

Light comes in a range of wavelengths. These wavelengths make up half of the energy spectrum reaching the earth – everything from radio waves, thousands of metres long, to gamma rays as short as a million-millionth of a metre. If X rays and gamma rays are absorbed by your cells they cause damage to DNA. Wavelengths of visible light from 400nm to 700nm are vital to the health of your body and psyche and the beauty of your skin. So are the infrared heat wavelengths as well as moderate doses of the ultraviolet radiation which we have been taught to fear.

'There is no more worthy, more glorious or more potent work, than to work with light.'

Omraam Mikhaël Aïvanhov

Our Genetic Need For Light

John N. Ott, time-lapse photographer and author of many books on light and health including *Light, Radiation and You*, put the study of photobiology on the map. Ott lived well into his tenth decade. In his later years he spent most of his time exploring the effects of various forms of light on the living body.

Ott's work with light parallels the recent work of paleopathologists on diet, who have laid bare important information about how our genetic inheritance throughout evolution determines the kind of food our bodies need for high-level health. Ott pointed out that animals, including ourselves, have been exposed to the sun – including ultra violet radiation – throughout the whole of evolution. As a result, we have highly developed genetic adaptive abilities to deal with it. Just as our bodies have become genetically adapted to the hunter-gatherer diet – masses of non-starchy vegetables, fruits and animal-based protein foods – we still need sunlight to thrive. Despite everything we have been told, we are genetically adapted to getting adequate UV light and need it for high level health of body and mind. In the past few decades, study of photobiology has charted the ways in which various forms of light radiation affect health. We know, for instance, that when we do not get adequate exposure to full spectrum light we become prone to seasonal affective disorder (SAD) – the depression experienced to a greater or lesser degree by many people, especially during the dark months of winter. We also know that the body and psyche thrive on full spectrum light thanks to its hormone-regulating abilities and that health eventually suffers without it. Even the academic performance of children and the productivity of workers is dramatically improved when the rooms they work in are lit with full spectrum lights.

'It sounds unbelievable, however, there is light in our body coming out from at least 60 billion cells. Every single cell emits light, which can be detected today with a sensitive photomultiplier system.'

Professor Hugo Niggli

LIGHT SUPPORTS SKIN

❏ Light from the sun activates the production of ATP, your skin's energy currency and raises cellular functioning to a higher level of vitality-feeding radiance.
❏ It increases the production of collagen fibres.
❏ It enhances functions of enzymes specifically involved in cell repair and regeneration.
❏ It helps the lymph system to clear wastes.
❏ It spurs the development of new capillaries.
❏ It enhances DNA and protein synthesis within the skin's cells.

Hormone Maker

The most powerful source of energy in our solar system, the sun gives off a wide spectrum of energy which penetrates the earth's atmosphere, fuelling life. Sunlight makes photosynthesis possible by which plants provide the organic molecules on which all living things depend. When UV light strikes the skin directly, it triggers the conversion of *dehydrocholesterol* – a derivative of cholesterol, the fatty substance out of which sex hormones are made – into *calciferol*, better known as vitamin D3. Calciferol is then carried in the blood to the liver and the kidneys where it is converted into other essential compounds. Although classified as a vitamin, calciferol and its by-products are, in truth, hormones in their own right – hormones essential for beautiful skin and strong bones.

'There are neurological channels from the retina to the pineal and pituitary glands, the master glands of the whole endocrine system that controls the production and release of hormones. This regulates your body chemistry and its growth, all organs of your body, including your brain, and how they function.'
Dr John Ott

INFORMATION CARRIER

Not only does light transmit energy to your skin and body, it carries information deep within it on a sub-molecular level. It is even the energy medium out of which your living matrix weaves its dynamic web to orchestrate cellular communication. All light travelling throughout your body carries the 'signature' of its source and each chemical reveals its nature through the light it gives off. As German expert in photobiology Rudiger Vaas says, "Every chemical element leaves a characteristic finger-print in its spectrum of light." For generations this awareness has been used in the cosmetic industry to analyse fragrances and other chemicals and identify the molecules out of which they are made. Healthy cells and tissues resonate with specific light wave patterns and manifest a high degree of order. When they lose their natural resonance, they lose order, vitality is under-mined and skin becomes prone to disease and degeneration.

Hormones For Beauty

Light even sets our biological clock in the brain. This clock adjusts metabolic events through circadian rhythms which regulate hormone production as well as the many functions of the skin. Skin's sebum production peaks at 1pm and is at its lowest at 4am – an important fact for any beauty therapist or doctor looking to alleviate acne. Treat acne at 1pm and it reduces the level of triglycerides which exacerbate the proliferation of bacteria, calming inflammation.

Skin experiences the greatest loss of moisture in the evening. So this is the time to apply more moisture-rich treatment products. Light-regulated DNA repair takes place primarily at night so use an antioxidant treatment cream. Night is also the time to make sure your body is supplied on an internal level with anti-ageing supplements to support DNA repair since it happens primarily during the hours of darkness.

LIGHT REPAIR

The DNA and RNA in the molecules of skin cells have the capacity to repair themselves. They do this due to the presence of enzymes which can only work thanks to light energy through a process called photo repair. In experiments with animals who were kept in light from which the UV part of the light spectrum had been removed, this repair process did not take place properly. Eventually the animals developed serious illnesses.

'Use the light that is within you to regain your natural clearness of sight.'

Lao-Lzu

See The Light

As sunlight enters through your eyes, its wavelengths are instantaneously transformed into bioelectrical impulses by light-sensitive receptors, then shunted along the optic nerve to areas of the brain where they act upon the whole body. They travel to the hypothalamus, a small area of the mid-brain active in regulating the autonomic nervous system (that part of the nervous system which regulates the body's processes without our having to pay much attention to it), thirst, appetite and hormones. The hypothalamus converts the light impulses it receives into neurochemical substances which it sends out to regulate physiological events from sexual responses to ageing, immune function, and mechanisms regulating the texture and function of muscles and skin.

Light impulses received through the skin and eye also travel via the limbic system, your brain's primitive centre of learning and emotion. Provided they are the right kind of light, they enhance the experience of positive emotions, making you feel happy and good about yourself and making you look more radiant. One of the first experiments by which light communication was discovered was this: two glasses of fresh animal blood were placed side by side. When a chemical was added to one glass, the blood cells within it rapidly produced antibodies. Almost immediately the same reaction took place in the blood held in the neighbouring glass even though no chemical had been added to it. When researchers carried out the same experiment but placed an opaque barrier between the two glasses, the light information needed to produce antibodies was not transmitted to the blood of the second glass, so no antibody reaction happened.

'The human photoreceptor molecules are not limited conveniently to the retina but rather are ubiquitous, being found in virtually every tissue.'
Orm Bergold MD

In experiments stretching over almost two generations, German biophysicist Professor Fritz Albert Popp and his colleagues demonstrated that measuring biophotons can give sensitive information about conditions within the cell and the functioning of its defence mechanisms. Philip Coleridge Smith, a surgeon at University Medical College in London, recently told the New Scientist he believes, in time, medicine may be able to use biophoton measurement as a diagnostic tool, for instance to identify inflammation in leg tissues to warn of an ulcer.

WHAT ARE BIOPHOTONS?

Biophotons are fine remissions of light which all living systems – from the cells of your skin to the cells of living plants – send out as well as receive. Biophotons cannot be seen by the naked eye. They *can* be measured by special equipment developed by a number of researchers throughout the world. Biophoton light is ultra-weak yet ultra-important. It is stored in the cells of your skin – within the DNA molecules of the nuclei and elsewhere in the living matrix. Scientists at the International Institute of Biophysics in Germany, in Japan and Russia have determined that biophoton emission is a ubiquitous phenomenon of living systems. This dynamic web of light released and absorbed may even turn out to be the primary means by which the biochemical processes of life are regulated. The intensity and order of biophoton emission and the ability of living cells to store light carry important information about the functional state of a living organism. The more light skin cells can store, the better. Diseased cells, such as cancer cells, do not have the ability to store light. They can even be damaged by it.

'Light,' says Popp, '. . . can initiate or arrest cascade-like reactions in the cells, and genetic cellular damage can be virtually repaired within hours by faint beams of light.' The more vital your skin and body, the more ordered is the activity of your biophotons and the longer your cells are able to store light. Even the food you eat carries light energy and information to the body. Research into biophoton emission is now used in industry and medicine – especially in the wellness movement where it is raising the whole approach to colour therapy to a new level of effectiveness.

'In the 1980s Fritz-Albert Popp, then a lecturer at the University of Marburg in Germany, became interested in the optical behaviour of cells. In a series of experiments Popp found that two cells separated by an opaque barrier release biophotons in uncoordinated patterns. Remove the barrier and the cells soon begin releasing photons in synchrony. The cells, Popp concluded, were communicating by light.'

Bennett David, *New Scientist*

Lighting Up For Beauty

Russian researchers at the Institute of Clinical and Experimental Medicine have discovered that acupuncture points on the skin are responsive to light, and that light information which enters the body during treatment can be carried along the energy meridians of acupuncture throughout the whole body. Acupuncturists, including those involved in using acupuncture in traditional Chinese 'facelifts without surgery', have long used light to influence the flow of Chi to rejuvenate skin and heal the body at the deepest levels. Light appears to be the primary source of regulatory information in all living systems. It brings about molecular change on a biochemical level as a secondary event.

'Photons participate in many atomic and molecular interactions and changes. Recent biophysical research has detected ultraweak photons or biophotonic emission in biological tissue. It is now established that plants, animals and human cells emit a very weak radiation which can be readily detected with an appropriate photomultiplier system. Although the emission is extremely low in mammalian cells, it can be efficiently induced by ultraviolet light.'

Professor Hugh Niggli

LIGHT ORDER AND COLLAGEN

At a microscopic level the strands of collagen which give skin its firm texture and hold it together are triple helical fibrils enclosed by thin sheaths of bound water molecules. They have a liquid crystalline structure with semiconductor properties. These collagen bundles act as a network of light-conducting pathways transmitting information to help regulate metabolic functions. When the physical order of collagen breaks down from chemical toxicity or the formation of AGEs and cross-linkage, their capacity to transmit information for skin beauty is undermined.

Eat Light

Many years ago, Nobel Laureate physicist Irwin Schrödinger insisted that living organisms are only able to maintain a high degree of health by 'sucking order' – that is drawing ordered information – from their environment. A fundamental way in which we do this is through the foods we eat. Dr Popp, together with Swiss biophotonic researcher Dr Hugo Niggli and their colleagues have taken Schrödinger's model and applied it specifically to the way in which biophotons behave. In the process they have discovered that fresh, healthy food uncontaminated by chemical pollution, transmits biophoton energy which carries a high degree of Schrödinger's 'order' on which health depends.

Foods grown in healthy soil, eaten in a fresh raw state, offer the greatest potential for creating order within the body's living matrix, in no small part thanks to the quality of biophoton energy they transmit to us. This is a major reason why for generations they have been used to trigger detoxification and healing in natural clinics in Germany and Switzerland. This is also why such foods form the core of the Living Matrix 21 Day Turnaround Programme, and why it is such a powerful method for arresting and reversing the signs of skin ageing (see Making It Happen, page 199).

Laser Light – Past Imperfect

On a completely different light note, for years light treatments from lasers have been used to resurface skin and treat extrinsic ageing. They are an alternative to chemical peels or old-fashioned physical dermabrasion. In the beginning dermatologists used the old CO_2 lasers in modified forms to vaporise microscopic layers of skin cells, so the depth of penetration could be controlled (see page 285). In recent years these are mostly being replaced by the Erbium: Yag lasers which act more superficially, are safer and present less danger of scarring.

The light from any kind of laser has a very specific wavelength designed for a specific purpose. It is also *collimated* light. This means that its waves, as sent towards your skin, run parallel to each other when they leave the light source. It is this collimated way of using light that gives laser its concentrated beam and intense burning capacity. Laser light is also *coherent*. This means the rays of light are in phase with each other. Finally, unlike sunlight or the light that courses through a living body, laser light is monochromatic. At the same time as being useful for very specific purposes, these characteristics also make lasers potentially dangerous – something to be used only with the greatest care – if at all.

'Few women see power as an end in itself. The point of power is the freedom to cultivate roses.'

Erica Jong

Light Rejuvenation At The Cutting Edge

The best of the new light therapies for skin rejuvenation are completely different. Used to create Intense Pulsed Light therapy, they are part of a new technology which involves the application of non-coherent, non-laser, broadened pulsed light to the surface of the skin. In pulsed light therapy, a light source is directed towards the surface of the skin. The kind of light it uses is not collimated, so it spreads in all directions. It is not coherent, so there is no danger of burning or scarring. And it is multi-chromatic, which means it encompasses a wide range of wavelengths – most often between 500 and 1200nm. The wavelength of light chosen by the therapist determines the depth of pulsed light penetration. This, together with the duration of each pulse, determines the effects which pulsed light therapy induce in skin. In the hands of a skilled operator, this new rejuvenation technology at the cutting edge can do some truly wonderful things for skin. But you do *need* a skilled operator. IPL Therapy also demands a series of treatments to get the best results.

LIGHT MIRACLE

Intense Pulsed Light technology offers unique light-driven power for skin to rejuvenate, not just superficially but at more fundamental levels. Used wisely, it may even enhance a cell's light-holding capacity. Unlike laser light, IPL supplies multi-chromatic light pulses adjustable both in duration and wavelength to perform a multitude of tasks not possible before through light therapy. In the hands of a skilled operator it can:

❑ Even out skin colouration.
❑ Mitigate UV damage.
❑ Clear blotches.
❑ Enhance elasticity.
❑ Firm skin.
❑ Treat large pores.
❑ Soften wrinkles.
❑ Restore radiance.

Four to six treatments given at three week intervals work best to produce long-term rejuvenation. There is no pain with the treatment and no 'downtime' needed afterwards.

'On average, patients considering intense pulsed light photorejuvenation therapy may be told that there is a 2 year perceived facial age improvement per visit.'
Daniel Lawry MD

IPL is a good example of the way beauty therapy has more than once pushed the envelope of scientific developments which, only later, become applied to medical treatments. Some of the best beauty therapists, plastic surgeons and dermatologists involved in 'appearance medicine' are forever on the lookout for cutting edge technologies which produce significant results. Photo-rejuvenation using pulsed light therapy is a major one. I find it the most exciting technology around. Sadly the equipment needed to give it is still very pricey. Also, as yet too few practitioners are familiar with what it can do.

Shards Of Light
The big cosmetic companies of the world – L'Oreal, Lauder, Unilever,

Shiseido – are also beginning to explore the effects of light on skin. Estée Lauder's Lightsource is a good example of a product which has come out of their creative light play. Based on NASA technology, and relying on microcrystals for its visual impact, the product attempts to make use of specific wavelengths of visible light to enhance the production of cellular energy in ageing skin. But light-based products which have appeared on the market so far look primitive in comparison with advanced light studies at the cutting edge of biophysics and the potentials that exist for skin regeneration coming out of a growing body of biophoton research.

Another exciting light-based technology has come out of Switzerland and Holland. The Miron company in Switzerland and VioSol in Holland have developed a dark violet glass which can be used to package top quality nutritional supplements and cosmetics. Thanks to the way their glass responds to sunlight, bottles manufactured from their special dark violet glass not only prolong the life of any product – so that a formula does not have to be riddled with chemical preservatives – it can use light from the environment to enhance a product's effectiveness.

Secrets Of The Mummys

This is perhaps not surprising, since in ancient times Egyptians stored their most precious essential oils either in gold or violet coloured pots. While our ancestors knew nothing about biophotons, they did know a great deal about the best way to preserve precious essential oils used for beauty and embalming.

DARK VIOLET POWER FOR BEAUTY

Violet light has the highest frequency of any visible light – 720 to 770 bio hertz. This frequency appears to activate and energise the molecular structure and healing energies of whatever is held within a dark violet glass bottle. This frequency is also believed to match that of the human nervous system. The brown, green and blue glass bottles traditionally used for medicines and cosmetics offer little protection from light degradation. They have far lower oscillation frequencies. Mixing special metal oxide pigments with glass in precise proportions protects whatever is contained within their violet glass containers from light frequencies that can degrade it, at the same time letting through higher frequencies to enhance the order of a compound's biophoton energies.

Swiss biologist Professor Hugo Niggli – a world expert in biophotons in relation to skin – tested the dark violet glass bottles and reported that, 'The test samples in the violet glass have a significantly higher quality after storage, a demonstrably more stable oscillation and showed the smallest energy loss.'

Living Nature's Professional which appears in Britain in September 2003, is the first international range of skincare products to have made use of this superb light-based technology at the cutting edge of skin enhancement. So good are the bottles that the last thing you want to do is toss them out when they get empty. Even water kept in this kind of glass and exposed to natural light tastes better and carries enhanced energy.

'And he was transfigured before them, and his face shone like the sun, and his garments became white as light.'

Matthew 17:2

HOW TO FEED ON LIGHT

The health and beauty of skin relies in so many ways on the life-supporting power of light that science is only beginning to chart them. Make use of what is already known and you can watch your own radiance grow by leaps and bounds:

❑ Forget the sunglasses, unless you are skiing or in the desert, to enhance hormone levels, balance mood and energise cells.

❑ Try the Living Matrix 21 Day Turnaround Programme and learn for yourself what ordered biophotons can do for your skin.

❑ Investigate what Intense Pulsed Light therapy in the hands of a competent practitioner can offer for your skin.

Now let's look specifically at sunlight. The news here is by no means all bad.

SUN MATTERS

spectrum secrets . . . make them work for you
not against you

We have inherited a fear of the sun. It has developed out of simplistic thinking and a commercially-fuelled set of false beliefs. Here's the inside story: ultraviolet light is *not* the *fundamental* cause of melanoma – the most dangerous form of skin cancer. Exposure to the sun is *not* the *main* reason that skin wrinkles happen. Most important, the chemical sunscreens we now use to protect ourselves from wrinkles and cancer will be contributing to both.

Rough, loose, creviced, wrinkled skin, complete with irregular blotches – is known as photo-damaged skin or extrinsically aged skin. It is always blamed on exposure to sun. It is not *exposure* that causes it, it is the *misuse* of sun coupled with exposure to the mounting levels of destructive chemicals which our skin is now experiencing that are the real culprits. To get a first-hand feel for what this looks like, take a look in the mirror at the skin on your bottom. It appears to be ten or twenty years younger than skin on your face. The difference speaks volumes about what extrinsic ageing looks like. How do you avoid it?

The ads tell us to smear on more sunscreens. The truth is far more complex. Extrinsic ageing means skin damage triggered by external factors – high exposure to UV light, chemicals in the environment, even products you use to protect yourself from them. To protect your skin from it, you are going to need more than a new sunscreen.

PROTECT YOUR DNA

Sunscreen chemicals which should protect your skin from damage may actually be causing it. They can use up your body's natural enzymes designed to guard against degeneration. A growing awareness of this in the cosmetic industry has led manufacturers to add free radical scavengers like vitamin A derivatives and phytonutrients to their sunscreen products. A bit like sweeping dust under a carpet, this only hides the issue. Chemicals used in sun products and other toiletries do not belong in our bodies. As Rachel Carlson insisted half a century ago, their ubiquitous presence in animal bodies undermines health, vitality and in this case, beauty too.

Cosmic Is Not Cool

The sun produces high energy rays from cosmic and gamma and X rays through longer, lower UV, infrared, microwaves and radio waves. Gamma and X radiation are mostly filtered out by the earth's atmosphere, although flying in jets at 35,000 feet exposes your body to them in big quantities. This is one reason we need extra antioxidant protection when boarding a long-haul flight. When gamma rays – which are also used to irradiate foods and sterilise medical equipment – hit water molecules in a living body, free radicals are generated in large numbers, important enzymes are destroyed and your skin's biophoton information loses its order.

BREAKING THE WAVES

The UV rays – most likely to trigger ageing in an unprotected or polluted skin with a compromised living matrix – span from 190 to 400nm. They come in three varieties:

❏ **UVA (320–400nm)** Deep penetrating 'silent-killer' ageing rays. UVA radiation can delve deep into the dermis and wreak havoc with DNA and collagen, triggering degenerative changes especially in white skin, messing up the skin's enzyme systems and cross-linking its collagen.

❏ **UVB (200–290nm)** Shorter, these guys penetrate more superficially. They can oxidise skin's natural oils, dry it out and undermine its ability to protect itself on the surface. UVB are mostly responsible for burning. They are what chemical sunscreens try to mitigate in an attempt to prevent sunburn.

❏ **UVC (280nm and shorter)** Highly dangerous to skin. Most of these are filtered out by the biosphere, but you can be subjected to them from most office lighting.

Facts And Fictions

Photo-ageing got its name because it often develops out of our exposure to UV radiation. You see it in sun-worshippers on the beaches of Australia's Gold Coast or California's Venice Beach. Extrinsic ageing mimics the destructive damage all skin is exposed to over time. This damage happens a lot faster when you hang out too long in the sun. Chemical pollution, long periods of intense physical activity, alcohol, cigarettes and drugs – just like excessive UV radiation – all generate high levels of reactive oxygen species in the skin – super oxides, hydroxy radicals and hydrogen peroxide. These cause free radical damage, degrade and cross-link collagen, and help produce wrinkles, sags and age spots. Like the rest of these onslaughts, big doses of sun also accelerate the formation of advanced glycosylation end-products (AGEs) to interfere with cellular functions and make skin lose elasticity. But the notion that sunlight is the bête noir in all extrinsic ageing is simply untrue.

'Mankind adapted to the full range of the solar spectrum, and artificial distortions of that spectrum – malillumination, a condition analogous to malnutrition – may have biological effects.'

Dr John Ott

EXTRINSIC AGEING – THE REAL CAUSES

Our ancestors were exposed to the sun's UV rays for over a million years of evolution. The human body is therefore genetically adapted to sunlight and well equipped to handle it. The exponential rise in skin cancers began in the twentieth century – not in all those years of evolution. What is happening? Two things. With each decade that passes we are bombarded by higher and higher levels of chemical aggression and forced to handle more electromagnetic pollution. Together they produce toxic build-up in our body stressing its natural antioxidant systems and undermining our immunity. This triggers degenerative processes and increases our skin's sensitivity to UV damage.

It also makes us highly susceptible to cancers. Meanwhile we continue to assault our skin with more chemicals in the form of irresponsibly formulated cleaning products, herbicides and insecticides, and to use skin and body care products to deliver yet more chemicals directly to the skin.

'There is a muscular energy in sunlight corresponding to the spiritual energy of the wind.'

Annie Dillard

How prone you are to *extrinsic ageing* depends on two things:

1. YOUR BODY'S BIOLOGICAL TERRAIN – the condition of the living matrix.
2. WHAT KIND OF SKIN YOUR ANCESTORS HAD.

Check Out The Terrain

The internal state of your living matrix determines how well your genes get expressed, how skin looks and how prone you are to rapid ageing. It is good to ask just how much antioxidant protection your way of eating and living provides you. If you eat a diet high in convenience foods, cooked grains and sugar, the answer is very little. The same is true unless you take great care over the kind of cosmetics, cleaning products and toiletries you choose in order to reduce levels of toxic build-up in your system. The living matrix loses its order and vitality when cells become insulin resistant so chronic high levels of glucose circulate in the bloodstream. As the body becomes depleted of the essential nutrients and co-factors the skin needs for health and beauty, genetic expression degrades and its susceptibility to extrinsic ageing increases. Drugs? Alcohol? Cigarettes? They further pollute the matrix, undermining the skin's ability to benefit from UV light and causing it to age faster.

The Living Matrix 21 Day Turnaround Programme not only cleanses your body, it rebuilds antioxidant protection, enhances immunity, and creates a high level of biophoton order in your cells. Making use of its principles provides you with a high level of protection from external aggression of all kinds. Carefully selected nutritional supplements, including antioxidant nutrients and immune-supporting plant factors, can make things even better. With the help of a good hat and sunblock – rather than a *sunscreen*, you can surf or play tennis with impunity.

'I find the less you focus on your flaws, the better off you are. Be yourself and be glad of who you are.'

Michelle Pfeiffer

HEALTHY CELLS FEED ON LIGHT

Biophoton research indicates that a healthy skin cell 'sucks order' from UV light. This improves its functions and increases skin beauty. A polluted or cancerous cell has not only lost the capacity to draw order from light, it perceives UV rays as dangerous. Once the body is detoxified the skin's natural ability to use UV light is restored and skin radiance returns.

Check Out Your Colour
The colour of your skin and whether or not you live in a climate in keeping with the amount of melanin its cells produce, matter in determining how your skin handles sunlight too. This has been determined by hundreds of generations of your own ancestors, what climate they lived in and how their skin adapted to it.

Take a pale Swede whose skin is low in melanin – the pigment that causes tanning and gives skin its colour. Set him down in the middle of the Sahara and make him live there hatless for twenty years. His skin will wrinkle, develop irregular pigmentation and dry out – like poor quality leather. Yet his black African counterpart can live to old age in the same environment with surprisingly few wrinkles.

'Age is an issue of mind over matter. If you don't mind, it doesn't matter.'

Mark Twain

Secrets of Colour
Resistance to photo-ageing depends a lot on how much melanin – the brown pigment – skin's melanocyte cells produce. We all have roughly

the same number of melanocytes. The big difference lies in the quality and quantity of the dark sticky stuff they pour out. Black skin churns out masses of melanin. Pale skin very little. High levels enable skin to absorb and reflect high levels of UV rays without damage. (Melanin is a great free radical scavenger.) Low levels of melanin means your skin is better adapted to living in Siberia or Finland where light is scarce.

It all goes back to human evolution. Black-skinned people originate in parts of the globe where exposure to sun is high. They don't need a lot of UV light to make the vitamin D they need for hormones and need little real protection against the sun's intensity. But move them to Northern Sweden and they become prone to loss of calcium from their bones since they find it hard to pick up sufficient vitamin D in a place where the sun is weak. Those of us from Britain, on the other hand, are incredibly prone to photo-ageing when we move to Southern Florida or Mexico. Our genetic inheritance has not prepared us for the onslaught. That is why you see so many wrinkled, half-baked thirty-year-old human alligators in bikinis lying on the beaches of Australia's Gold Coast. These days we all move about like migrating birds. The saying 'mad dogs and Englishmen go out in the midday sun' is absolutely true. The people with dark skins who live in hot countries cover themselves up, they don't have a tradition of lying around in bikinis.

THE BLACK AND WHITE OF IT

In simple terms, the lighter your skin the more susceptible it can be to photo-ageing. Bad news for white Europeans. But there's good news too. Light coloured skin is less prone to scarring and damage from skin peels, laser treatments, or cuts. So where your black brother gets away with wrinkle-free skin at the age of sixty, he can suffer permanent damage to his skin from trauma. He is not immune to sunburn either.

I learned this firsthand as a child from singer Nat Cole who had beautiful blue-black skin. He and my father, American jazz musician Stan Kenton, often worked together. I spent my childhood hanging out in jazz clubs and concert halls and Nat became one of my pals. One night he was complaining of being sunburnt. 'How can you possibly be sunburnt?' I wanted to know. 'Black skin burns too,' he said. 'And the hell of it is that you never get any sympathy when it does 'cause nobody can see it's happened.'

'The sun, with all those planets revolving around it and dependent on it, can still ripen a bunch of grapes as if it had nothing else in the universe to do.'
Galileo Galilei

Know Your Skin's Capacity

It was Thomas Fitzpatrick MD who created the classification system for skin used throughout the world to determine susceptibility to photo-ageing based on skin colour and ethnic origin. It looks like this:

SKIN TYPE	COLOUR, TONE AND ETHNICS	BURN TIME	RISK FACTORS FOR SCARRING, PEELS AND LASERS
TYPE 1 Celtic Northern European	Fair, freckled, Blond hair, blue eyes	Burns easily does not tan	Low risk
TYPE 2 Nordic, Semetic, Native American	White skin with sandy or brown hair blue/green eyes	Usually burns then tans with difficulty	Low risk
TYPE 3 Central European, Mediterranean	White to olive, medium brown hair, brown eyes	Sometimes burns but will tan	Moderate risk

TYPE 4 Oriental, Filipino, Polynesian, Central and South American	Olive to light brown, medium skin brown hair and eyes	Rarely burns	Significant risk
TYPE 5 African, Middle East, Arab	Dark brown, black hair, black eyes	Very rarely burns	High risk
TYPE 6 Ebony skin	Black, black hair and eyes	Almost never burns	Very high risk

Buying Into Skin Damage

The standard protocol for sun protection is to smear on more chemical sunscreens. Selling them is a $2.5 billion a year business and growing rapidly. We fear ageing and skin cancer so we keep buying. The trouble is, much of what we buy may be seriously contributing to the damage we are trying to prevent.

'No commercial sunscreens have been proved safe. Their chemicals penetrate the skin into the circulation and add to the burden of toxins to be detoxified.'
Joseph G. Hattersley

Sun protection products come in two forms – *chemical sunscreens* and *physical sunblocks*. A few products contain both. The physical block products literally create a physical barrier of fine, non-reactive minerals on the surface or your skin, rather like micro-fish-scales. They *reflect* excess UVA and UVB back into the atmosphere instead of letting skin absorb it. Using them is like wearing a hat or a veil so the sun's rays don't penetrate at all.

Chemical sunscreen products – and most sun protection products fit into this category – are different. They do not reflect. They *absorb* UVB and UVA rays allowing them to penetrate your skin. More chemical screens these days have begun to target UVA radiation as well, but the 'sun protection factor' (SPF number) you read on a product's label will have been calculated entirely by how much UVB radiation the chemicals it contains are able to absorb.

'Technology . . . is a queer thing. It brings you great gifts with one hand, and it stabs you in the back with the other.'

Carrie P. Snow

Most widely-used chemical sunscreen products are based on compounds like these or chemicals similar to them:

❑ *Dibenzoylmethane* related chemicals (Parasol) – for UVA.
❑ *Methyl-methoxycinnamate* – primarily UVB with some UVA absorption.
❑ *Bensophenones* and *cinnamates* – believed to be less effective UVB absorbers and to extend to around 320nm so they target most UVA too.

CHEMICAL SCREENS – NOT GREAT FRIENDS OF SKIN

There is something you need to know about chemical sunscreens before you rush out to buy the latest product which promises to keep the wrinkles away and to protect your skin from cancer. Unlike physical sunblocks, chemical sunscreens 'absorb' the UVB radiation in an attempt to neutralise. They are rapidly used up in the formation of new chemical compounds which your skin then has to find ways of detoxifying from your system.

'Unfortunately, the scientists have not yet come up with any magic molecules that we can do what we want and these massive SPF products don't protect the skin nearly as much as the public believes.'

Dr Des Fernandes

Chemical Cascades

What are the implications of the absorption and all these chemicals for the skin? Nobody knows for sure. What we do know is that once inside, active ingredients in sunscreens do react within your skin to form new compounds. This is a major reason that sunscreen products often sensitise skin. They make your skin more prone to 'allergic reactions'. And, this is why many people find they can no longer use them. Chemicals in sunscreen products can become like the proverbial straw that breaks the back of what the skin's biological terrain can manage.

We also know that the UV screening capacity of these products is rapidly used up by chemical reactions within the skin. This is why many cosmetic companies are moving away from chemical screens. The more that skin is exposed to these chemicals, once commonly added to foundations and moisturisers, the more likely your skin is to become highly reactive and inflamed. This is why chemical sunscreens are now disappearing from many products.

In any case, UVA rays, the wavelengths which primarily trigger extrinsic ageing, are not neutralised by most chemical sunscreens. So while you may apply a sunscreen product frequently enough to stop burning, you can get little assurance that it will help prevent wrinkles. Also, chemical screens get used up so rapidly that the product you slather on at 10am may offer no protection at all by noon.

INSIDIOUS INVADERS

Every month another chemical sunscreen is banned in one country or another as a result of its mutagenic properties – that is its ability to distort genetic information, inviting cancer and ageing. Throughout a million years of human evolution we have never been exposed to such chemicals. Most are man-made. They never existed before. Like most drugs, our bodies do not have the enzymic abilities to clear them from our living matrix. Some screw up DNA. Some other compounds they form through reactions with each other get stored in skin tissues, adding to the build-up of toxic waste to undermine skin radiance and spur rapid degeneration. The increasing use of chemical sunscreen products parallels the rapidly rising incidence of skin cancer. The very chemicals we are drawing into our skin to protect us appear, to a significant degree, to be welcoming it.

Big Problems

Many studies show that chemical screens affect skin negatively. Research carried out in the Department of Physics at the University of Alabama to find out if the sunscreen *octyl methoxycinnamate* binds to skin DNA is a good example. 'Sunscreens are designed to prevent skin cancer by absorbing ultraviolet radiation from the sun before it gets to the DNA in skin cells,' scientists reported. 'The purpose of this work is to determine whether or not oxtyl methoxycinnamate, an active ingredient in many sunscreens, will bind to DNA. If so, the sunscreen could transfer energy [ultraviolet radiation] to the DNA and cause damage . . . We concluded that octyl methoxycinnamate can indeed bind to DNA in aqueous solution.'

In other words, the chemical used to neutralise the free radical potential of UV light may instead be delivering it to the skin's DNA where it can do the worst damage of all.

'Mounting evidence indicates that many of them [sunscreens] contain carcinogens and that the rise of skin cancers parallels the increase in sunscreen usage.'

Lita Lee PhD

OTHER THINGS YOU SHOULD KNOW ABOUT SUN PROTECTION PRODUCTS

❑ Regardless of skin type, there is up to a 30–fold difference between individuals in the number of free radicals and other photo-products generated through sun exposure depending on the state of the living matrix and your genetic sensitivity to sun.

❑ How much sunscreen protection you get from any product is highly individual regardless of what protection factor is written on its label. It is also *independent* of how much DNA damage your skin suffers from exposure.

Both of these things are largely determined by the order and health of your skin's biological terrain. Alter that by detoxifying your body and enhancing immunity with the Living Matrix 21 Day Turnaround Diet, and you establish the highest possible level of protection from UV damage as well as developing your skin's ability to feed on light energy at a cellular level. Then what happens? Your skin becomes more beautiful with each passing month.

'Women are most fascinating between the ages of thirty-five and forty, after they have won a few races and know how to pace themselves. Since few women ever pass forty, maximum fascination can continue indefinitely.'

Christian Dior

WAY TO GO

To protect yourself from ageing (as well as cancers) supply your skin with all it needs to function in the best of all possible ways. Limit your use of chemically-based sunscreens. Better still, throw them out. Go for a mineral-based sunblock or use one of the new mineral foundations every day. Based on physical agents like titanium oxide and zinc oxide, these products reflect the light instead of relying on chemicals to 'absorb' and trans-mute it. They are safe, inert and protective. Physical screens are commonly used by surfers, skiers, cricketers and tennis players. But choose your product carefully. Unless the mineral fragments have been milled into micro particles, they can make you look a bit like Marcel Marceau.

Next let's look at how not to become part of the epidemic of skin ageing and skin cancers. It is easier than you think.

WIPE OUT THE EPIDEMIC

ageing and skin cancer . . . past history

Skin cancer became rampant at the end of the 20th century. It was rare before that – found primarily in white farmers and sailors. Given the million years of genetic evolutionary practice our bodies have had in dealing with the sun, and the fact that it is only in the last 50 years that skin cancers have escalated to epidemic proportions, it is worth asking 'why?' What is so different now compared to our grandparents' time that is making us so susceptible to melanoma and other forms of skin cancer?

Cancer anywhere in the body can only develop when mutated DNA duplicates itself more rapidly than our body's antioxidant mechanisms and immune functions can counter. The implication from many recent studies on skin cancers of all kinds, are that both very high and very low exposure to UV light can be harmful, while moderate exposure is health-enhancing. Even more surprising is growing evidence that moderate exposure to full spectrum sunlight actually *lowers* the risk of most internal cancers. Mortality from breast cancer, for instance, declines with increasing sunlight intensity. A study of prostate cancer in the US shows similar correlation as does a study carried out on colon cancer.

A Quick Look At Skin Cancers
There are three kinds of skin cancer: basal cell, squamous cell and melanoma.

BASAL CELL CANCER: the most widespread, this form of cancer has more than tripled in Europe in the past fifteen years. In the US 1.2 million cases are diagnosed each year. Basal cell cancer tends to show up on the face, and in farmers and fishermen the back of the neck – wherever skin is most exposed to sun. Growths are usually small and red. They are often mistaken for persistent pimples. This kind of cancer rarely spreads to the inside of the body and is relatively simple to excise.

SQUAMOUS CELL CANCER: this form of malignancy also turns up mostly on sun-exposed areas of the body. It looks like scaly or hard patches which won't heal. In a recent ten-year period the incidence of squamous cell cancer increased by 65 per cent. This kind of cancer is more inclined to spread internally than basal cell cancers.

MELANOMA: the least common of the skin cancers, melanoma is also the most deadly. Statistics estimate that as many as one in 75 Americans – and a far greater number of Australians – are likely to develop it now. A melanoma looks like a dark or multicoloured growth. Unlike the other two cancers, it is *not* most prevalent on the face or where skin sees a lot of sunlight. In fact it occurs mostly on areas of the body which are only intermittently exposed to sun: the bottom of the feet, the lower legs, the back of the neck. A bad sunburn in childhood increases your risk of melanoma, which is now striking ever younger people. More than a quarter of those expected to develop it in the next year will be under 39. The mysterious melanoma is much more common in Scotland than in England or Wales yet less common in Northern Ireland.

Shun The Light

Like extrinsic ageing, skin cancers are wrongly blamed on sun exposure alone. Research, including a large study carried out by the United States navy, shows that most people who fell prey to melanoma work indoors. Melanoma incidence is correlated to exposure to artificial UV from lying on sunbeds and to working under bright halogen lights which give off some dangerous UVC rays. It is also linked to working for long stretches underneath fluorescent lights, and to exposure to high levels of cathode rays from TV sets and computer terminals.

'Emissions from [fluorescent] light extend into the potentially carcinogenic range.'

A. R. Kennedy

GET SAVVY ABOUT THE SUN

Here are some important things to remember about tanning and how to protect your skin from extrinsic ageing and cancers:

- ❑ There is no way to get a safe tan.
- ❑ *Never* use a sunbed. They filter out UVB burning rays but let the UVA in deep. They are nothing more than automatic ageing machines and increase your risk of melanoma.
- ❑ SPF numbers don't tell you about UVA protection from wrinkling and ageing. Most only deal with UVB protection against burning.
- ❑ For the safest protection from ageing and burning read labels. Shun chemical sunscreens in favour of physical sunblocks – products based on micro minerals such as titanium dioxide or zinc oxide which do not absorb the sun's rays or react with your skin.
- ❑ Apply a sunblock quarter of an hour before going out into the sun.
- ❑ Water resistant products are not what they seem. Their effectiveness is compromised by sweat and swimming. Reapply them often.
- ❑ If you are or have been using any kind of AHA's, Retin-A or Renova or any other pharmaceuticals on your face, cover it with a hat as well as a physical sunblock and don't spend a lot of time outdoors.
- ❑ Never get sunburnt – the damage it causes continues to get worse for 24 hours after the initial burn appears and when the burn has been severe, can last a lifetime.
- ❑ If you are determined to tan, use masses of internal antioxidants from vitamins and trace elements as well as potent anti-ageing external skincare products such as Living Matrix Mist™, Estée Lauder's Night Repair, and Environ (see Resources).
- ❑ Think twice before taking oral contraceptives or HRT. Use of these hormone-based drugs is correlated with a three times greater risk of melanomas in women under 40. They make you highly prone to irregular pigmentation – age spots – as well.

❑ Take a tip from the Arabs who know a lot about sun protection. Cover your body well when you plan to spend long hours outdoors. Always wear a hat.

❑ Use one of the excellent new non-reactive, mineral-based makeup products on your face (such as Jane Iredale, see Resources) which lasts all day, looks natural and covers your skin and reflects UV rays for extra protection.

'You yourself, as much as anybody in the entire universe, deserve your love and affection.'

Buddha

How About Fake Tans

Despite claims on the labels, all self-tanners are based on pretty much the same ingredient: dihydroxyacetone (DHA). DHA is a simple sugar involved in carbohydrate metabolism. The colour that you get from using self-tanning products containing it depends on how your skin reacts to this chemical. It browns your skin by interacting with the amino acid arginine found in the skin's surface cells. Unlike a natural tan from the sun, the tanning effect of these products offers no protection from UV exposure.

HOW TO USE ARTIFICIAL TANNERS

Success with artificial tanners depends on your skill in applying them, not on how much you pay for a product. Here are the keys:

❑ Exfoliate skin first using a loofah or skin brush to prevent uneven colour.

❑ Moisturise your skin being careful to include the dry body areas of knees, elbows and ankles.

❑ To prevent uneven darkening on bony areas like your knees, elbows and ankles, remove excess moisturiser with damp cotton or a damp flannel.

183

❑ Layer the product on. Use fewer layers where you want less colour and use less where your skin is thicker since the colour stays longer on these parts of the body.

❑ Wash your hands immediately after applying a product to avoid orange palms.

❑ Wait to dress for 30 minutes after applying a self-tanner to avoid staining your clothes (or longer, read the pack carefully).

❑ Wait an hour or two after applying a product before showering or bathing (again, read the pack carefully).

❑ Reapply regularly to keep the colour.

How fast DHA works on your skin depends on how much of this chemical the product you use contains. A self-tanner which takes several applications will give a better effect since it gives you more control over how dark your skin gets. What product you buy at what price is pretty irrelevant. Results depend primarily on how carefully you apply it. Colour changes start to occur within an hour. Maximum darkening happens somewhere between 8 and 24 hours later and will last for 5 to 7 days. As far as dangers are concerned, a few people experience allergic reactions to self-tanners. But the real concern is how DHA may interact with other chemicals in the product or within your body. About this there is still too little information available. The general consensus seems to be that DHA is safer than most other common chemicals in cosmetics and toiletries.

Look To Your Lifestyle

Neither chemical nor physical sun products can protect you from extrinsic ageing. For that, you need to address inside issues. If you don't, it becomes a bit like sticking a plaster over an unhealed wound. That's where antioxidant vitamins, minerals and phytonutrients come in. The Living Matrix 21 Day Diet is full of them. Equally important, thanks to its high raw content, the programme is also full of skin-enhancing, ordered biophoton energy to help detoxify your body of chemicals long waiting to be eliminated before they can trigger more age-related changes.

TOP UP ON ANTIOXIDANTS TO SUPPORT THE MATRIX

Free radical scavengers protect from oxidation damage caused by excess exposure to UV, chemicals and pollution. To look after your immune system, your body needs a high raw diet of fresh foods and possible supplements of specific nutrients to make the most of its antioxidant potentials:

❑ Get into the Living Matrix programme for high level, on-going protection.
❑ Drink no more than a glass of wine a day – two at the most.
❑ Don't smoke and stay away from passive smoke exposure, both of which burn up your body's antioxidant potentials and cause free radical damage, inflammation, and age skin fast.
❑ Take no unnecessary drugs – prescription or recreational.
❑ Use extra antioxidant nutrients and plant factors regularly:

Vitamin E: an active oil-based free-radical scavenger, vitamin E potentiates the effects of sun protection. It can even be used to quell sunburn after the fact.

Vitamin C: offers anti-ageing protection to the water-based elements of skin and synergises the age-protecting capacities of other antioxidants.

Carotinoids and Flavonoids: plant-based free radical scavengers, these phytonutrients are useful in creating a high level of anti-ageing synergy with vitamins and minerals. Eat lots of fresh vegetables and low-sugar fruits like blueberries and strawberries for a good supply of them.

Seleno-methionine: a trace mineral, it not only protects your skin internally from UV damage and cancer, it can be applied externally in the evening to be absorbed through the skin's surface and protect it inside and out.

'I refuse to admit that I am more than fifty-two, even if that does make my sons illegitimate.'

Lady Nancy Astor

UV Damage Deficiency Disease

South African plastic surgeon Des Fernandes is not only one of the most creative plastic surgeons in the world, he is a pioneer in skincare. His Environ range is one of the most active and effective on the market. It continues to become more advanced, sophisticated and effective with each year that passes. Fernandes looks at both intrinsic ageing – once believed to be caused by nothing more than the passing of the years – and extrinsic or photo-ageing, as unnatural. He considers both disease processes which, he says, can and should be treated. I could not agree more since exposure to strong UV radiation, just like exposure to chemical toxins, literally uses up your body's antioxidant supplies. 'Few people understand that photo-ageing is almost entirely a manifestation of vitamin deficiency in the skin,' he says. 'The most important vitamins are light sensitive ones and the antioxidants A, C, E and the carotinoids.' Add that to a *Skin Revolution* way of living that maximises vitality, enhances biophoton order and improves the functioning of the living matrix itself and you have a prescription for beautiful skin that knows no age. Go for it.

HEAT WAVES

radiant energy helps clear cellulite

For more than 100 years, infrared energy has been used in Europe to treat everything from skin ailments and athletic pain to cancer. Widely researched in the past quarter of a century, in its latest incarnation infrared energy is delivered in the form of a sauna, like none other you have ever seen. Nature's most powerful force for clearing toxic overload, it is also an effective and delightful method for healing, regenerating and rejuvenating skin. And it can enhance the order of the living matrix.

Of all the wavelengths emitted by the sun, some of the most beneficial for skin lie within the infrared spectrum. IR radiation makes up over half of the light energy we receive. It consists of wavelengths from 0.076 microns, known as 'near' IR, through to 1000 microns, at the 'far infrared' range which occurs just below or 'infra' to red light, the next lowest energy hand. (A micron equals 1/1,000,000 of a metre).

'The last place we tend to look for healing is within ourselves.'
Wayne Muller

Deep Heat
IR radiation is a unique form of *radiant heat*. It was discovered two hundred years ago by Britain's most famous eighteenth century astronomer, William Herschel. Measuring temperature at many points along the prismatic spectrum, Herschel discovered that while ordinary light transmits some heat, the sun's heating effects become more marked once you move towards the red end of the spectrum and beyond. That's how 'infrared' energy got its name.

Exposure to infrared energy light carries none of the dangers that too much UV light can. And the kind of warmth it imparts bears little resemblance to ordinary heat. Heat from common sources heats the air, IR heat radiates deeply into living cells. When skin – in fact the body as a whole – is exposed to IR rays their radiant energy warms the tissue itself without significantly affecting the air. You can experience the infrared heat phenomenon when you go out and stand in the sun on a crisp winter day. Although the air is cold your face is warmed by the sunshine. IR radiation penetrates your body to a depth of 1½ inches or more. In ways which are, as yet, by no means fully understood, its beneficial physiological effects can be carried deep into the body's organs and systems to act on them in a health-enhancing way.

Natural Healer

IR energy is particularly good for skin. It has also been used successfully for more than a century in the treatment of soft tissue sports injuries. Infrared lamps have also long been favoured by beauty therapists wanting to increase the penetration of active ingredients they apply to their client's skin. This it does with ease. For almost fifty years, IR lamps were used widely in hospitals and European natural clinics for relieving stress, enhancing the uptake of medicinal compounds, relieving pain and speeding healing. Then, in the sixties, in the face of mounting disregard in orthodox medical circles for simple natural treatment, its use gave way to drug-based methods of treatment.

'Several studies have implicated infrared signals (heat) in therapeutic touch (eg Schwartz et al. 1990, Chien et.al. 1991). This is important because some practitioners of therapeutic touch and related methods do not experience Mesmer's magnet-like sensation, but rather a sensation of warmth during their work.'

James L. Oschman PhD

Matrix Communication

As far back as 1923 a Russian biologist named Gurwitsch observed that infrared energy is one of the ways in which cells communicate with each other through a process known as *biological induction*. In the 1950s German scientists confirmed his findings. They discovered that IR light is actually absorbed by an animal's living tissues in the same way plants feed on the sun's energy during photosynthesis.

It was not until the early eighties that researchers came to realise that it is possible for abnormal cellular functioning to be normalised with the help of polarised monochromatic infrared light. This discovery remains the main biological basis for the use of infrared light nowadays. It is supported by widespread clinical reports from practitioners making use of it both medically and cosmetically.

Deep Acting

Infrared wavelengths stimulate cell metabolism in ways which go far beyond what can reasonably be expected from an energy which only penetrates the human body an inch or two. It can bring about improvements in digestion, increased energy levels, and heightened resistance to illness.

'I used to hesitate to recommend something that seemed so expensive, but when you realise the lifelong incapacity and expense of diseases such as heart disease, chemical sensitivity, chronic fatigue, fibromyalgia, chronic pain syndromes, migraines, Alzheimer's or any others caused by chemical and metal toxicity, a sauna is cheap.'

S.A. Rogers MD

CHECK THE BENEFITS

❑ Immune enhancement and greater protection from skin sensitivities and inflammation.
❑ Increased circulation – essential for glowing skin.
❑ Effective detoxification of wastes and chemicals, giving a higher protection from age-related degeneration and improving the functioning of the living matrix.
❑ Improved cellular exchange of nutrients and oxygen and elimination of cellular waste.
❑ Help clearing cellulite.
❑ Elimination of waterlogging in the tissues and the slack or puffy skin that goes with it.
❑ Better cellular metabolism.
❑ Enhanced production of ATP – the body's energy currency.

Out In Space

In the early eighties NASA developed enthusiasm for IR radiation as a means of keeping astronauts fit and healthy on long space flights. NASA researchers discovered that IR energy enabled astronauts to maintain a good level of cardiovascular fitness during long space flights where regular aerobic exercise was not possible. This was a major finding. It confirmed, as clinicians using it have long claimed, that bene-fits from IR radiation can be profound. IR can even be used to improve cardiovascular fitness in ways that before were believed only possible through sustained physical exercise.

'Americans got caught up in a fitness boom, but probably just as many fell by the wayside. As we've reported, recent research shows that you don't have to run marathons to become fit – that burning just 1000 calories a week ... is enough. Anything goes, as long as it burns these calories.'
                                    Wellness Letter, University of California

Here's how it seems to work: your body reacts to all kinds of heat by cooling itself. It shunts blood from internal organs towards the outside – into limbs and muscles. This increases your heart rate in the same way that running or rowing can. It also increases metabolic rate as well as the rate at which blood pumped by the heart flows through the body. This phenomenon appears to be only one of many deep acting effects from exposing the skin to infrared light regularly. It also stim-ulates repair, relieves pain and encourages healing to areas deep enough in the body that they lie far beyond the level to which its radiant energy penetrates the body's surface.

Your Own Healing Radiance
So natural is IR radiation and so welcome are the effects it exerts on living systems that it may come as no surprise that our bodies not only welcome its energy, we actually generate infrared radiation in our own tissues. A living body continuously radiates IR energy through the surface of the skin at between 3 and 50 microns with most of its output hovering around 9.4 microns. A young body sends out a great deal of infrared power. One which is ailing or which has lost some of its vitality as a result of high toxicity or degeneration, loses much of its ability to emit IR waves.

The palms of your hands emit IR energy somewhere between 8 and 14 microns and a number of researchers have measured and recorded IR radiation from the hands of natural healers, body workers and talented beauty therapists. They believe that an increase in the level of infrared radiating from the healer's palms as he works is the major cause of the warming phenomenon which healer and healed report during treatment. IR triggers the body's own infrared energy healing processes. Many IR researchers insist that IR radiation is selectively absorbed by the tissues which have the greatest need for it.

'Seek healing, a refilling of energy and spirit, as soon as you see that you
need it. You don't have to push yourself to give, do, or perform when what
your body, mind, soul and emotions need is to heal.'

Melody Beattie

A GIFT OF ENERGY

Studies have been carried out in an attempt to quantify the
beneficial effects of IR light on a cellular level. Scientists find
that within the cell's energy factories – the mitochondria – IR
stimulates the production of ATP – the energy currency on
which all our metabolic processes depend. This may be a major
reason why exposure to IR energy improves the look and function of skin. Like the rest of the body, skin needs a constant,
fully adequate supply of energy to heal damage to its DNA,
regulate the production of collagen and elastin, give birth to
new cells, and eliminate waste. These are many of the most
important processes on which beauty depends. When your skin
lacks energy, its cells function poorly and become prone to cell
suicide, known as *apoptosis*.

'Just standing around looking beautiful is so boring, really boring, so boring.'

Michelle Pfeiffer

Mounting scientific interest in infrared and the growing number of
clinical reports celebrating its benefits, have led to the development of
new infrared techniques and technologies which offer exciting new
ways of using it. As a result it is already used widely in China, Japan,
and Germany, Switzerland and Austria. These methods range from
wearing specially woven fabrics for sports gear designed to attract IR
from the environment and channel it into the body, to lamps and hand
held devices. Over 750,000 IR thermal systems have been sold in the
past five years in the Orient for whole body treatments. In the past
two decades some 30 million people have already received localised

IR therapy in one form or another. The crowning glory of new IR treatment technologies is the far infrared sauna.

Treat Yourself

Many of the best IR saunas come from Austria where the fascination with and appreciation of the benefits of radiant heat treatment has never diminished. If you have not yet tried an infrared sauna you have a delight in store. I have long respected IR treatment. It is a traditional part of the standard therapeutic fare in European natural medicine centres. But, until I tried it for myself, I was totally unprepared for the benefits this new form of sauna has to offer for the skin, for fat loss, for cellulite and for heightening vitality. Completely different than a conventional sauna which over-heats the air, can interfere with breathing and is, most definitely, the wrong kind of heat to subject delicate facial skin to regularly, an infrared sauna enhances body health and skin beauty in many ways.

'The infrared energy . . . may induce up to 2 – 3 times the sweat volume of a traditional hot-air sauna while operating at a significantly cooler air temperature.'

Dr Aaron M. Flickstein

Cool Heat

A conventional sauna relies on *convection* as its heat source. The skin is heated by direct contact with the hot air its element produces. But this requires very high ambient temperatures – between 185° to 235°F to accomplish. A conventional sauna is also costly to run and requires a warm-up time of between 30 to 90 minutes. In a far infrared sauna less than 20 per cent of the heat produced by its elements heats the air. The rest penetrates the body. Instead of the air temperature in a sauna becoming unbearably hot, it remains somewhere between 95° and 130°F – 50 to 125 per cent lower than a conventional sauna so the whole experience of using it is a great deal more pleasant.

Because IR so closely approximates the body's own energy our skin can absorb more than 90 per cent of what reaches it. Lower heat is also safer for anyone with a cardiovascular problem or skin prone to broken capillaries. Infrared thermal saunas heat up much more rapidly – in 10 to 15 minutes. But it was the reports of so many health benefits from IR saunas which encouraged me to experiment with them. The benefits to my skin and health with regular use of an IR sauna have been good. I use mine once a day.

IR energy enhances order in the living matrix. It rebalances hormones, energises the body, clears toxicity and even antidotes the negative effects of both electromagnetic and chemical pollution in the environment. IR energy is even useful in counteracting the negative effects of sun on skin. According to the Ninth Edition of Clayton's Electrotherapy: 'Infrared radiations are the only antidote to excessive ultraviolet light.'

HOT TIPS FOR A COOL SAUNA

Here are some important ways to guarantee you get the best possible benefits from an IR sauna:

- ❏ Drink an 8 to 12 ounce glass of pure spring or filtered water before entering the sauna and take another big glass in with you to sip when you feel thirsty. Without water neither waste elimination nor fat burning can take place effectively.
- ❏ Make the best of infrared's ability to enhance skin penetration by covering your face with a good treatment product or mask.
- ❏ Massage your body with organic coconut oil, essential oil based products or anti-cellulite creams and lotions while in the sauna.
- ❏ Make your first sauna a fifteen to twenty minute affair, then work up as you come to enjoy the experience to between thirty and forty-five minutes at a time.
- ❏ After a sauna, shower using a skin brush to further enhance lymphatic drainage, slough off dead cells and clear away waste through the skin.
- ❏ Apply a good body oil based on essential oils or a top quality lotion or cream *after* your shower. Your skin is now in prime condition to soak up whatever you put on it and to reap the benefits.
- ❏ If you have easy access to an IR sauna or decide to put one in your own home, experiment to see how often sessions work for you to bring you the best results. I use mine daily, sometimes even twice a day when I am working hard. It takes away the shoulder aches that develop from hours in front of a computer typing and relaxes me after long, hard work.

'Women are never what they seem to be. There is the woman you see and there is the woman who is hidden. Buy the gift for the woman who is hidden.'
Erma Bombeck

Double The Benefits

Another method for delivering IR energy is through a light-emitting diode which transmits via low-energy light (known as both IR and low energy photon therapy or LEPT). LEPT delivers a super-luminous low-level laser like red light. Together they increase the strength and extensibility of collagen, improve blood flow, eliminate waterlogging and puffiness and restore good skin muscle tone.

LEPT AND INFRARED LIGHT – A POWERFUL DUO

❏ Encourage the creation of new capillaries which in turn enhances oxygen supply to living cells.

❏ Stimulate the production of collagen by activating fibroblast activity in the skin.

❏ Stimulate the production of ATP, your body's energy currency on which health and beauty depend.

❏ Increase lymphatic activity to eliminate oedema and clear toxic substances.

❏ Enhance repair to as well as the production of new DNA and RNA.

❏ Induce a thermal effect on tissues supporting the immune system and improving cellular metabolism.

❏ Stimulate the release of the brain chemical acetylcholine to help counter stress.

'The near-infrared light emitted by these LEDs seem to be perfect for increasing energy inside cells. This means whether you're on Earth or in a hospital, working in a submarine under the sea or on your way to Mars inside a spaceship, the LEDs boost energy to the cells and accelerate healing.'

Dr Harry Whelan

Antidote To UV Damage

A body absorbs what it wants from any IR and LEPT light offered and simply does not seem to take what it doesn't need. Laboratories in Russia and the United States are busy exploring the benefits of this combination. Meanwhile, military units like the US Navy SEALS continue to use it to accelerate healing. It is not yet widely available, to my knowledge, no beauty therapists are yet using LEPT together with IR. IR saunas are a different story. They are becoming widely available both in salons and also in kit form which makes them easy to assemble in a room in your house. All you need is an electric socket.

Best Kept Secrets
There are many beauty secrets still locked within the infrared wavelengths. We already know that IR used regularly helps clear cellulite from thighs and bottoms, counteracts dandruff, detoxifies and firms skin, and encourages the healing of scars and burns. After a long haul flight, an IR sauna helps clear jetlag. Regular use creates a smoother, finer skin texture. IR saunas even encourage effective fat burning during weight loss. The way in which an IR sauna helps counter the disastrous effects of stress is believed to be thanks to radiant heat's ability to act upon the autonomic nervous system by helping the body rebalance its hormones. An extra bonus too: IR saunas don't wipe you out the way conventional saunas can. They can be both energising and relaxing simultaneously.

'Miracles don't come from the cold intellect. They come from finding your authentic self and following what you feel is your true course in life.'
Bernie S. Siegel

BURN FAT

Far infrared saunas generate two to three times the sweat produced in hot-air saunas with far greater comfort. And they help trigger fat-burning, clearing out lipophilic toxins stored in the body's fat cells. Once the store of these pollutants has been diminished, weight loss becomes an easier process. Raising body temperature with infrared energy enables it to remain raised for hours after the sauna has finished heightening thermogenesis for fat burning. While weight reduction which occurs as a result of water lost through sweat is of no consequence, the heat conditioning which results from regular use of a far infrared sauna enables the actual burning of calories to take place more easily both while in the sauna and for hours afterwards.

Take Care

Wonderful though IR saunas are with their myriad of therapeutic benefits, there are some important cautions to pay heed to:

❑ If you are using prescription drugs of any kind check with your doctor beforehand and get his OK.

❑ If you have any chronic health condition, be sure to get your doctor's approval first.

❑ Saunas are never recommended for pregnant women or women who suspect they may be pregnant.

❑ IR energy is reflected by surgically implanted metal rods or pins but silicon implants from breast surgery are heated by IR radiation. Check this out with your doctor before a sauna if you have silicon implants. Silicon melts over 200°C so there should be no problem as IR radiation never heats anywhere near that. But get medical support to be safe and sure it is OK for you.

❑ Do not use an IR sauna for the first 48 hours after an injury until the heat and swelling have subsided. After that, IR is great to speed healing.

❑ Anyone predisposed to bleeding such as a haemophiliac should never use any kind of sauna.

❑ Heat on the lower back of a woman during her period may increase menstrual flow. Some women are pleased with this claiming it helps clear congestion and back aches. You should be aware of this so you can make your own choices.

❑ Never use infrared treatments in an attempt to treat any disease unless you are under the direct supervision of a doctor.

'If we could learn to like ourselves, even a little, maybe our cruelties and angers might melt away.'

John Steinbeck

MY FAVOURITE AROMATHERAPY RECIPES

Here are some suggestions for sauna potions you can make
yourself to use in the sauna.

Single Oils: Mix a few drops of one or more of these together
with 2 ounces of almond or walnut oil as a carrier. Spread the
mixture on your skin to enhance elimination, increase circulation and tone skin: cineol, cypress, grapefruit, spearmint, lemon-
grass, tangerine or cedarwood.

Cellulite Helper: Mix five drops of rosemary and lemon with
five drops of grapefruit and 2 of cypress in 2 ounces of jojoba
or another carrier oil and massage into cellulite areas before
and during your sauna.

The only problem I have found with using a far infrared sauna is
that the practice has become highly addictive in my family. We all like
it so much and make use of ours so often that it has become like a
good friend. Sometimes I wonder how much less pleasant life would
be without it.

PART FIVE:

MAKING IT
HAPPEN

never-ending rejuvenation and regeneration

LIVING MATRIX 21 DAY TURNAROUND

the ultimate wrinkle-cure programme

Now you have all the savvy you need to commit yourself to your own 21 Day Turnaround Programme. You have got the principles of matrix nutrition under your belt, know about magnum force supplements if you choose to use them, the importance of clearing toxic overload, and all the rest. It is time to put all this into practice.

Here you will find an easy to follow plan complete with suggested menus, how to shop for and prepare matrix foods – even some of my favourite recipes for living salads, protein dishes, breakfasts and drinks. You are about to enter a whole new world of radiance, good looks and vitality. Let's get started.

QUICK GUIDE TO MATRIX LIVING

Living Matrix Turnaround eating is a simple, natural way of transforming skin and vitality easily, deliciously and fast. Here are the basic principles:

❑ Choose your foods for two reasons: 1. because they are irresistibly delicious and 2. because they can supply your skin with the highest possible support biochemically (through the nutrients and plant factors they contain) and energetically (because they offer optimal biophoton order).

❑ Eliminate grain-based carbohydrate foods – at least for the 21 day period – including flour, starchy vegetables like potatoes, white rice, sugar and other sweeteners. Afterwards, if your body feels it needs it, add brown rice.

❑ Eat masses of natural, fresh, organic, non-starchy vegetables and low-sugar fruits. Non-starchy vegetables high in phytonutrients and antioxidants are your primary source of carbohydrates.

❑ Eat two big salads a day. Not the usual thing made from lettuce and tomatoes and the odd cucumber but powerhouse medleys of biophoton order complete with sprouted seeds and a great variety of fresh herbs, not to mention crunchy peppers, carrots, apples and beetroot, as well as anything else beautiful you can lay your hands on or grow on your kitchen counter.

- ❏ Stay away from soft drinks, packaged fruit juices, alcohol (a glass – at most two – of wine a day if you must) and all processed drinks.
- ❏ Use cold-pressed, extra-virgin olive oil, walnut oil, and flaxseed oil on salads and coconut oil or olive oil for cooking. Never heat flaxseed oil.
- ❏ Enrich your diet with omega-3 fatty acids by eating fatty fish at least three times a week.
- ❏ Stay away from margarine and other processed oils or any sauces or salad dressings which contain them.
- ❏ Eat good-quality protein like fresh fish, free-range chicken, eggs, game, organic meat and low-carb soya products at lunch and dinner.
- ❏ Eliminate coffee or at the very least have only one cup a day. It dehydrates and damages skin.
- ❏ Stay away from commercial foods.
- ❏ Take a multiple vitamin including all the B complex daily.
- ❏ Practice yoga or strength training if you can get into them three days a week for 30 minutes at a time, to enhance lean body mass as your face and body are restructuring themselves.
- ❏ Walk briskly for 20 to 30 minutes each day to counter insulin resistance, enhance energy, bring radiance to skin, help clear cellulite and maintain good emotional balance.

Now let's get down to making it happen.

Clear The Junk

First order of the day is to empty your cupboards of all those skin-threatening foods – biscuits and pasta, breakfast cereals, jams and jellies, convenience foods – and the fridge of ice creams, packaged fruit juices and ready-in-a-minute frozen meals as well as anything else which might tempt you in the first few days to fall back into old habits. Living Matrix eating is great for your family too. If they want noodles or pasta, cereals or wholemeal toast at breakfast keep a special place for their foods. Give them cooked vegetables but let them sample some of your powerhouse salads too. Even meat and potato types have been known to fall in love with them. Everybody is better off without convenience packaged foods.

Remember you can eat as much as you like of Living Matrix foods so you will not go hungry. Every one of the volunteers who tested out the programme for me reported back – usually in amazement – 'All of my cravings for sugary and high-carbs stuff completely disappeared after the first few days.' More than a few of them – especially women – had this to add: 'It's a miracle!' This is because your body acts quickly to stabilise blood sugar levels and as it does, you tap into high levels of energy. At the same time skin loses its puffiness as excess water in the tissues is released as part of the detoxification process. And – joy of joys – addictive eating completely disappears in most people. Be aware that it usually takes three to five days on matrix eating for your body to adjust. If during your first few days you discover that cravings temporarily get stronger, eat more protein foods as snacks or at mealtimes, rest a bit while your body is making the changeover and be patient. Soon all things will not only be well, they will be terrific.

RAW ENERGY FOR GREAT SKIN

On the Living Matrix 21 Day Turnaround Programme about half of your foods will be eaten raw and as many as possible will be living foods – sprouted seeds and legumes with all the biophoton order they impart to your skin. Raw foods have rejuvenating and regenerative powers. This is why they are used throughout the world at the most famous natural clinics and spas for beauty as well as for healing chronic and acute illness. Uncooked foods improve cellular functioning, enhance the energy and biochemistry of the matrix, and provide high levels of antioxidant and immune enhancing plant factors. Making a high percentage of what you eat raw increases overall energy and stamina too and makes skin radiant.

Next Agenda – Matrix Shopping

The most important foods for your Living Matrix Turnaround will be fresh non-starchy vegetables, low-sugar fruits, and proteins like meat, seafood, eggs and game, as well as maybe a little unprocessed cheese and soy proteins like tofu if you're vegetarian. The healthiest, freshest, and the most natural foods are found around the outside edges of the supermarket.

These include crunchy fresh vegetables and fruit, fresh game and meats, sea foods, eggs and low-fat cheeses. These natural, wholesome foods are perishable and therefore have to be replaced often, unlike the ready-in-a-minute, pre-made stuff that you find in the inner aisles. You will be shopping 'at the edge' in another way too: you'll be looking for foods as close as possible to those our ancestors ate. You'll want to choose a wide variety of vegetables and fruits which you can eat raw. Here are some shopping lists and suggestions to take with you when you go:

NOTHING BUT THE BEST

❑   Your foods will be natural whole-foods.
❑   They need to be as fresh as possible and eaten as close to a living state as possible. This allows little time for the deterioration which occurs as a result of oxidation.
❑   All the foods you eat will be non-toxic and non-polluting to your body. They should contain no synthetic flavours, colours, preservatives or other additives used to cosmetically 'enhance' them.
❑   Try to vary the foods you choose from day to day and week to week. Down through evolution the human body has adapted to a wide range of foods which offer a broad spectrum of nutrients.
❑   Use fresh garlic and herbs often. They bring high level support for skin regeneration.
❑   Eat what you enjoy and enjoy what you eat.
❑   Say goodbye to addictive eating forever. Once your body clears itself of the residues of starchy grain-based foods and sugar all those cravings that can make you feel you have no willpower vanish.

LIVING MATRIX VEGETABLES

Full of biophoton order, phytonutrient power and just plain delicious, these fresh living foods are the best you can get.

CHOOSE FROM:

Vegetables
Avocado
Bean sprouts
Beet greens
Beetroot
Broccoli
Cabbage
Carrots
Cauliflower
Celery
Chickpea sprouts
Collards
Courgette
Cucumber
Endive
Escarole and other dark green lettuces
Garlic
Kale
Lettuce
Mushrooms
Mustard greens
Onions
Peppers
Radishes
Rocket
Romaine lettuce
Spinach
Swiss chard
Tomatoes
Watercress

Fruits
Apples
Apricots (fresh)
Berries – blackberries,
   blueberries, raspberries
   strawberries
Cantaloupe
Citrus fruits – lemons,
   oranges, mandarins,
   tangerines, grapefruit
Honeydew melon
Kiwifruit
Peaches
Pears
Plums
Rhubarb
Tomatoes

SAY YES TO COLOUR

The more vibrant and beautiful the colours of your vegetables and fruits are, the greater the immune-enhancing and antioxidant phytonutrient energy they carry. Bright blueberries or strawberries, deep green leafy vegetables such as spinach and rocket, tell us that the food we are about to eat is brimming with polyphenols, helpful in preventing diseases including cancer and heart disease, as well as countering Syndrome X and protecting skin from early ageing.

You will want to look for vegetables that are particularly health-enhancing, such as garlic and onions – great when finely grated in a salad or used when cooking your protein dishes.

Fresh Herbs Help Your Body

Make good use of the wonderful culinary herbs available: caraway, fennel, dill, chervil, parsley, lovage – the Umberiferae; summer savory, marjoram, the mints, rosemary and thyme – the Labiates which have a strong aroma and are particularly useful for seasoning; the Liliaceae such as garlic, onions, chives and leeks. These three are my favourites: basil, tarragon and horseradish.

Herbs have a special role to play in Living Matrix eating. They contain pharmacologically active substances such as volatile oils, tannins, bitter factors, *secretins, balsams, resins, mucilages, glycosides* and organic vegetable acids, each of which can contribute to overall health in a different way. The *tannins* in common kitchen herbs are astringent. They exert an anti-inflammatory action on the digestive system. They help inhibit fermentation and decomposition. The *secretins* stimulate the secretion of pancreatic enzymes – particularly important for the complete breakdown of proteins in foods to make them available for bodily use. *Organic acids* in herbs have an antibiotic action and are helpful in the digestion of fats. So are the bitter factors – found in good quality rosemary, marjoram and fennel. They also act as a tonic to the smooth muscles of the gut and boost secretion of digestive enzymes. Use herbs lavishly in your meals and you will find you can create the most remarkable combinations of subtle flavours and aromas.

Buy Organic

Whenever possible, go organic. Not only do organic vegetables taste better, the organic matter in healthy soil is nature's factory for biological activity and biophoton order. Organic brings your skin a superb balance of minerals, trace elements, vitamins and phytonutrients and vitamins which we cannot get any other way. The organic matter in soil is built up as a result of the breakdown of vegetable and animal matter by the soil's natural residents – worms, bacteria and other micro organisms. The presence of these creatures in the right quantity and type – which you never find in factory farming – gives rise to physical, chemical and biological properties which create fertility in our soils and make plants grown on them highly resistant to disease. This resistance to illness and degeneration is then passed on to us when we eat the foods. Destroy the soil's organic matter through chemical farming and, slowly but inexorably, you destroy the health of the people and animals living on the foods grown on it.

Natural food emporiums are great places to find good organic vegetables and other produce, as well as eggs, meat, dairy products and fish, from animals that have not been stuffed full of antibiotics, dipped in chemicals or treated with hormones. Try to shop as much as possible in stores that offer organic produce and untreated food.

Simply The Best

When selecting meats and fish, there are two major considerations: make sure it's fresh and as unprocessed as possible. Buy fresh fish and seafood instead of processed forms such as smoked fish, crab cakes or breaded fish. There's no harm in having the odd slice of smoked salmon, especially if it is naturally smoked. But the more a fish is processed, the less quality it brings you in terms of high-level health. (And these days, sadly, most smoked salmon has sugar added to it.)

Eat oily fish at least three times a week but every day if you can. Pre-formed omega-3 fatty acids DHA and EPA are fantastic for skin. The omega-3s in wild salmon, mackerel, sardines, tuna and herrings can be absorbed by your body without conversion to make it usable. Omega-3s help balance hormones, protect from degeneration, and have powerful anti-inflammatory properties. Flaxseed oil is also a good source of omega-3 fatty acids. It is great used on its own or with extra virgin olive oil to dress your salads. But it differs from fish oil in a couple of significant ways. Flaxseed contains a lot of linolenic acid, which is the precursor to DHA and EPA, but the problem is that your body needs to convert the linolenic acid to DHA and EPA. Some people can't make this conversion, especially if they have eaten a lot of trans fatty acids and an overabundance of omega-6 fats in the past.

Get Ultra Fresh

The key to good fish is to buy it fresh. Always ask the person serving you which fish is the freshest and what days of the week different kinds of fish arrive in the shop. You can tell a lot about the freshness of fish just by its smell and look. Really fresh fish does not smell like fish at all. It smells more like the salty bite of a sea breeze. If it's a whole fish you are looking at, pull back the gills. They should be bright red. The moment they go pale pink or grey you know the fish has been sitting in the shop too long. Try poking the flesh of the fish with your finger as well. If it springs back instead of forming an indentation then you're likely to have a piece of fresh fish. Check out the eye of the fish. It should be dome-shaped and clear and not sunken and murky. Because I live a fair way from the centre of the city where I buy my fish, I always protect it when I buy in quantity by taking a chill-box with me. That way it stays ultra fresh until I can get it home, bag it and freeze whatever I am not going to use immediately.

Go For Organic Meat

The meats we get today are a far cry from those our Paleolithic ancestors ate. Probably the closest you can get to those today is by buying wild boar, rabbit, buffalo, venison or kangaroo. These meats are higher in protein and lower in fat, which makes them healthier. That being said, all organic red meats like beef and lamb are excellent sources of zinc, a mineral that's enormously important not only for insulin balance and weight loss but also for skin and the reproductive system. Organic meats are guaranteed to be free of antibiotics, steroids, herbicides and pesticides. One exciting development in the meat in some countries such as the United States is that some farmers are beginning to feed their animals on foodstuffs rich in omega-3 fatty acids, so within a few years we may have meat available with a healthier fatty acid profile than the meats we have today. (It may well cost a fortune too!) Free-range and organic meat is far better than factory farmed in every way, including the protection it offers from BSE.

When choosing dairy food, it is good to remember that butter, although it is not a source of essential fatty acids, is a perfectly respectable food – far better than any margarines, no matter how fancy or how sophisticated is their formulation. When choosing other dairy foods, try to go low-fat. Look for low-fat cottage cheese, ricotta, mascarpone, and unsweetened yoghurt. Eat a bit of cream or sour cream as a special treat now and then. Stay away from flavoured cottage cheeses, yoghurts and other dairy products which are almost always chock-full of sugar or other kinds of sweeteners, as well as questionable flavourings.

LIVING MATRIX PROTEINS

Fish and Shellfish
Bass
Trout*
Sole
Sardines*
Herring
Mackerel*
Salmon*
Tuna, fresh*
Tuna, tinned in water
Tarakihi
John Dory
Cod*
Haddock
Halibut
Snapper
Swordfish
Green-lipped muscles
Calamari
Oysters
Clams
Crayfish
Lobster
Crab
Scallops
   * rich in omega-3 essential fatty acids

Meats
Organic beef
Organic pork, bacon and ham
Organic lamb

Game and Poultry
Organic or free-range chicken
Turkey
Wild duck
Pheasant
Quail
Rabbit
Venison
Wild boar

Eggs
If possible, buy organic, if not at least free-range. Eat them any way you like: soft- and hard-boiled, in omelettes, poached, scrambled or fried.

Cheese

An occasional treat, limited to 4oz a time. Be sure to check any carb content.

- ❑ Parmesan
- ❑ Camembert
- ❑ Feta
- ❑ Cottage cheese
- ❑ Ricotta
- ❑ Mozzarella

Vegetarian Options

- ❑ Tofu, tempeh, miso and other soya products – but check carb content on label.
- ❑ Microfiltered whey protein – this is the highest value biological protein in the world. It's *great* for non-vegetarians too when you need to make a quick breakfast drink. If you are a vegetarian, use plenty of it to make sure you get enough complete proteins.

As far as drinks are concerned, the best you can find is pure water. Buy it plain, sparkling or even flavoured, so long as there are no artificial sweeteners in the product. These days you can find a huge selection of good herbal teas, as well as organic green tea. Rich in antioxidants, green tea is the best drink around for skin. Coffee is a major contributor to skin inflammation and blood sugar disorders. It also dries out your skin – even oily skin – making it prone to wrinkles. Avoid it altogether if you can. If not, limit yourself to one cup a day. You don't want coffee to undo all the good that Living Matrix eating is doing for you.

LIVING MATRIX DRINKS AND EXTRAS

WATER POWER

Water plays a major part in digesting your food and absorbing nutrients thanks to its role in helping your body create enzymes needed for digestion. When you don't drink enough water between meals your mouth becomes low in saliva and skin shows it. Water is the medium through which wastes are eliminated from your body. Each time you exhale, you release highly humidified air – about 2 big glasses worth a day and carried on it, metabolic wastes. Your kidneys and intestines eliminate another 6 or so glasses of water and waste every 24 hours, while another 2 glasses worth are released through the pores in your skin. That makes 10 glasses a day – and this is on a cool day. When it gets hot, when you are exercising, or when you are working hard, the usual 10 glasses lost in this way can triple.

On average, in a temperate climate – when you are not sweating from exertion or heat – you need about 3.5 litres or 6 pints a day for optimal health, although few of us consume as much as one third of that. The important thing to remember is that how thirsty you are is *not* a reliable indication of how much water you need to drink. Do as French women have done for decades. Keep a large bottle or two of pure, fresh, mineral water within easy reach and make sure you consume your quota of this clear, delicious health-giving drink.

Drinks

❑ Use filtered or spring water – drink 8 to 10 glasses a day.
❑ Herb teas, flavoured mineral water (although only those with no sweeteners or calories) and organic vegetable bouillon or broth.
❑ Drink vegetable broth if you fancy it made with broccoli, cabbage, cauliflower, bean sprouts, asparagus, mustard greens, spinach, watercress, ginger, garlic or any combination thereof is good. Bring to the boil and simmer for 15 minutes. Season with herbs and sea salt and store in the fridge, reheating as needed.
❑ Avoid all alcohol if you can. In any case no more than a glass of wine a day – two at the very most.

COOL THE BOOZE

Alcohol is another substance you want to go easy on. Not only is it high in empty calories and pretty useless in terms of nutrients, alcohol causes your liver to produce one of the most potent cross-linkers known for skin – acetaldehyde. The more acetaldehyde in your body, the faster skin ages. Hard liquor like whiskey, gin and vodka raise insulin levels. It is best avoided. A glass of dry white or red wine with one of your meals does most people no harm. It may even have a beneficial effect. A number of studies indicate that red wine, in particular, increases the body's sensitivity to insulin and carries some antioxidant power too. If you choose to have a glass or two, make sure you only drink **good** wine. Run of the mill *vin de table* is full of toxic substances which your skin can do without.

Seeds For Sprouting

These make great sprouts. Grow them in bowls on your kitchen sink. Always buy organic if you can:

- ❑ Mung beans
- ❑ Chickpeas
- ❑ Marrow fat peas
- ❑ Adzuki
- ❑ Black lentils
- ❑ Brown lentils
- ❑ Raw buckwheat

Secrets Of The Coconut

When it comes to sauces for your protein foods, make your own if you possibly can. As far as oils are concerned, extra-virgin olive oil and flaxseed oil are best for salads. You can also use olive oil for wok frying. Coconut fat is good for this too, and for searing meat or fish, since being a saturated fat it is very stable. Coconut oil has some other important attributes too. It supports the thyroid, activates metabolism and is a fine source of just plain energy when you need it. Coconut oil is rich in medium chain triglycerides (MCT) which have been shown to reduce body fat, reverse arteriosclerosis, improve glucose metabolism, and even lower serum and liver cholesterol.

LIVING MATRIX FATS

The fats you'll eat on Living Matrix Turnaround are the healthiest available. Most can be used in salad dressings or for cooking proteins. Eat about a tablespoon or so per meal from the list below. In addition to the fat you get from food, use 2 teaspoons of flaxseed oil every day on your salads and consider using a good supplement of omega-3 EPA and DHA fish oils.

- ❑ Almonds and almond butter
- ❑ Avocados (and guacamole)
- ❑ Coconut oil
- ❑ Extra-virgin olive oil
- ❑ Macadamia nuts and macadamia butter
- ❑ Olives
- ❑ Tahini

LIVING MATRIX EXTRAS

How about the rest? See below.

Salad Dressings and Sauces
You can make these with walnut oil, extra virgin olive oil or flaxseed oil together with lemon juice, Champagne vinegar, red wine, balsamic or apple cider vinegar.

Herbs and Spices
Use all spices and fresh herbs.

Fibre
The raw vegetables you will be eating in your salads are full of wonderful fibre. So is sprouted buckwheat. You can also add some whole or ground flaxseeds to salads and mueslis for extra fibre.

Sweeteners
The best sweetener in the world is stevia. Sadly it is not available in the EU for rather silly regulatory reasons to do with the lobbying power of the big chemical companies which sell artificial sweeteners like aspartamine and saccharine. Artificial sweeteners are foreign chemicals and not good to use at any time. Many studies show that they can have a dangerous effect on living organisms when used regularly. If you can

get stevia, use it. It is 300 times sweeter than sugar itself and good for you. It comes in many varieties, the best is the organic Stevita Spoonable Stevia which can be used just as you would use ordinary sugar, although you will need a great deal less of it.

Manuka honey is another alternative for sweetening. Used in moderate amounts it does not have the same insulin unbalancing effect that other honeys, sugars, malt extracts and the rest do. Manuka honey has far greater molecular density than any other form of honey. It is this that makes it behave differently in the body. It also has remarkable anti-bacterial and anti-viral properties. Mixed with papaya it makes an excellent face-mask.

Nutritional Supplements
Take the following daily:
- ❑ A good multiple vitamin including phytonutrients and B Complex (see Resources).
- ❑ The three magnum force nutraceuticals – if you feel your skin needs them – carnosine, nicotinamide and MSM.
- ❑ 1000 – 3000mg omega-3 EPA and DHA fish oils in capsule form if you eat fatty fish at less than once a day.

For information on other supplements, see Magnum Force page 80.

Flavour Is Everything
When it comes to seasonings in Living Matrix eating, the more the better. I love fresh herbs best but when I can't get them I use a wide variety of dried herbs. Buy organic whenever you can, since herbs and spices in a supermarket are most often irradiated in order to give them a longer shelf life, and you want to avoid irradiated foods whenever possible. Irradiation can be a cover-up for spoilt food. There are a wide variety of other wonderful foods – from Indonesian fish sauce to Mexican chillies – that you may not be used to eating, most of which are available in natural food emporiums and really good delicatessens. Get to know them, experiment and see how many can make Living Matrix meals even more delicious. Now let's look at some Living Matrix menus.

FIRST RATE POWER FOR TRANSFORMATION

Following these guidelines will automatically provide you with skin transformation of the highest order. It is a diet rich in the biophoton order necessary to maintain a high degree of resistance to skin reactions and degeneration. Provided your foods are fresh enough, and provided you eat at least half of them raw, you will also benefit from all the phytonutrients they bring to your skin.

MATRIX MEAL SUGGESTIONS

Let's look at some typical meals for Living Matrix breakfast, lunch and dinner and some good snacks too if you want them. The menus that follow are great for getting you started on this new way of eating. They will help you grasp what skin revolution living is all about. You will be forging for yourself a whole new way of eating and thinking about food. If, like me, you like to jump into things feet first, spend a day or two cleaning out your cupboards and refilling the fridge with matrix supporting foods, then launch into the programme for 21 days with unbridled passion. The meals can be as simple as a piece of grilled fish, liver or steak with a salad, or as complex and indulgent as you wish to make them. Be sure to check out the recipes in the next section if you decide to get fancy. It's fun and you will be delighted with the changes you experience. Some of the suggestions listed below refer directly to recipes supplied. Others, like 'grilled fish' leave you to your own devices.

START WITH SOMETHING RAW

Try to begin a meal with something raw. This helps avoid something called *digestive leucocytosis* – an immune reaction which has white blood cells rushing to the lining of the stomach when we eat cooked foods before raw. Have a few mouthfuls of salad or a slice of melon before moving on to the fish. You could even start with raw oysters if you are lucky enough to find fresh ones.

Revolutionary Breakfasts:

- **Berry Bliss Smoothie** (see recipe, page 225) made with 20 to 30 grammes of microfiltered whey protein powder, a teaspoon of flaxseed oil, and an apple, pear or a handful of berries blended with a few ice cubes. It will have you out the door in a New York minute. Herb tea or green tea.
- **Instant Omelette** (see recipe, page 222) with fresh sprouts. Cook your omelette in olive oil and toss in chopped tomatoes, peppers, spinach – what-have-you. Serve with a slice of melon (not water-melon). Herb tea or green tea if you wish.
- **Live Muesli** (see recipe, page 220) made with coconut oil and soaked or sprouted raw buckwheat, apples, pears or berries. Herb tea or green tea.
- **Grilled Fish** – salmon is especially good with garlic and sweet onions plus a bowl of mixed berries. Herb tea or green tea.
- **Blueberry Curds and Whey** (see recipe, page 222) a delicious new twist on an old-fashioned dish. Herb or green tea.
- **Sunday Morning Hand-Made Sausages** (see recipe, page 226) make ahead of time for a lazy morning under the duvet. Serve with finely grated raw apples, carrots and beetroot dressed with the juice of an orange and some curry powder. Herb tea or green tea.
- **Vanilla Nutmeg Smoothie** (see recipe, page 225) another instant blender meal, rich and creamy with a spicy overtone. Herb or green tea.

Lunches:

- **Chicken Kebabs** skewered with onion pieces and mushrooms dipped in olive oil and seasoned with herbs and fresh lemon juice. A rocket and black olive salad dressed with extra virgin olive oil and lemon.
- **Crudités** served with **Fish Dip** or **Seafood Pâté** (see recipe, page 243). Half a rock melon.
- **Fresh Spinach Salad** with slivers of white meat – chicken or turkey – slices of yellow, red and green peppers and sweet red onions and sliced fresh mushrooms topped with grated hard-boiled eggs. Toss with olive oil and Dijon mustard dressing.
- **Steamed Sea Bass** smothered in **Live Pesto** (see recipe page 237). A salad of radicchio with fresh herbs.
- **Nut Crusted Tuna** (see recipe, page 248) on a bed of rocket, with

black olives and herbs. Mixed sprout salad with **Easy Mayonnaise** (see recipe, page 238).

- Salad dressed with olive oil, balsamic vinegar and garlic dressing.
- **Big Greek Salad** with left-over chicken or lamb made with lettuce, cucumber, tomato wedges, sprinkled with sunflower seeds and a teaspoon of pumpkin seeds, Greek olives and 2 teaspoons of feta cheese – olive oil and lemon dressing.
- **Curried Chicken** (see recipe, page 249) served with **Caesar Salad With Hard Boiled Croutons** (see recipe, page 232). Slices of fresh kiwi fruit, apples, and oranges.

Dinners:

- **Powerhouse Salad** made with everything you've got that is fresh and looks delicious dressed with **Basil and More Basil Dressing** (see recipe, page 244) and topped with chicken slices or grated hard boiled eggs – lots of them.
- **Sautéed Mackerel** with garlic, fresh tomatoes, slivered olives and fresh garlic. **California Sprouted Salad** (see recipe, page 231). Strawberries with fresh lemon juice and mint.
- **Bunless Turkey Burger**: combine minced turkey with finely chopped green onions or scallions and red pepper. Grill with onion slices and a Portobello mushroom or two. Top with **Biophoton Salsa** (see recipe, page 238). Serve with **Fresh Strawberries** dipped in finely ground almonds.
- **Crudités** – cucumbers, tomatoes, celery, and crunchy lettuce with **Curried Avocado Dip** and **Light Mayonnaise** (see recipe, page 238) **Grilled Wild Salmon** seasoned with fresh ground pepper and capers. Serve with a mixed sprout salad dressed with **Curried Avocado Dip** (see recipes, page 242).
- **Rocket Salad** with Greek olives. **Grilled Prawns** served with aioli. Fresh blackberries and raspberries.
- **Chef's Salad** (see recipe, page 233). Sliced oranges topped with shredded coconut and grated ginger.
- **Red Cabbage Coleslaw** with onions, garlic and an apple dressed with homemade mayonnaise. **Stir Fried Chicken** with pak choy, bean sprouts, ginger, green onions, garlic, water chestnuts cooked in coconut oil with a coconut cream sauce sprinkled with toasted sesame seeds. Watermelon balls with ginger.

Snacks:

Eat snacks only if you feel the need. Most people find they feel better simply eating three meals a day. But if you love snacks, here are some suggestions.

HOW ABOUT SNACKS

Judge for yourself whether or not snacks work for you. For some people they are terrific, for others eating more often than every 4 to 5 hours increases insulin resistance and leads to food cravings. You need to play it by ear and find out which works best for you. Here are some suggestions for good quality snacks:

❑ Half a chicken breast.
❑ An apple, an orange, a pear or a few strawberries.
❑ Half a cup of unsalted walnuts, cashews, almonds, or brazils.
❑ A few crudités dipped in salsa.
❑ A handful of sunflower seeds.
❑ A hard-boiled egg.

Make Way For Radiance

Living Matrix eating can not only make your skin more beautiful. It can be the beginning of a whole new way of living. You become more alert and more active. You may sleep less – yet far better than before. This is because your body clears itself of toxic build-up. You can deal with stress better than before and feel calmer yet stronger. 21 Days on the Living Matrix Turnaround programme can bring inner light and outer beauty together creating your own brand of unmistakable charisma and authenticity. Meanwhile your skin glows and your vitality radiates. It's what I call deep beauty of the highest order. Enjoy it and all around you will delight as well.

REVOLUTIONARY BREAKFASTS

break the mould

The Living Matrix 21 Day Turnaround Programme is easy to follow and demands little food preparation to enhance your living matrix, fight free radical aggression and follow a path to keep skin ageless, year after year.

You will be eating protein, vegetables and fruits every day. If you want to keep time in the kitchen to an absolute minimum, you can grill your meat and fish or steam it and make a one-bowl meal of all your delicious raw vegetables. If you want to explore the outer reaches of delicious matrix eating, you might like to follow some of the simple recipes that follow. Better still, take them as a starting point and create your own magic with the wonderfully nourishing foods that are part of the living matrix life.

Into The Kitchen

In the beginning, switching over from conventional eating to Living Matrix breakfast can seem a bit of a stretch. I guess it's partly because we get set in our ways. Most have come to think of breakfast as a grain-based meal complete with toast, a muffin, or one of those packaged cereals every chubby kid in Steven Spielberg's movies spoons enthusiastically into his mouth.

It is mostly our passion for the conventional convenience food breakfast which has us reaching for another sticky bun or cup of coffee mid-morning to keep going. Come join the revolution each morning as you head into the kitchen. Take a breath and open wide the doors of possibility. You might be surprised at just how simple, delicious and energising it can be.

My mother had an attitude towards breakfasts that I used to think kind of weird. Now I've come to embrace its weirdness fully. She could never figure out why anybody wanted to eat conventional foods at breakfast time. Her idea of a delicious breakfast was some spicy Italian dish or left-over bouillabaisse from the night before. I've recently taken to heart her fascination with unusual breakfasts.

I sometimes find myself preparing a salad rich in phytonutrients, based on sprouted seeds and grains. I crush a clove of garlic, and chop some rocket or radicchio, then add some cubes of left-over chicken or fish cooked the day before. If I am really in a hurry, I toss it all into a square plastic container, pour on the olive oil, squeeze some lemon juice, season with a dash of Worcester sauce, salt and pepper. Then I put the lid on and give it a toss within the container. I either eat it immediately or take it with me. When my 22-year-old son Aaron saw me doing this recently he found it curious. One morning he thought he'd try it for himself. Like me, he found the occasional weird breakfast so refreshing and uplifting that he has since begun making them himself, usually at the weekends after a night out.

Quick And Easy

I have never been one for breakfasts which take a long time to prepare. I have more interesting things to do at the beginning of the day – including sleeping late on Sundays when I can get away with it. So let me share with you some of the phytonutrient-rich, quick things I make myself as part of my own matrix living.

LIVE MUESLI
Serves 1

Live muesli is what I most often make for breakfast. Everybody loves it – even children raised on sugar crunch convenience foods. When it comes to health and good looks nothing carries revolutionary breakfast power to the living matrix like a bowl of fresh raw muesli. Not only are live mueslis higher in essential nutrients than their grain-based counterparts, the quality of the phytochemicals they contain is the best in the world. Contrary to what a lot of people think, raw fruits and vegetables are also easy to digest. Each fruit or vegetable, fish or seed carries within it the exact enzymes necessary for us to digest it efficiently and fully. Bircher muesli was created by the great Swiss physician Max Bircher-Benner who first healed himself of what was apparently an incurable condition using a high-raw diet and then went on to heal hundreds of thousands of others in the same way. Bircher muesli is so delicious that even died-in-the-wool junk food eaters fall for it. This recipe – my family's favourite breakfast – calls for an apple. But you can use almost any fruit – strawberries, peaches, apricots, cherries, pears – whatever is inexpensive and in season. The recipe serves one, but can just as easily be made for twelve. This particular form of muesli is dairy-free. If you prefer to use dairy products you can use plain low-fat yoghurt in place of soy milk. The raw buckwheat has been soaked overnight so that enzymes break down the hard-to-digest starches making them taste sweeter while being much easier to absorb. It is even better if you let it sprout for two or three days before you use it. You can always use steel-cut organic oats if you like, but buckwheat is far better as it is a living plant, and as a living plant it brings a high level of biophoton order to the body.

WHAT YOU NEED
2 dessertspoons of raw buckwheat soaked overnight in water or sprouted
2 teaspoons of coconut oil (it is hard when room temperature is below 76°F – this is the usual way I make use of it)
1 apple or fresh apricots – chopped or grated
the juice of 1 orange or tangerine
1–2 teaspoons Manuka honey (optional)
½ teaspoon of powdered cinnamon or nutmeg or some fresh grated ginger

HERE'S HOW
Mix together the soaked buckwheat with the coconut fat using a fork to cream it all together. Combine with the fruit and juice, yoghurt or soy milk and sweeten with the honey if you like. Sprinkle with cinnamon or ginger. Serve immediately.

OTHER WAYS TO GO

FRUIT JUICE MUESLI: substitute some fresh fruit juice, such as apple, orange or grape, for the soy milk or yoghurt. To thicken the juice blend with a little fresh fruit in season such as a pear, or apple.

SUMMER MUESLI: add a handful of fresh or frozen strawberries, blackberries, loganberries or raspberries, or pitted cherries to the basic muesli, or substitute a finely diced peach or nectarine for the apple.

BLUEBERRY CURDS AND WHEY
Serves 1

Blueberries are richer in phytonutrient power than any other fruit. Besides, they are delicious. This is an old-fashioned recipe, just about as old-fashioned as you can get, but with a new twist: it is enriched with microfiltered whey protein and almonds. You can substitute walnuts, pecans, or even macadamias if you prefer to make a highly-satisfying one-bowl meal that is refreshing, sweet and delicious. You can use frozen blueberries if you can't get fresh or for a change use raspberries or strawberries instead. You can also add 1 tsp of flaxseed oil for extra omega-3 support.

WHAT YOU NEED
100 grammes of creamed cottage cheese
50 grammes of fresh blueberries, strawberries, or raspberries
1 scoop of whey protein (optional)
1 tbsp chopped almonds or other nuts that have been toasted over a high heat in a dry frying pan
Manuka honey to taste (optional)
1tsp flaxseed oil (optional)

HERE'S HOW
Chop and toast your nuts beforehand. Store toasted nuts in a refrigerator for use in this recipe or any other recipe where you want to use them as a topping or a crust. (Toasted chopped nuts will keep for 2–3 weeks in a fridge.) Using a food processor or a hand blender mix all ingredients except nuts and berries together with creamed cottage cheese. Fold in the sliced berries. Sprinkle with the toasted nuts and serve immediately.

OMELETTE ON THE RUN
Serves 1

I don't know why people make such a palaver out of omelette making. It's about the easiest thing in the world. I learned this from Paul, the father of my youngest son, who turned out omelettes-to-die for in less than two or three minutes. The key is having the right pan to cook it in. Years ago I bought myself a French crêpe pan – a cast iron flat round pan which is about the best thing in the world for omelette making. You can make this omelette either with whole eggs, or with one whole egg and 3 egg whites, depending upon how fluffy you like to go. I make mine with whole eggs.

Eat it on its own, or fill with grated cheese, salsa, or chopped garlic, tomatoes, onions and green peppers. This way it turns into what I call a salad omelette, namely an omelette full of beautiful fresh crunchy vegetables. You can even fill it with left-overs from the day before.

WHAT YOU NEED
2 to 3 eggs beaten until light and fluffy, or alternatively 1 whole egg and 3 egg whites
50 grammes of left-over ham or chicken – finely chopped (optional)
1tbsp grated cheese i.e. Parmesan, Ricotta, Mozzarella (optional)
dash of Mexican chilli seasoning
cracked pepper to taste
1 medium tomato
2 cloves crushed garlic
½ of a green or red capsicum
1–2 tsp of extra-virgin olive oil
Salt and ground pepper to taste

HERE'S HOW
Oil the pan and sauté the stuffing ingredients – ham, chicken, tomatoes, garlic, what have you – until they are warmed through. Pour the egg mixture over the top. Let it set, using a spatula to tilt the liquid egg to the edges of the pan. After it has set completely, sprinkle the surface with cheese (if you are using cheese) and fold in half. Cover with black pepper and seasoning and serve immediately. If you are making a stuffing-free omelette, then simply pour your eggs directly into the pan once the oil has heated. Use a spatula to tilt the liquid egg to the edges of the pan. When almost set, roll up and serve sprinkled with salt and other seasoning.

SCRAMBLED TOFU
Serves 1

Lighter and more delicate in texture than scrambled eggs, tofu works well for breakfast provided you season it richly, for tofu has almost no flavour of its own. If you add a pinch of turmeric, you will create a 'vegan scrambled egg' in a rich yellow colour just like the real thing.

WHAT YOU NEED
1 tbsp of extra virgin olive oil
2 cloves of garlic, crushed or chopped
2 green onions, chopped fine
pinch of turmeric (optional)
sea salt to taste
fresh ground black pepper to taste
Mexican chilli powder to taste
½ cup of grated Parmesan (optional)
½ tsp of curry powder
½ tsp of cumin powder

HERE'S HOW
Heat the oil in a heavy frying pan and sauté the green onions and garlic until they are soft (2–3 minutes). Mash the tofu then stir it into the pan with the turmeric. Add your other seasonings and any other herbs you want. Cook over high heat, turning frequently until tofu goes firm. This takes about 2 or 3 minutes. Sprinkle on the cheese if you are using it. Season with salt and pepper and serve immediately.

QUICK SHAKE
Serves 1

If you like chocolate, this is one of the fastest recipes I know for breakfast. I use it often. It makes the best quality protein breakfast you can find in less than two minutes. You can also make it with vanilla flavoured powder or any other flavoured microfiltered whey.

WHAT YOU NEED
1–4 scoops of microfiltered whey protein or whey protein isolate powder – enough scoops to yield 20–30 grammes of protein
1 tsp flaxseed oil
1 cup of cold water
2 tbsp unsweetened organic cocoa
3 ice cubes
1–2 heaped tsps of ground flaxseeds (optional)
1–2 teaspoons of Manuka honey

HERE'S HOW
Pour all ingredients into a blender or food processor. Blend until smooth. Serve immediately.

VANILLA NUTMEG SMOOTHIE
Serves 1

This breakfast-in-an-instant is based on the traditional egg-nog that people used to drink at Christmas. In fact the egg is optional, you can make it with or without. If you decide to put the egg in – I like to do this because it gives more flavour – make sure your egg is free-range or organic. You don't want to mess around with battery laid eggs eaten raw. There is always the danger of salmonella.

WHAT YOU NEED
200ml of cold filtered or spring water
6 ice cubes
1–2 scoops of natural or vanilla flavoured microfiltered whey protein or whey protein isolate powder – enough scoops to yield 30 grammes of protein
1 egg (optional)
1 tsp of vanilla essence or several drops of natural vanilla oil
a pinch of freshly grated nutmeg to taste
Manuka honey to taste (optional)
1 tbsp of flaxseeds (optional)

HERE'S HOW
Place all the ingredients in a blender and blend vigorously until combined. Be careful not to blend for more than 20 seconds, however, since this can change the nature of the microfiltered whey protein. Sprinkle a little extra grated nutmeg on top and serve immediately.

BERRY BLISS SMOOTHIE
Serves 1

WHAT YOU NEED
50 grammes of fresh or frozen raspberries, strawberries, blackberries, loganberries or a mixture
100ml of plain live yogurt

Manuka honey to taste (optional)
2 tbsp of flaxseeds (optional)
3 ice cubes (optional)
tsp of lemon zest (optional)

HERE'S HOW

Put all ingredients into a blender and blend well but not for more than 20 seconds. You can add more or less water if you want a slightly thicker or thinner shake. Serve immediately.

SUNDAY MORNING HAND-MADE SAUSAGES
Serves 4

I adore sausage. Yet the sausages that you buy are full of all sorts of artificial flavourings and colourings, not to mention carbohydrate 'stuffers' which you don't want to eat. This is an old-fashioned pattie sausage which you can vary depending upon your taste, and what herbs and meats you have available. You can make it with pork, venison, chicken, lamb, beef or wild boar. I mix the ingredients together the night before, then put them in the fridge to chill and absorb all the flavours. Eat within 3 days.

WHAT YOU NEED

350 grammes of lean minced pork, chicken, lamb, beef, venison or wild boar
1 tsp sea salt
2 tbsp of oat bran preferably soaked overnight
4 cloves of garlic (optional)
2 tbsp of chopped fresh parsley, coriander or sage
½ large onion chopped fine

HERE'S HOW

Combine all your ingredients in a big mixing bowl and mix thoroughly with your hands. Refrigerate until well chilled, then separate into four patties and cook in an oiled skillet until crunchy on the surface and done through.

POWERHOUSE SALADS

biophotons and phytonutrients lead on

The quickest and easiest way to get phytochemical-rich biophoton-ordered skin transformation is a delicious nutrient-dense powerhouse salad twice a day to complement your top quality protein dishes. Forget the limp lettuce leaves and tomato fare. I'm talking green mesclun and bright flowers, wild herbs, fennel, rocket, ruccola, colourful Swiss chard, almonds and bright peppers, as well as vegetables that most people don't even think to put into a salad, such as cauliflower and broccoli.

That is one style for a whole meal salad. The other is rich and crunchy made from sprouted seeds and legumes – embryonic plants at the height of their enzyme activity and life force, all of which provides your skin and body with a high level of energy and order. Powerhouse salads are the order of the day for skin regeneration and rejuvenation. They will detoxify your body and bring vitality to your whole life.

The Art Of Ordering

Preparing a gorgeous salad is more art than science. For me it is like meditation. I set aside 10 minutes as a break from my busy work life to see what I can create from the freshest ingredients I happen to have in my fridge or in my garden. Often people say to me, 'I'd love to eat more salads but I don't have time.' I know they still have a lot to learn about how easy salads are to make and how quick. I can make a protein-rich salad that is a whole meal for four people and have it on the table in 10 minutes. Even better than popping something in the microwave. (I don't even own one.) There are no statutory controls in any country on microwave leakages and the last thing skin needs is more microwave ionising radiation. Besides, everything I have ever tasted that was cooked in a microwave has tasted 'dead' to me and I love the rich flavours of wonderful fresh foods.

Shop For Skin Beauty

To make a quick, irresistible, delicious salad is easy. The process begins in the shopping stage. Buy what's most beautiful. Forget the rest. Bring home your vegetables, wash and dry them thoroughly. Put them in a vegetable bin in the refrigerator. When you shop once or twice a week for fresh vegetables, do this as soon as you get home, then you are all set for instant salad meals. The key to keeping your vegetables fresh for a whole week once they've been washed is to store them in plastic bins in the fridge that are covered by big plastic bags. This keeps things fresh and crisp for so long it always surprises me. When it comes to fresh herbs, such as basil, parsley and coriander, I place them in a sealed plastic bag into which I have sprinkled several drops (not more) of pure water. This way they too stay fresh for the week.

For efficient salad making you need to have all your vegetables ready to go. For preparation is what takes all the time. Then when you come into the kitchen you simply pull out two, three or four bins full of lovely bright coloured fresh foods and dive into salad making. I love working with whatever is there. You can make a fabulous salad from a bunch of rocket with some gorgeous black olives, and fresh slivers of Parmesan cheese. Delicious and especially nutrient-rich salads are easy to make. Use shredded raw broccoli and cauliflower, red and yellow capsicums, chopped red onion, and slivers of Chinese cabbage, smothered in a creamy home-made mayonnaise made with extra virgin olive oil or an irresistible curried avocado dressing.

Instrument Of Torture – Couldn't Live Without It
The one piece of kitchen equipment I never want to be without is a mandolin. These remarkable vegetable shredders are so different than the usual graters you find in most stores. The tiny knives they contain make perfect slices of whatever vegetable you like. Stainless steel mandolins are not only expensive, they are virtually useless. The best are cheap and made from plastic. They have a V shaped blade, into which plastic inserts fit, each of which has different sized knives. You can julienne, make chip size chunks, slice thin or thick. Unlike the conventional grater which mashes vegetables and fruits, a mandolin slices them clean and sharp. Be sure to use the hand protector device which comes with every model. If you don't – and I know this from bloody experience – what you end up with is shredded fingers instead of shredded cabbage.

I try to mix between two and five vegetables together to make a salad. Not only do I combine varieties of vegetables, I also mix textures, using fine julienned celeriac, for instance, together with a coarsely grated red cabbage, plus slivered green onions. It's the mixture of colours and textures that makes it all work. Let your imagination take over. Feel and taste the ingredients you are using. Treat the whole process of salad making as you would that of painting a picture or making a sculpture. Have fun. Make it a delightful experience and you can't miss.

Phytonutrient Delight

Any salad made from fresh vegetables and fruits which carry a high degree of biophoton order can also be chock-full of flavonoids, carotenoids and sulphoraphanes – the phytonutrients that offer the best you can get for high-level health as well as protection against premature ageing. Sounds like it should be a salad that tastes bad, but you eat it knowing that it's going to do you good? Wait until you taste one for yourself.

For a long time I was troubled by how to make salads tasty when using vegetables which are particularly rich in phytonutrients like broccoli and cauliflower. Then I discovered the way to do this: simply shred them very, very fine using a mandolin, so that you get small crunchy pieces. This adds texture and richness, while giving your salad great nutrient density. At first when I began experimenting with this I thought that no-one but me would eat my offerings. I soon discovered otherwise. My friends loved them – especially when they are tossed with a rich home-made mayonnaise or avocado dressing. Now I grate broccoli and cauliflower into many of the salads I make day after day.

Oh So Lazy

Lazy about salad dressings, I usually make my salad in a large flat bowl. Then, instead of mixing the salad dressing separately, I dress the salad right then and there. A few tablespoons of extra virgin olive oil, some chopped fresh herbs, crushed raw garlic, a dash of Worcester sauce, some Maldon salt, the juice of a lemon or a couple of tablespoons of wine vinegar or balsamic vinegar, some home-made Cajun seasoning from the fridge or a dash of the powdered variety from the market. To top it off I use some freshly ground coarse black pepper. I like to grind peppercorns with a mortar and pestle because it tastes so much better that way. I sprinkle this all on top and toss. Ready in an instant. Sometimes I top off salads with seeds like pumpkin, sesame or sunflower. On others, I scatter chopped fresh garlic or shredded wild garlic leaves when they are growing down the path near where I live. When they are to be found in the garden, I even add some fresh edible flowers like marigold petals or heartsease.

It's What You Do With What You Got

Of course you need none of these things to turn a simple salad into a masterpiece. What you do need is a child's sense of experimentation, plus plenty of love. For it is that ingredient which makes every meal a joy: it's not just what you make but how you make it that matters, it's also your attitude to what you are doing in the kitchen. Years ago in India I discovered that the best foods are those you buy in the cheapest cafés. They have been made with love and joy, sometimes with humour too. The word café is really a euphemism for these places which are often little more than a few stones within which a fire has been built for cooking. Yet the foods they sell are infinitely better tasting, more nourishing and safer – less likely to cause Delhi Belly – than all the fancy foods you can get in expensive restaurants. It doesn't matter how skilful or how knowledgeable and important a cook is, if he doesn't invest the food he gives you with affection then it's dead food, not energy food. This affection cannot be faked or disguised. Have fun, experiment with the energy and colour of living foods. You can't help but create something wonderful and infinitely nourishing. Here are a few of my own suggestions to help inspire you but really the process is so simple that the last thing you need is a recipe. Let's look at sprout salads first then some of the whole meal dish salads I love which are quick to prepare, travel well if you are going to take your lunch to work and are always satisfying.

How To Sprout A Seed

Yes, they are easy to find in supermarkets but they are so much better when you sprout them yourselves. Sprouts are vegetables which grow in any climate, mature in 3–5 days, can be planted any day of the year, need neither soil nor sunshine, and are some of the richest sources of antioxidant vitamins, minerals and phytonutrients in the world. Grow them in jars in your kitchen or the airing cupboard. They are the perfect compromise between the agriculture of years gone by and the 'just add water' mentality of the 20th century. Sprouts are full of anti-cancer properties and anti-ageing properties. The vitamin content of a seed increases phenomenally when it germinates. The vitamin C in soya beans, for instance, multiplies five times within three days of their germination. In fact, a mere tablespoon of soya bean sprouts contain half the recommended daily adult requirement of vitamin C – provided of course that they are fresh. Sprouts are also rich in chlorophyll, known to have anti-cancer and anti-ageing properties. Researchers have discovered that when they expose bacteria to carcinogenic chemicals in the presence of extracts taken from lentil sprouts, mung bean sprouts and wheat sprouts, that cancer development is inhibited by 99 per cent.

I have recently developed a really simple way to grow these little living foods which are so delicious.

After you have assembled your seeds – from mung beans and adzuki to marrow fat peas, buckwheat and lentils (no alfalfa please), pour each variety into its own small bowl and cover it with two or three inches of clean water, place a plastic bag over the lot and forget them for 24 hours. Then, once a day at the same time each day, drain each dish into a sieve or colander, rinse the seeds under running water, rinse the bowl and return the seeds to the bowl they were soaked in. (If you live in a very hot climate you will need to do this twice a day.) Cover the lot with a damp towel and then with a piece of plastic or a plastic bag laid over all the bowls and forget them again until the next day when they will need the next wash. After two or three days you will have delicious sprouts ready for eating. Rinse them a final time, place them on a tray and pop them into the fridge then cover again with the damp towel and a piece of plastic over the top. They stay fresh for three or four days while you are using them up for your salads.

Sprout-Based Meal In A Moment Complete With Proteins

My favourite quick salad with sprouts is this: I take a handful of three or four varieties, put them in a bowl, chop a tomato or add an avocado or maybe grate some bright red sweet pepper and sprinkle some nori seaweed strips over the top. I then pour on half olive oil and half flaxseed oil, squeeze the juice of a fresh lemon and season with fresh herbs, chopped garlic and any other spices that take my fancy. To this I add my protein foods – some diced chicken or lamb, chopped hard-boiled egg or occasionally slivers of Parmesan cheese. It makes a quick meal which has everything I need in it to keep me going for hours and hours and I love the chewy crunchiness it has.

You can also combine sprouts with raw vegetables for the best of both worlds.

CALIFORNIA SPROUTED SALAD
Serves 2

This salad relies heavily on sprouted seeds and grains. Sprouts taste delicious and make absolutely wonderful California-type health salads.

WHAT YOU NEED
½ cup chickpeas
½ a small tomato, sliced
1 tbsp of green peppers, chopped fine
2 cloves of garlic, crushed or chopped
1 avocado, sliced
½ bulb of fennel, sliced
½ cup mung bean sprouts
½ cup brown lentil sprouts
Maldon sea salt to taste
Freshly ground pepper to taste

HERE'S HOW
Slice the tomatoes, peppers, fennel and avocado and place in a bowl.
Add the chickpeas and sprouts, crush the garlic over them, add salt
and pepper, toss and pour over your favourite dressing.

CAESAR SALAD WITH HARD BOILED CROUTONS
Serves 2

Instead of croutons made from bread, use rashers of lean organic bacon,
diced and fried crisp, then drained on a paper towel, or a couple of
hard-boiled eggs grated coarsely or chopped. My preference is a couple
of hard-boiled eggs. The good thing about the bacon is it gives that
crunchy texture. But the eggs add a rich creaminess which contrasts
beautifully with the light crunchiness of raw vegetables. So take your
pick. Anchovies are a great source of omega-3 fatty acids as well as
being rich in the nucleic acids, DNA and RNA, which some experts in
human biochemistry believe may help prevent premature ageing. To
this Caesar salad you can also add slices of left-over chicken or fish or
turkey to create a delicious whole meal in a bowl.

WHAT YOU NEED
For the salad
1 head of cos or romaine lettuce
50g of Parmesan cheese, shaved, not grated
6 –12 anchovy fillets, drained and cut in thirds
300 grammes of cooked chicken in chunks (optional)
Seasoning to taste

For the croutons
2 rashers of lean bacon, diced, fried and drained or
2 hard-boiled eggs roughly grated or chopped

For the dressing
1½ medium sized lemons, juiced
2 cloves of garlic, chopped fine or crushed in a mortar and pestle
2 tbsp of extra-virgin olive oil
several dashes of Worcestershire sauce
1 free-range organic egg

HERE'S HOW
To prepare the dressing
In a small bowl mix together the lemon juice, garlic, olive oil and
Worcestershire sauce, break the whole egg into the bowl and whisk
with a fork to blend well.

To prepare the salad
Wash and dry the lettuce leaves, then tear them into chunky morsels.
Wrap them in a clean towel and chill in the fridge until you need them.
Place the lettuce leaves in a large flat salad bowl, add the cooled 'crou-
tons' and pour the freshly made salad dressing all over, add the anchovies
and season. Toss and serve up with shaved Parmesan.

CHEF'S SALAD
Serves 2

A chef's salad is one of those perfect meals you can not only order in
a restaurant, but also make yourself – provided you have plenty of left-
overs.

WHAT YOU NEED
1 head of the most beautiful lettuce you can find (any kind) torn into
bite size pieces
½ cucumber, cubed
4 hard-boiled eggs, halved
100 grammes of ham, sliced in strips
100 grammes of cooked chicken, sliced in strips
50 grammes of Parmesan cheese, in julienne strips
1 small tomato, cubed

2 tbsp of lemon juice
2 tbsp of extra virgin olive oil, or half olive oil and half flaxseed oil
1 tbsp of balsamic vinegar
dash of Worcestershire sauce
2 cloves of garlic, crushed or chopped fine
3 tbsp fresh parsley, basil or coriander, chopped
Mexican chilli seasoning

HERE'S HOW
Arrange lettuce, cucumber and tomato in a big flat salad bowl and sprinkle on the fresh herbs. Pour the oil, lemon and vinegar over the top and season and toss. Arrange eggs, chicken, ham and cheese on the top of the salad. Shake Mexican chilli seasoning over all and serve immediately.

GREEK SALAD
Serves 1

So simple, this salad is such a delight. It too is pretty readily available in restaurants. But I prefer to make my own.

WHAT YOU NEED
100 grammes of dark lettuce leaves, spinach or rocket torn into bite size pieces
1 small Spanish onion, sliced in rings
80 grammes of feta cheese, cubed
a handful of fresh, black olives, drained
1 small tomato, wedged
½ a green capsicum, julienned
50ml of extra virgin olive oil
50ml of balsamic vinegar
juice of half a lemon
season to taste with sea salt and ground pepper.

HERE'S HOW
Lay all ingredients in a large salad bowl and pour over the olive oil, vinegar and lemon. Toss well and serve immediately.

MESCLUN AND FLOWER SALAD
Serves 2

Mesclun is that wonderful mixture of delicate salad leaves, including such things as curly endive, romaine, radicchio, flat leaved parsley, dandelions – even purslane. All are brimming with phytonutrients. These leaves are not only easy to grow, you harvest them by cutting a few leaves at a time and letting the plants go on reproducing yet more beautiful leaves. Nowadays mesclun is pretty easy to find in supermarkets, often washed and ready to eat. I like to serve this salad with a fish soup, roast or lobster because it is so light and uplifting. The flowers are not absolutely necessary but they add such beauty to the dish that I can never resist.

WHAT YOU NEED
For the salad
50–75 grammes of three or four of any mesclun leaves: romaine lettuce, dandelion leaves, radicchio, rocket, lamb's lettuce, oakleaf lettuce, purslane, curly endive
½ a ripe avocado, sliced
a handful of fresh mushrooms, sliced
50 grammes of celery, finely sliced
10–12 bright coloured nasturtium flowers (optional). You can also use marigolds or heartsease, the gorgeous little pansy-like flowers that have a reputation for easing heart-ache.

For the dressing
2 cloves of garlic, chopped fine
½ tsp Dijon mustard
50 grammes of walnut oil
1 tbsp of white wine vinegar
1 tbsp lemon juice
1 tbsp of chervil, chopped fine
1 tbsp flat leaved parsley, chopped fine

HERE'S HOW
Put all of the mesclun leaves plus the other salad ingredients into a big bowl. I like to use glass bowls because the leaves are so beautiful it's a shame to conceal them. Then, for the dressing, put all the ingredients into a screw top jar and shake vigorously to blend. Sprinkle delicately over the leaves, toss lightly and serve.

WILD SALMON SALAD
Serves 4

My favourite salads are whole meal salads where you pick your vegetables and then add to them ready cooked protein foods: tofu, which has been fried in coconut oil and seasoned with Cajun seasoning, flaked cooked salmon, cooked chicken, small cubes of left-over lamb roast, left-over wild duck, even hard-boiled eggs. This salad is ready in a minute, easy to prepare and is delicious.

WHAT YOU NEED
500 grammes of cooked or canned wild salmon, flaked
4 large stalks of celery, sliced thin on a diagonal using a mandolin
3 tbsp of fresh coriander, chopped fine
½ a small red onion, chopped fine
a small finger of fresh ginger, shredded fine
2 tbsp of fresh lemon juice
½ cup of mayonnaise (preferably home-made)
4 glorious lettuce leaves

HERE'S HOW
Combine the flaked salmon (or whatever else you're using) with the celery, coriander, onion and other ingredients. Drizzle with lemon juice and mix in the mayonnaise with a fork. Spoon onto a plate covered with 4 large lettuce leaves and chill for half an hour before serving.

DRESS IT OR DIP IT

delicious any way you go

This the area of the Living Matrix Programme which feels delightfully self-indulgent. Make great dressings for salads, dips for crudités and sauces of all sorts to go with your meals. Here are some of my own favourite recipes.

LIVE PESTO

Probably my favourite sauce of all time is Italian pesto. I grew up eating it over pastas and for a time missed it terribly when I wasn't eating pasta. Then I realised that the same sauce, which is low-carbs, goes brilliantly on fish, green beans, spaghetti squash – even a salad of buffalo mozzarella and thin sliced tomatoes. I make this sauce in a blender and store it in the fridge, and use it up within 2 days. I am notorious for buying huge bunches of fresh basil and making masses. When I want to freeze pesto, I make it without the cheese and then add the cheese to it when I defrost it. It keeps very well this way.

WHAT YOU NEED
½ cup of extra virgin olive oil plus ½ cup of flaxseed oil or
1 cup of extra virgin olive oil
4–6 cloves of garlic, crushed or chopped
a huge bunch of fresh basil leaves, about as much as you can gently pack into 3 big cups
70 grammes of pinenuts, macadamias, or even almonds
70 grammes of freshly grated Parmesan cheese

HERE'S HOW
Put the olive oil and flaxseed oil (if you're using it) into a blender. Add everything except the cheese. Blend until smooth. Pour into a bowl and stir in the cheese. This recipe makes about 12 servings.

BIOPHOTON SALSA

I adore salsa. It's such a great way to add zing to anything from salad to fish. You can eat this salsa hot or cold. I like to spoon it onto omelettes for brunch or breakfast and to eat it with crudités. This recipe is all raw. It makes the best possible use of the phytonutrients in the herbs and vegetables that go into it. I like to cut my salsa rougher than most so you get a great mixture of textures as well as flavours. Make it in the food processor, as far as I'm concerned, and you turn a salsa into a gazpacho which is all very well if that's what you are after.

WHAT YOU NEED
2 cloves of garlic, finely chopped
½ a red onion, finely chopped
a handful of fresh coriander, chopped
a handful of fresh basil, finely chopped or 2 tbsp of fresh mint, chopped
a handful of broadleaved parsley, chopped
green or red chilli pepper, roughly chopped (after removing the seeds)
1 large tomato, roughly chopped
1 large green pepper, roughly chopped
Maldon sea salt to taste
freshly ground black pepper to taste
3 tbsp of extra virgin olive oil
3 tbsp of lemon or lime juice

HERE'S HOW
Mix everything together in a bowl and chill in the refrigerator. It takes this chilling process to let the ingredients in salsa meld properly. I like to eat my salsa fresh and would never keep it in the fridge for more than 48 hours.

EASY MAYONNAISE

Mayonnaise is not as difficult to make as everybody makes out, particularly since the advent of high-speed blenders and food processors. It does take a little bit of patience and a little bit of practice. If by any chance you don't succeed with your first emulsion, simply wash out and *dry* carefully your blender or food processor then use the 'unemulsified emulsion' to drop back, drop by drop, into a new supply of egg yolks as though it were oil itself. Go through the process all over again. Naturally you will have to add a bit more seasoning as you'll end up with a bit more mayonnaise. If at first you don't succeed, try again. You will. This mayonnaise is made with extra virgin olive oil. You have the option of making part of the oil that it contains flaxseed oil as well. You can do all sorts of wonderful things to it, like add nuts, garlic, herbs, mustards, virtually the sky is the limit once you get the basic principles of how to do it. Commercial mayonnaise – the kind you buy in jars in the supermarket – is something you want to avoid as much as you can. These products are full of trans-fatty acids and made from the cheapest, nastiest forms of hydrogenated junk fats. Mayonnaise you make yourself will keep for 4–5 days in the coolest part of the refrigerator. Here's my basic recipe plus some suggestions on how to vary it.

WHAT YOU NEED
275ml of extra virgin olive oil
2 yolks from large eggs
2 tbsp of cider vinegar
2 tbsp of lemon juice
½ tsp of dry mustard
sea salt to taste
freshly ground black pepper to taste

HERE'S HOW
Put the egg yolks in a blender or food processor and begin to blend on a low setting. Very, very gradually add your oil – literally drop by drop as the blender is running until you see an emulsion beginning to happen. When this begins you will no longer be seeing liquid swirling round and round, but something thicker with the consistency of a light face cream. Continue slowly to add oil to the mixture in a thin stream, all the while keeping the blender low, until you have added half the contents of the oil. Then put in the vinegar, mustard, salt and pepper as well as the lemon juice, all the while continuing to blend. Finally, slowly add the remaining olive oil. Taste and adjust seasoning. This recipe makes about 300ml.

VARIATIONS ON A MAYONNAISE THEME

Flax It
Replace a quarter of the olive oil with flaxseed oil.

Go For Garlic
Add 2–4 crushed cloves of garlic when you are adding the lemon juice for an intense garlicy mayonnaise – excellent with fish soup.

Nuts Are Great
Add 70 grammes of chopped walnuts when putting in the lemon juice.

Orange Zest
Take one cup of your home-made mayonnaise, but leaving out the garlic and mustard, and add to it 2 tsp of grated orange zest as well as a tbsp of fresh orange juice and 2 tbsp of finely chopped fresh mint leaves.

Curried Mayonnaise
Take one half cup of your home-made mayonnaise and add to it a tsp of mild to medium curry powder as well as a tsp of finely grated fresh ginger.

TOFU MAYONNAISE LITE

This mayonnaise, instead of being made with oil, is made with tofu. You can use it for salads and dips as well as sauces to go on cooked vegetables. It's easy to make and light as air to eat. Like conventional mayonnaise, you can vary this recipe by adding garlic, Cajun seasoning, mustard or fresh herbs to give a totally different look and flavour to your mayonnaise.

WHAT YOU NEED
450 grammes of soft tofu, drained
50 grammes of granular lecithin
3 tbsp of lemon juice
1 tsp of fine lemon zest
a small pinch of stevia (optional)
50ml of flaxseed oil or extra virgin olive oil
1 tsp of vegetarian broth powder

Maldon sea salt to taste
freshly ground black pepper to taste

HERE'S HOW
Put the tofu into a blender and add the lecithin granules, lemon juice, stevia and broth powder as well as half of the oil. Blend well until thoroughly mixed. Now slowly, drop by drop, add the remaining oil and blend again for 2–4 minutes until the mixture grows thick and creamy. Finally stir in the lemon zest. This mixture will keep in the refrigerator for 5–6 days.

SOUTH PACIFIC CURRY SAUCE

This sauce I learned from my friends from the Cook Islands who seem to use coconut for everything with marvellous results. It's easy to make and will turn meat, fish or chicken into a delicious meal. If I'm feeling really energetic, I serve it over a bed of unsweetened hand-shredded coconut in place of rice.

WHAT YOU NEED
1 tin of unsweetened coconut cream
½ an onion, chopped fine
2 tsp of mild, medium, or hot curry powder
3 cloves of garlic, crushed
a pinch of turmeric (optional)
1 tbsp coconut fat

HERE'S HOW
Place the onions and garlic in a pan (I often use the pan that I have stir-fried whatever meat, fish or chicken that I'm going to use in the curry so that after I have cooked the protein and removed it from the pan, the crispy crunchy bits and pieces carry the flavour over into the curry sauce).

Add the coconut fat to the frying pan and brown garlic and onions, picking up any left-over residue from protein foods you have cooked. Pour on the coconut cream and add all the other ingredients. Bring to a gentle simmer, and simmer for a minute or two, then it's ready to serve. This recipe makes enough sauce for a curry to feed 4–6 people.

CURRIED AVOCADO DIP

This dip is great for crudités. I serve it together with a platter of fresh phytonutrient vegetables such as endive, bulb fennel, crunchy lettuce, celery, slices of red, green, and yellow capsicum and anything else I happen to have around. It's a huge hit with everybody. If you make it a little thinner by adding a bit of water to it, you can also use it as a dressing on a salad.

WHAT YOU NEED
2 large ripe avocados, peeled and cubed
3 cloves of garlic, chopped
3 tbsp of lemon juice
1 tsp of vegetarian broth powder
⅛ tsp of Cajun seasoning
Maldon sea salt to taste
freshly ground black pepper to taste
1 tsp of mild to medium curry powder
1 tbsp of lemon zest

HERE'S HOW
Add chunks of avocado plus garlic, lemon juice, broth powder and other seasoning to the food processor – everything except the lemon zest. Blend until creamy and add lemon zest and serve. This recipe makes about 1 cup.

TERIYAKI MARINADE

I love teriyaki but so often the marinades that are made to soak fish, chicken and meat in to get a teriyaki taste are full of sugar and saké, both of which raise insulin far too high. This is my alternative. It's equally delicious, easy to make and very low in carbs.

WHAT YOU NEED
100ml of tamari or soya sauce, with no sugar added
2 tbsp of soy oil (or olive oil in a pinch)
30ml of spring or filtered water
2 tsp of wine vinegar
1 finger of fresh ginger, grated fine
2 cloves of garlic, crushed or chopped
1 to 2 teaspoons of Manuka honey (optional)

HERE'S HOW

Combine all your ingredients in a flat, low pan then marinate your beef, pork, chicken or tofu before teppenyaki grilling or stir-frying or barbecuing. If you are stir-frying, you can pour the remainder of the sauce into the pan once the meat and vegetables are cooked to further season the food. This recipe makes about 125ml.

FISH DIP OR SEAFOOD PÂTÉ

I discovered this recipe one night when I happened to cook too much fish and didn't know what to do with it. So I put it into a blender and began adding various ingredients. I ended up producing a fish pâté or dip so delicious that the whole thing disappeared before I had a chance to store it overnight for the next day's lunch. You can make it with just about any kind of light tasting fish you can find. I even use smoked salmon but if you do this make sure you buy a form of smoked salmon that doesn't have sugar in it. I love to eat it as a meal in itself – something to dip crunchy crudités into. It travels well for lunch or dinner on the go.

WHAT YOU NEED

450 grammes of cooked white fish or smoked salmon
50 grammes of mayonnaise (home-made)
a handful of chopped fresh parsley, coriander or basil
1–2 tsp of vegetable bouillon powder (to taste)
2–5 tbsp of filtered or spring water (play this by ear, watch the consistency)
dash or two of Worcestershire sauce
2 tbsp of extra virgin olive oil or half olive oil and half flaxseed oil
2–4 cloves of fresh garlic, crushed

HERE'S HOW

Place all the ingredients in a blender and blend until smooth. If you need a little more water, add it here remembering that once you have chilled the pâté it's going to go firmer in the refrigerator so you need to make allowances for this. If you are using it as a dip, naturally you use more water. If you are using it as a pâté you will use less. Turn off the blender and adjust the flavouring. Be creative about this, put anything else in that you think might be nice such as part of a chopped onion perhaps – this is best blended in by hand afterwards to keep the onions from going liquid, for their crunchiness is a wonderful part of the texture of the pâté itself. Remove from the blender and pour into ramekin dishes. Cover and chill. This will keep in the fridge for 2 to 3 days.

DEVILLED EGGS

I grew up on devilled eggs. It was one of those American dishes always served at barbecues and get-togethers in the country. I associate it with beautiful summer afternoons and young girls in gingham dresses. Devilled eggs are not only great garnishes for salad dishes and make good hors d'oeuvres, they are also an excellent snack food that you can carry with you during the day.

WHAT YOU NEED
6 large organic or free-range eggs, hard-boiled
12 black olives, chopped
2 tbsp of minced red onion
3 tbsp of mayonnaise (preferably home-made)
1½ tsp of Dijon mustard
Maldon sea salt to taste
freshly ground black pepper to taste
80 grammes of finely chopped celery
Mexican chilli powder as a garnish

HERE'S HOW
Slice the hard-boiled eggs in half lengthwise. Take out the yolks, put them in a bowl and smash them. Stir in all your other ingredients except the olives, then spoon into the egg whites and garnish with the olive slices, lightly doused with Mexican chilli powder and serve.

BASIL AND MORE BASIL DRESSING

Since basil is my favourite herb I'm occasionally accused of overdoing it, but so far as I'm concerned there is nothing more uplifting than a basil dressing on a magnificent salad of green leaves. My favourites are rocket – especially wild rocket – and lamb's lettuce or *mache* as the French call it.

WHAT YOU NEED
100ml of extra virgin olive oil
3 tbsp of fresh lemon juice
25–50 grammes of fresh basil, chopped
1 tsp of vegetable bouillon powder
freshly ground black pepper to taste

HERE'S HOW
Mix all the ingredients in a food processor until smooth. Adjust the flavour as necessary. Use immediately or store in a container in the refrigerator for up to two days.

MATRIX PROTEIN DISHES

architectural beauty starts here

Matrix protein dishes are as simple as can be to prepare. At home it usually takes us no more than 10 minutes to prepare a delicious meal for four people and get it on the table from scratch. Both lunch and dinner are made up of either a gorgeous salad of mixed vegetables or one made of a variety of home-grown sprouts with an apple or an avocado, with perhaps some fresh herbs and olives tossed in.

Our protein foods are usually steamed or barbecued. I love barbecues. I have had one for years yet hardly used it because it took so long to get started. So after wrestling with my self-righteous, politically correct view that barbecues should always be carried out the old-fashioned way, I broke down and bought one of those light-the-gas-and-there-you-have-it varieties. I now use it several times a week. I keep it on the porch outside my kitchen door so I can use it even when it's raining. It starts instantaneously. I can toss onto it a piece of organic lamb's liver, fish, a steak or chicken and by the time I have made the salad it is all ready. If I am feeling broody and want to make a more elabo-rate meal for guests, I just follow the Living Matrix eating principles and either add my protein foods directly to my whole meal salad or make a protein dish as simple or elaborate as I like.

Here are favourite recipes I use when I get into 'spend time in the kitchen' mode. Most of the time I am so lazy that I just do it the easy way.

My son and I sometimes make ourselves a huge salad with fresh fish (usually left-over from the night before) or chicken for breakfast. This gives us lots of phytonutrients, a sense of lightness and a wonderful supply of protein to carry us through the morning. Don't be afraid to experi-ment. It's only the Western diet based on convenience foods that has had us eating refined carbohydrates alone for breakfast. In traditional soci-eties, breakfast is much more like meals eaten later on in the day. It is often a large meal, while tea, dinner or supper are light and eaten early.

I find that this way of eating works extremely well. You have energy when you need it and don't end up going to bed at night with a heavy stomach hoping that you will be able both to digest your food and sleep at the same time. What appears below are some of my favourite recipes for main meals. I sometimes make extra in the evening to take with me for lunch the next day when I am out. The best recipes are the ones that you make up yourself. Here are some of mine to give you some ideas.

SAUTÉED SEA BASS WITH GARLIC
Serves 2

Great for any fish – sole, halibut, cod, salmon, tuna, whatever, this recipe is quick and easy to prepare.

WHAT YOU NEED
450 grammes of sea bass fillets or other boneless white fish
1 tbsp of coconut oil
4 gloves of garlic, chopped
½ a red onion, diced fine
2 tbsp of fresh coriander or broad leaved parsley, chopped fine
the juice of one large lemon

HERE'S HOW
Melt the coconut oil on a tepenyaki grill or heavy frying pan. Add the fish and sauté for 5 minutes, turning over only once. Remove the fish from the pan and pour in all the other ingredients, allowing them to heat through. This takes about a minute and a half, then pour these other ingredients over the fish and serve immediately.

OLD-FASHIONED MEATBALLS
Serves 3

Meatballs is a traditional favourite of my friend Belinda Hodson, for people of all ages. This recipe is simple to prepare, tasty, and the meatballs will go well with a number of different sauces. These meatballs are also great for picnics and barbecues.

WHAT YOU NEED
750 grammes lean mince (beef or lamb)
½ teaspoon of garlic powder
pepper and salt
4 cloves garlic, finely chopped
1 egg
1 large onion, diced
1 tbsp of fresh parsley, finely chopped
1 tbsp of fresh thyme, finely chopped
1 tbsp of fresh marjoram, finely chopped
1 tbsp of fresh sage, finely chopped
1 dsp of coconut oil

HERE'S HOW
Heat the oil in a frying pan. Mix the remaining ingredients together in a large mixing bowl and form into balls. Spoon the balls of meat into the frying pan and cook gently for 20–25 minutes.

Drain meatballs on paper towels then serve with your favourite sauce.

NUT CRUSTED TUNA
Serves 1

This is a wonderful way of cooking fish steaks, whether they be salmon, swordfish, tuna or any other kind of large fish. You can use almonds, pecans, walnuts or macadamia, whatever you prefer.

WHAT YOU NEED
150 grammes of boneless fish steaks
2 tbsp of melted coconut oil
2 tbsp of melted butter
Maldon sea salt to taste
freshly ground black pepper to taste
120 grams of chopped nuts (the best way to do this is in a coffee grinder)
2 tsp of fresh chopped parsley

HERE'S HOW
Pre-heat your oven to 220°C. Grease a baking sheet. Mix the chopped nuts together with the seasoning and put them onto a plate. Melt the coconut oil and butter in a pan. Remove from the heat. Dip the fish in the oil/butter mixture and then into the nut mixture, pressing down to

make sure the nuts hold. Place the nutted fish steaks on the baking sheet and pop them into the oven for 6–10 minutes until cooked through.

TEPPANYAKI TOFU
Serves 4

A great vegan form of protein, tofu is something that all of us should have in our diet on an ongoing basis. The problem with tofu or soya bean curd is that it has no flavour of its own. So you need to marinade it well before cooking it. I like to cook a lot of tofu in strips or chunks some of which I can eat immediately, some I store to be used the next day at another meal, or eaten cold as a snack. You can add these tofu strips to a phytonutrient rich salad.

WHAT YOU NEED
450 grammes of firm tofu

Marinade
60ml of tamari or soya sauce (without sugar)
1 tbsp of extra virgin olive oil or coconut fat
4 cloves of garlic, crushed
1 small finger of fresh ginger, shredded fine
1 tbsp of lemon juice
½ tsp of wasabi or 1 tsp of Meaux mustard
1 tsp of Manuka honey

HERE'S HOW
Slice the tofu into long strips. Separate them and lay them in a shallow baking pan. Mix together the marinade ingredients and pour over the other ingredients. Allow to marinate for an hour or two (best overnight). Remove the tofu strips and fry on a teppanyaki grill or in a heavy frying pan using coconut fat or extra virgin olive oil, turning gently until lightly browned on all sides.

CURRIED CHICKEN
Serves 4

Curried Chicken is a dream to make. It comes creamy thick, full of spices, with a rich fragrance and flavour. You can make it on the stove or the lazy way in the oven: I take a chicken cut in pieces, and put it into a large cast iron pot with a lid. I then toss in all of the ingredients, pop them into the oven with the lid on, and cook for about an hour at 200°C. Turn the chicken so that the sauce covers it and cook for another 15 minutes. This way you end up with curried chicken pieces rather than a true curry but it is so quick to prepare – in all it takes about 5 minutes – and once it's done you have got a dish to use any time you want for snacks or main courses. Here is my recipe for a more conventionally made chicken curry.

WHAT YOU NEED
1 large chicken, skinned and de-boned and cut into bite size pieces
2 tbsp of coconut oil
6 cloves of garlic, chopped
1 good sized finger of fresh ginger, sliced fine
2 tsp of mild to medium curry powder
1 large can of coconut milk
3 tbsp chives
a handful of fresh parsley, chopped
1 tablespoon Manuka honey
a pinch or two of cayenne pepper
a pinch of turmeric
2 tbsp of chopped green onions
Maldon sea salt to taste
freshly ground black pepper to taste

HERE'S HOW
Melt your coconut oil in a heavy pot. Add the chives, garlic and ginger and lightly brown. Toss in the curry powder and spices. Put in the chicken pieces and coat them with the sauce, allowing them to cook lightly for 2–3 minutes. Now cover and turn the heat down until the chicken pieces cook through, stirring every 5 minutes to make sure that nothing burns. Finally, pour on the coconut milk, add a little water if you need more juice, bring to a sizzle and cook gently for another 4 minutes, season with chilli, parsley and honey and serve.

SALMON DELIGHT
Serves 2

Another recipe from my friend Belinda. Salmon is such a delightful fish with a unique and delicate flavour. I really love this dish because it is easy to prepare and very tasty. The marinade enhances the natural flavours of the fish and the spring onion really gives it its own special zest.

WHAT YOU NEED
2 fillets of salmon
the juice of 4 medium sized lemons
2 large spring onions
pepper and salt
1 dessertspoon of coconut oil
the zest of 1 lemon, 2 lemon wedges and parsley (for garnish)

HERE'S HOW
Finely chop the spring onions and place in a mixing bowl. Add the lemon juice, pepper and salt and blend. Place the salmon fillets into the marinade (pink side face down) and leave for 45 minutes. Turn the fillets onto other side and leave for a further 15 minutes.

Heat coconut oil in a fry pan. Drain the fillets and place in pan. Sauté the fillets until tender then serve with a garnish.

PART SIX:

SKIMMING THE SURFACE

the icing on the cake

Jesse Kenton-Smith BSc (Hons), MBBS, FRCS, FRACS (Plast)

ERASING AGE SIGNS

beauty through a surgeon's eye

Let me state my values up front: as a surgeon I have always been fascinated by what can be done to help a child with a cleft palate or someone with a deformity caused by disease or accident. I like to help them look better, feel better about themselves and lead a happier life. As far as beauty is concerned, I believe there is nothing wrong with growing old gracefully. I look at ageing from both an aesthetic and a technical point of view. If there is something you want to improve, or you want to look fresher and possibly younger, there are a number of viable options.

GO FOR HARMONY

Whatever method you choose for external facial rejuvenation, it should aim to create natural looking results. It should also render your face more harmonious. Much of what you see in magazines looks overdone. Puffed-up lips or cheeks, or too much Botox around the eyes and forehead will make you look artificial – like a badly ageing Hollywood blonde in a TV soap. It will not make you look better, younger, healthier. Go for a fresher, natural looking harmony.

Aesthetic techniques range from the use of injectable fillers, and skin resurfacing to cosmetic surgery. First let's look at the way in which skin ages. Then we can consider what professional treatments can help to counter the superficial traces of time.

'I don't regret anything. Everything happens for a reason – it's part of the healing process. Life is a healing process.'

Richard Gere

Two-Faced Ageing

Skin ages in two ways: from the inside, called *intrinsic ageing* and from the outside, known as *extrinsic ageing* or photo-ageing. Intrinsic ageing occurs as we get older leading to thinning of the epidermis and dermis, loss of elasticity, decreased metabolic activity and diminished vitality. Fibroblasts – the cells responsible for producing collagen – become fewer in number and less active than when the skin was young. Less collagen is produced. This creates a thinner, more lined skin.

Extrinsic ageing takes place as a result of damage inflicted by environmental aggression, especially over-exposure to the sun's UV rays. When combined with the effects of intrinsic ageing, it can make your skin rough and dry with poor elasticity. It can also induce destructive vascular changes as well as damage to the DNA. The skin becomes more prone to pre-cancerous growths so that wrinkles, blotches, blemishes and scaly skin may become an unwelcome reality.

GET SAVVY

Rejuvenation technologies can be bewildering – a minefield for the uninitiated. It is fruitless to pursue treatments that can never give the results you want, or to undergo procedures where results fall short of your expectations or where the risk of a bad outcome is higher than you are willing to accept. What I want to give you here is an understanding of what medical treatments – from skin peels to facelifts – can and cannot accomplish. Then you can decide for yourself what each technique may have to offer.

Wrinkles Come In Three Forms

Let's start by looking at wrinkles first. Lines are like canyons in the skin. They come in three varieties: static, dynamic and skin folds. Static wrinkles are with you all the time – even when your face is at rest. Dynamic wrinkles appear only when your face is moving – for instance when you frown or smile. Many wrinkles are a combination of static and dynamic. Lines which occur as a result of sagging when the outer skin and the soft tissues beneath have lost elasticity, are known as skin folds. Drooping eyebrows, baggy upper and lower eyelids, jowls and deepening nasolabial folds – the smile crease between the side of your nose and the corner of your mouth – are the most common skin fold wrinkles. Let's look at how all three kinds form.

'A woman can keep one secret, the secret of her age.'

Voltaire

New Shoes – Old Shoes

Imagine you have just bought a beautiful pair of new shoes made of the finest, softest, most supple leather imaginable. Something so fine it would make your last pair of Manolo Blahnik's look like flip-flops. This is very much the way skin looks and feels when you are born. Take your new shoes and put them on. When you walk and flex your feet, creases appear in the leather. When your foot is flat on the floor, these creases disappear. Because they only appear when you move, they are dynamic wrinkles. It is the same on your face. When you scowl, raise your eyebrows, squint or smile, lines – dynamic wrinkles – appear. The muscles in your face are attached by one end to the bones beneath, and to the other to the skin itself. Pull on the muscle, it creases the skin, and creates dynamic wrinkles.

We all have dynamic wrinkles. Even my one-year-old daughter has them when she smiles. When you smile or frown, the muscle contracts, again and again, eventually creating a dynamic wrinkle. Dynamic wrinkles can be temporarily ironed out using Botox or resurfacing techniques (see page 257). Over time, a dynamic wrinkle becomes deeper, so eventually it remains present even when the muscle is not working. In short, it turns into a static wrinkle.

'When I passed forty I dropped pretence, 'cause men like women who got some sense.'

Maya Angelou

Shoe Trees And Weathering The Storm

We can take the shoe analogy even further. Continue walking in your new, beautifully supple shoes and creases get deeper. After a while, you notice that they are still partly visible even when you take the shoes off. They have turned into static wrinkles. They can be helped by using a filler such as collagen, Restylane or Hylaform to fill in the indentation that creates the wrinkle (see page 273). This kind of treatment is a bit like storing your shoes with wooden shoe trees inside, to fill out the creases.

As your shoes get older, they become even more weathered. They lose their once smooth, supple appearance and begin to take on a crinkled look. This state of affairs can be improved by various creams designed to nourish, restore and rejuvenate the leather – at least to a certain extent. In a similar way, moisturisers, alpha hydroxy acids or tretinoin can help smooth out fine lines on the face and support the skin's elasticity. Or, if the leather of your shoes were thick enough, you could peel off the top few layers to expose newer, better looking layers underneath. This would get rid of the deeper cracks, clear the blotches and refine scuffed areas. In much the same way, chemical peels, dermabrasion and laser resurfacing can enhance texture and remove irregular pigmentation on the surface of your skin.

'Beauty is a mystery. You can neither eat it nor make flannel out of it.'
D.H. Lawrence

Clearing The Statics

Static wrinkles vary greatly in their severity. So do treatments for them. Isolated wrinkles of any depth respond well to filling agents. Injected either into or under the skin, they plump up a trough or furrow, smoothing out the line. The most common filling agent is collagen, although newer products like Restylane and autologous fat injection – using tissue taken from your own body – often give longer lasting results. Fine wrinkles are improved with the use of tretinoin and alpha hydroxy acids. But you can only achieve a more profound reduction in generalised wrinkles by resurfacing. The deeper the treatment, the better its potential results. But here is the down side: the deeper you go, the higher the risk of scarring and complications. After all, if you were to take too many layers of leather off a fine shoe, you could end up with a hole.

Finally, if your much worn shoes become loose and baggy, you might take them to an old-fashioned cobbler to have them reshaped and tightened up. In the case of living skin, this is when surgery comes into play.

'Friendship with oneself is all important, because without it one cannot be friends with anyone else in the world.'
Eleanor Roosevelt

The Ageing Face

Before we investigate professional anti-ageing options in depth, let's examine some of the most common age-related problems and begin to point the way to some possible solutions. We'll start at the top of the face and work down describing the changes. Then we can take a look at possible solutions. In the next chapter we'll explore treatments in more detail. This will give you a better idea of what kind of help you may want to seek. It may help you become more savvy about what will and what will not work. No matter how much expensive 'lifting serum' you spread on your face, you are never going to completely get rid of your jowls. Only surgery will do that.

HIGHBROWS

Brows which rise gracefully above the bony socket of the eye and are higher at the sides than the middle, are considered beautiful. Women are taught to pluck eyebrows from underneath since this 'raises' the brow and opens up the eye area. With time skin loses elasticity. Eyebrows slump, leading to a hooding of the upper eyelid which can make a face look tired. The forehead compensates for this by pulling the brow up, but this only causes a furrowed brow. In mild to moderate cases of brow descent and forehead furrowing, Botox can help. More severe descent can be dramatically improved through brow repositioning – a brow lift. Hooding and upper eyelid bags may need an upper lid lift or *blepharoplasty*.

FROWNS AND SCOWLS AREN'T GREAT

Lines get etched in the brow when frown muscles are 'overactive'. This causes vertical and horizontal wrinkles in the *glabella* region – between the brows. This can make you look grumpy, angry or worried. It is the effectiveness of Botox in this region which has made it all the rage. Really deep lines may also need filling (see chapter 270). Brow lifting surgery can remove or weaken these muscles permanently.

THE EYES HAVE IT

With age, the skin around our eyes loosens and sags. Bags under the eyes and 'crow's feet' appear. Or the upper eyelids become hooded and bulge as underlying fat deposits around the eye get weighed down by gravity.

AT THE FOOT OF THE CROW

Crow's feet form over time as a result of the muscle which encircles the eye having to contract when you blink or squint. Smoking not only makes skin sallow and grey, it also makes crow's feet much worse. Botox can partly alleviate the dynamic aspect of these wrinkles, while the fine wrinkles or 'crow's feet' can improve with creams containing tretinoin or hydroxy acids. So can resurfacing, using chemical peels or laser light. Deeper static wrinkles may need filling.

OUT WITH THE BAGS

Lower eyelid bags can form over time where skin and soft tissue grow lax, causing the fat around the eye to pouch. Excess lower eyelid skin can be tightened with resurfacing procedures, but they may need surgery – *blepharoplasty* – on the lower lids.

'I never feel age . . . if you have creative work, you don't have age or time.'
Louise Nevelson

Gaunt Skin Folds

When your skin loses elasticity, it also loses fat. This causes cheeks to shrink and can create a gaunt appearance. The descent of the cheek can deepen the *nasolabial fold* between the outside of your nostrils and the corner of your mouth creating a major skin fold wrinkle. Facial tighteners you see advertised so convincingly on TV which promise to return your face to more youthful contours through passive exercise can't solve this for you, although the expense of buying them can make you a lot poorer.

Nasolabial folds and gaunt cheeks can be softened using fillers like collagen and Restylane or more permanently with fat grafting. Certain types of facelift can raise the cheeks and minimise nasolabial folds. Resurfacing with chemical peels, dermabrasion and laser treatments can offer little in improving these skin folds.

'Beauty of whatever kind, in its supreme development, invariably excites the sensitive soul to tears.'
Edgar Allen Poe

Lips Are Full

Ageing has a profound effect on mouths and lips. Thinning – a loss of volume in the lips – is one of the first signs of age. A youthful lip is a full lip. Plumping up the lip can reverse thinning and fill out the lines around the mouth. Personally I dislike enormously the current fashion for 'Hollywood lips' – a mouth which looks like it has been attacked by a swarm of killer bees. Don't over-do it or you risk looking ridiculous!

A loss of fullness can develop at the junction between the red portion of the lip and the lip skin. This is known as the 'white roll' – a tiny ridge at the entrance of the mouth. When firmness fades in this area, lipstick gets harder to apply. It can bleed into the fine lines which radiate from the mouth.

Both thin lips and fine lines respond well to fillers, fat grafting and dermal grafts. A good moisturiser can improve fine lines around the mouth. Wrinkles which do not respond to filling can be treated with resurfacing techniques like dermabrasion, laser or chemical peels.

'I am odd-looking. I sometimes think I look like a funny Muppet.'
Angelina Jolie

From Jowl To Jaw
Jowls are skin fold wrinkles formed as soft tissues of the lower cheek get drawn down by gravity to produce a poorly defined jaw line and skin pouches. Early jowls can be improved with liposuction followed by fat grafting to help define the jaw line. The treatment of choice for jowls is a facelift.

Neckscapes
The neck is a hard area to treat. Neck skin is very different than the skin on your face. Over time, it can become crepey and loose. Bands called 'turkey gobbler' bands (platysma) form vertically at the front of the neck as the body ages. They become more noticeable in your fifties and beyond. These represent the front edge of the platysma muscle. When it contracts, the bands become more prominent. Some clinicians are willing to use Botox to make moderate improvements here. But when it comes to reju-venating a neck by external means, a neck lift combined with a facelift works best. It gets rid of the platysmal banding, redefines a youthful neck contour and removes loose skin. Necks do not respond well to resurfacing as they have a much lower ability to heal themselves without scarring. Laser treatments, dermabrasion and deep peels on the face don't work the same way for rejuvenating necks. A line of demarcation is often left

between the treated face and the neck, despite efforts to blend it in. Good skin care products can help somewhat with neck ageing.

Lend Age A Hand

It is not just how your face looks that matters. The hands are a total give away when it comes to how old you appear. When the dermis thins, the skin on the back of the hand can become so fine it is almost transparent. Often there is also a loss of fat from beneath the surface. This makes the tendons which extend fingers prominent. Hand skin can become loose, blotchy and show signs of sun damage, like scales or lesions.

A good hand cream hydrates the skin, reducing its dry, scaly appearance, and helps to improve the look of the ageing hand. Blotchiness often yields to bleaching agents such as hydroquinone or to light to medium chemical peels. But peeling must be done gently since the skin on your hands does not possess the same ability to regenerate as does the skin on the face. Peeling can also improve scalyness associated with sun damage, once the possibility of skin cancer has been eliminated.

A new and exciting advance in hand rejuvenation is the practice of fat grafting. A surgeon harvests fat, usually from the front of the belly under local or general anaesthetic, and then transplants it in very small parcels into the back of the hand. This puffs out wrinkly skin and makes veins and tendons on the back of the hand less visible. Your surgeon can then minimise prominent veins using sclerotherapy – where he or she injects the veins with a substance to shrink them. This is much the same kind of treatment which is used to clear minor varicose veins.

'When I dream, I am ageless.'

Elizabeth Coatsworth

CHECK OUT YOUR FACE

Now that we've looked at how a face ages, it is time to look closely at your own face. Try not to be hypercritical of what you see in your mirror. Beauty is very much in the eye of the beholder and we are always our own worst critics. Look at your face dispassionately and with compassion. This way you are likely to see things with greater clarity.

Seeing The Future

Take a close look at the skin on your face, neck and hands then ask yourself these questions. What do you like about them? What would you like to change? Does one or another area have a youthful appearance? Deep or fine lines? How about the colour of the skin? Uniform or patchy? Look to your forehead, brow position, frown lines, eyelids, cheeks, mouth, jaw line, neck and hands. Discuss your feelings with your partner or a close friend. Tell them what you like and don't like then ask their opinion. It may be the one thing you dislike about yourself, they love. My wife, Donna, loves the darkness beneath my eyes – something I inherited from my mother. Donna thinks it looks mysterious whilst I would love to get rid of this. The very fact that she finds charming what I dislike, makes me feel better about myself.

When carrying out this exercise it is important that you do it with compassion – a commodity easier to show towards others than oneself. Anyone can make particularly critical judgments about their looks. To do so is just as an unrealistic way of appraising things as looking at yourself through a pair of rose coloured glasses.

Find The Best

One of the most important factors in achieving good results from any medical treatment including surgery is taking care when choosing your practitioner. Many so-called 'cosmetic surgeons' are not surgeons at all. That some hold their heads up and claim that they can safely perform delicate cosmetic surgery quite frankly scares me. A good plastic surgeon will have spent many thousands of hours in the operating theatre refining his skill and techniques. A doctor without this kind of training who sets himself up as a cosmetic surgeon may have as little as 10 hours' operating experience. If you are lucky, he may have done a few weekend courses. Choose your practitioner carefully.

Some dermatologists have taken up cosmetic surgery. A dermatologist is an expert at diagnosing and treating skin conditions and may well be good at resurfacing as well. He is someone to consult about skin treatments, skin problems or disease conditions. Surgical experience, however, is limited amongst dermatologists.

Calm Cool And Collected

You want to be realistic about what can be changed. Unrealistic expectations of what can be achieved by a treatment can bring unnecessary disappointment. Don't let pie-in-the-sky ideas raise your expectations beyond what can reasonably be accomplished. You can certainly fill in your wrinkles, but this will not fill in cracks in your relationships. You also need to consider how much time you will need for recovery in the case of each treatment. Ask questions about medical risks and the degree of physical discomfort and be clear about how much a particular procedure is going to cost before you begin. Your friends and family may not be supportive or understand why you wish to seek improvements. But only you can decide what is right for you.

'Autumn is a second spring when every leaf's a flower.'

Albert Camus

CHECKLIST FOR CHOOSING A PRACTITIONER:

❑ Check on your practitioner's training and qualifications. Beware 'cosmetic surgeons' who may have little training or experience. In some countries any doctor can call himself a 'cosmetic surgeon'.
❑ Discuss the range of possible outcomes with your practitioner. Look at before and after photos of his work, and be wary, for you may see only the best results.
❑ Shop around to find a surgeon or physician you feel comfortable with and trust.
❑ Follow your instincts – if you have a bad feeling or find communication between you difficult, move on. This is not the right professional for you.
❑ Discuss fees, payment of fees, medical risks and expected recovery time before you undertake any treatment.
❑ Check out personal recommendations. They too can be useful in finding the right practitioner.
❑ Ask your trusted GP for a recommendation.

To get the best possible advice and outcome, make sure you see a trained professional. Now let's look at the treatments available and what they can do to rejuvenate your skin and add more vitality to your life.

FILLERS AND FREEZERS

grow-your-own cell therapy

No matter how young or healthy you feel, and no matter how radiant your skin looks, wrinkles, blemishes, imperfections or abnormalities can undermine your wellbeing and sense of self. When this happens it may be time to seek help from a professional – a surgeon, dermatologist or highly trained practitioner in aesthetic medicine.

'You know you're getting old when all the names in your black book have M.D. after them.'

Harrison Ford

The tools, techniques and procedures of aesthetic medicine have never been more sophisticated and they are getting better by the year. The knowledge, experience and skill of the professional are the most important factors in the success of the outcome of any cosmetic procedure. Investigate carefully the qualifications of the practitioner and listen to the recommendations of others. But trust your own gut feeling about him or her too. Always ask questions about why they recommend a particular procedure for a specific problem. Find out the down side too. Will you be able to carry on with your life in a normal way afterwards or do you need a time of retreat for healing, as you would after a deep peel? Make sure you understand the procedure before you undertake treatment. Here are some of what are considered to be the most valuable non-surgical procedures for countering age-related damage, how they work and what you should know about them.

'Alas, after a certain age every man is responsible for his face.'

Albert Camus

WHAT TO ASK

These are some of the questions useful to ask your plastic surgeon or dermatologist when considering aesthetic treatment:

❏ What kind of treatment do you think will work best for this problem and why?

❏ How long will the results last?

❏ Will the treatment need to be repeated and if so how often?

❏ How long will it take before I experience the full measure of improvements?

❏ Does the fee you are charging include the cost of any touch-ups if needed a week later?

Clearing Lines

One of the simplest and most effective non-surgical procedures for smoothing out expression lines is Botox. Its results are subtle. It is relatively affordable compared to other treatments and appears to be safe. 'Botox parties' have taken over from Tupperware. For a while, even Boots the Chemist was offering Botox injections at some of their stores. So much has been written about the miracle of Botox that some people feel left out if they haven't had it yet. Let's take a look at what it is and what it can achieve. Then judge for yourself.

A substance produced by a *Clostridium botulinum* bacteria, Botox is one of the most deadly substances known to man. It is the same toxin that produces botulism, an often fatal form of food poisoning. In the light of this, you might think that all those movie stars, models and society women who have embraced Botox early on must be completely mad. (They may well be, but not for trying Botox.) By now, literally millions of tiny doses of this drug have been injected with minimal side effects. This gives Botox one of the best safety profiles of any drug. Injected, Botox does not travel throughout your body, nor does it remain there indefinitely.

'Botulinum toxin has been used since 1980 and its whole history has shown it to be profoundly safe. The doses that are used for cosmetic purposes are a miniscule fraction of what's required for any systemic effect. In small amounts, the poisonous component is essentially not present.'

Andrew Markey MD

Controlled Paralysis

Botox injections paralyse the facial muscles, softening and eliminating dynamic wrinkles. But it is only suitable in certain areas of the face. When injected into the small muscles of the face they stop working for about 3 months. It is the movement of these small muscles of facial expression that cause the dynamic and eventually static wrinkles to form. The injections are relatively painless and cause no change in sensation or numbness. Here are some of the improvements Botox can make.

❑ **Frown Lines**

Here Botox shines: it is most useful for the region between the eyebrows – the glabella – where frown lines appear. Lines here are caused by 3 small muscles called *procerus, depressor super-cilli* and *corrugator supercilli*. Like most of the muscles of facial expression, one end of these muscles is attached to bone with the other to skin. When the muscles contract, your skin is pulled towards the bone causing the creases that make people look stressed, tired, worried or angry. Injected here, Botox gets rid of frown wrinkles, but not the wrinkle that is visible when at rest (static wrinkle). To treat a static wrinkle, you need a filler as well.

'People say that you can tell when someone's had treatment, but it's not true. If you've had it done by someone good, you can't tell.'
Dr Neil Walker FRCD

❑ **Forehead Lines**

Botox injections improve the horizontal lines on the forehead as well. The forehead muscles – *frontalis* – are important in stopping the eyebrows and upper eyelids from drooping. As you age, the brow tends to slump over the top of the eye sockets, leading to hooding of the upper eyelids. The frontalis muscle counteracts such 'brow slump' by contracting, etching the horizontal lines in the process. Short of hanging upside down permanently and learning to walk on your hands to stop forehead wrinkles, Botox is your best bet for eliminating them. For mild and moderate forehead lines, Botox is commonly injected in a 'V' shape running from above the glabella, to weaken the muscle. More severe forehead lines, especially when associated with a very slumped brow and hooded upper eyelids, may need a surgical brow lift.

❑ **Crow's Feet**

Contractions of the *orbicularis oculi* muscle, which encircles the eye allowing it to close (and squint and scrunch up), produce crow's feet. The aim of using Botox here is to weaken but not fully paralyse this muscle, thereby reducing creases at the outer edges of the eyes. An injection of Botox just below the outer portion of the eyebrow and just outside the eye socket can lift the outer brow, giving the face a younger appearance by weakening the downward pull of this muscle.

'If you don't like something, change it. If you can't change it, change your attitude. Don't complain.'

Maya Angelou

Botox – What's Entailed

Using a very fine needle, injections of tiny quantities of Botox are directed into specific facial muscles, to weaken or temporarily paralyse them. Beforehand, the practitioner will have applied ice or anaesthetic cream to lessen any discomfort, especially if multiple site injections are planned. To treat glabella frown lines he or she is likely to use five injections. For the forehead, crow's feet and platysma bands of the neck, about 3 injections are used on each side.

The effect of Botox takes up to a week to kick in, in some people two weeks or even longer. You may experience minor bruising from the treatment. If you do, be patient for a few days to allow it to settle. Sometimes 'touch ups' are required a few weeks later. Following treatment you can go about your daily business almost immediately although it is best to avoid doing anything too strenuous on the day of the procedure. It you don't like the muscle paralysing effect in any area of your face, the good news is it wears off in a few months. If you do like the effect, the bad news is the same. There is some evidence that a memory response may develop with repeated treatments, so you get a gradual lengthening of the time between treatments to maintain the results.

BOTOX FACTS

- ❑ Given by injection to paralyse facial muscles.
- ❑ Effective for 3 to 6 months.
- ❑ Suitable only for certain areas of the face and neck.
- ❑ Safe and relatively affordable.
- ❑ Relatively painless.
- ❑ Low risk of complications.

Proceed With Caution

Botox is a drug with a good safety profile. Most people experience no side effects at all. It is, however, a paralytic agent. If it ends up in the wrong place, this can temporarily paralyse muscles not intended to be affected. Injections into the glabella and forehead may track the Botox into the eye muscles causing a very droopy upper eyelid and giving you a half-asleep look. This usually lasts 3 weeks. The use of special eye drops during this time may help counteract the droopy upper lid. Over-treatment – too much Botox unwisely injected – can lead to a mask-like, expressionless face. When Botox is injected into the platysmal bands of the neck – a procedure not often followed – this may cause temporary weakening of the voice or create problems swallowing. This is why many people are not happy to offer Botox in the neck.

'There is no excellent beauty that hath not some strangeness in the proportion.'

Sir Francis Bacon

COMMON SENSE CAUTIONS

The effect of repeated doses of Botox remains unknown. As yet, no long-term hazards have been identified. Nevertheless, it is not recommended that you use Botox during pregnancy or when nursing a baby, as possible effects on the foetus or child remain uninvestigated.

Fill The Gap

There is a host of substances on the market which people are willing to inject into their skin to fill out static wrinkles and concave scars. Many of them I would not touch for safety reasons or because the long-term effects remain unknown. Let's look at what is available. Fillers come in two forms:

- ❑ Those made from your own tissue, known as *autologous*.
- ❑ *Exogenous* substances like bovine collagen or Dermalogen taken from the skin of a cadaver.

Before you have any kind of filler injected, you need to be clear whether you want the effects to be temporary or permanent. The advantage of using a temporary filler is that if you do not like what you see, the effect gradually disappears. With permanent fillers, it will not. Fillers can be used either to fill in static wrinkles or to augment – that is to build up – certain areas, most commonly around the mouth and cheeks. Wrinkles on the frown lines of the glabella, the forehead, crow's feet around the eyes, the nasolabial fold and around the mouth – all respond well in the hands of a skilled practitioner. For filling out the soft tissues on the back of the hands, fat transfer works better.

'I see my body as an instrument, rather than an ornament.'
Alanis Morissette

TEMPORARY FILLERS

There is a big distinction between foreign substances – *exogenous* – and one's own tissue – *autologous*. Foreign substances implanted permanently near the skin surface have a history of working their way out, causing scarring or foreign body reactions called granulomas. In trying to rid the body of foreign material, the body's immune defences set up an inflammatory response, causing pain and swelling. Let's look at temporary fillers first.

THE FOUR FACES OF COLLAGEN

Collagen for line filling comes in four forms:
- **Bovine:** extracted from cow skin, then purified, sterilised and turned into liquid form, this is the most common form of collagen. It requires allergy tests – injecting a small amount on the arm – before using it on the face. Allergy occurs in less than 5 per cent of the population.
- **Dermalogen:** taken from the skin of a human cadaver, this collagen is sterilised, purified and rendered liquid for use.
- **Autologen:** taken from your own skin, this form of collagen is harvested from previous surgery then processed into liquid form for injection.
- **Isologen:** this is composed not of collagen itself but of the live cells from your own fibroblast cells which manufacture collagen. They are removed from your own skin, cultured or cloned in a lab and turned into a liquid for injection. (More about Autologen and Isologen later.)

Help From The Cow

The gold standard injectable is bovine – cow – collagen. It can be injected into the dermis of the skin. Some practitioners feel that nothing else handles quite like it. Unfortunately, in many people collagen only lasts about 3 months before it needs repeating, although in some it can last from 6 to 9 months.

'I'm not interested in age. People who tell their age are silly. You're only as old as you feel.'

Elizabeth Arden

Allergy Tests Essential

Skin testing is essential before using bovine collagen to ensure you have no allergic reaction. Often, a second test is advised a week or two later. Even after 2 skin tests, about 3 per cent of people still have an allergic reaction – usually swelling and redness at the injection site. Reactivation of oral herpes simplex (cold sores) can occur, so if you are at risk, it is advisable to take oral prophylaxis such as acyclovir to prevent this. A rare complication is skin loss leading to scarring, usually in the glabella region. Collagen injections can be carried out in a doctor's office. They usually take around half an hour. You can return to your normal activities right away but you may get mild swelling, irritation or redness for a day or two.

BOVINE COLLAGEN

❑ Injected under wrinkles to fill them out or plump up lips.
❑ Effective for about 3 months.
❑ Skin testing essential.
❑ Complications include reactivation of oral herpes simplex virus or, on rare occasions, skin loss leading to scarring.

Dermalogen

This is a temporary foreign injectable containing human collagen derived from the skin of human cadavers (dead bodies). The material obtained is screened for AIDS viruses and other viruses, and undergoes processing to inactivate viruses. So far, no viral transmission has been recorded. Allergic reactions are rare, but skin testing is advised. It may be used in patients allergic to bovine collagen.

DERMALOGEN

❑ Temporary injectable made from human cadaver collagen.
❑ Allergic reactions are rare but skin testing advised.
❑ Can be used by patients allergic to bovine collagen.

'I used to be Snow White, but I drifted.'

Mae West

The Hyaluronics

These temporary injectable fillers last from 6 months to a year – in most people they last longer than collagen, but this differs from person to person, and in some people collagen can last longer. They have been used on over 500,000 people so far in Europe, Canada and Australasia. They are not licensed for use in the US. It is my belief that these injectables have significant advantages over collagen.

Both Restylane and Hylaform are composed of chains of hyaluronic acid, a substance found in the living material of skin itself, where it plays an important role in keeping skin moisturised. Skin testing is not required since allergic reactions are very rare. The molecule in these injectables are identical in all species. They are also found in all tissue types – quite clever really. When long chain hyaluronic acid breaks down, it attracts water so bulking up the molecule, making the filler effect last longer.

HYALURONIC FILLERS

- ❑ Injectable fillers.
- ❑ Last from 6 to 9 months.
- ❑ Skin testing not required.
- ❑ Three products exist in the Restylane range for superficial, medium or deep wrinkles, augmentation or filling.

'Women are not forgiven for aging. Robert Redford's lines of distinction are my old-age wrinkles.'

Jane Fonda

The Restylane and Hylaform hyaluronic fillers each come in three forms with different particle sizes for different purposes: fine molecules are used for superficial wrinkles and fine lines around the eyes and mouth, medium-sized molecules for moderate wrinkles, and an even larger particle size for plumping lips. A practitioner may use a combination of these products. Since fashions for natural beauty change over time, unlike permanent fillers, hyaluronic acid-based fillers leave you the option of changing with them. You can opt for a touch-up or re-evaluate the need for further treatment.

CAUTION – PERMANENT FOREIGN FILLERS

Historically, permanent implants of foreign fillers have had fundamental drawbacks when used just under or within the skin. These substances may work their way to the surface over time causing infection, scarring or allergic reactions. If an allergic reaction occurs to a temporary foreign implant e.g. collagen, the problem will, by nature, be limited since the offending substance slowly disappears. With a permanent foreign implant, the material will not disappear. This may lead to a chronic cycle of inflammation, infection and scarring.

'People try to drag you down and shatter your dreams a lot of times. Maybe because their own dreams haven't been fulfilled.'

Mariah Carey

Liquid Silicone

A few decades ago injecting liquid silicone was all the rage. We now know silicone can set off a foreign-body reaction where the body tries to wall off or 'eat' the foreign material using its macrophages – white blood cells designed to ward off attack by invading bugs. The body cannot remove the silicone. A nasty inflammatory process is set up, causing swelling, pain, skin erosions and scarring. The only way to deal with the problem is surgically to remove the implant. If it has been injected into your lips or part of your face, the treatment can be worse than the problem. Silicone is not licensed by the FDA in the United States for soft tissue injection.

Now, liquid silicone injections are undergoing a resurgence with the claim that, if an experienced practitioner performs the procedure, the risk is low. Since it can take 10 years or more for the silicone to become a problem, I fail to understand how such claims can be made. With the other permanent methods now available such as *silastic hydroxyapatite* and the widely used Goretex and Artecol, my advice would be: don't do it.

Goretex

A cross between rubber and cloth, this filler – often used for replacing arteries in bypass surgery – can be placed under the skin of the lips to produce a pouting look and to rejuvenate ageing thin lips to their former glory. Its technical name is *expanded poly-tetra-fluoro-ethyline*. Small cuts are made in the corners of the lips and the Goretex threads are passed through. For a few years Goretex was very popular, but long-term – as tends to happen with permanent material placed close to the skin – many of the implants became infected requiring removal. This is not an easy job. I personally suggest that you limit the Goretex you own to that in your breathable raincoat.

'It gives me a deep comforting sense that things seen are temporal and things unseen are eternal.'

Helen Keller

Artecol
Used for filling lines, lip augmentation and filling nasolabial folds, Artecol consists of tiny spheres of *polymethylmethacrylate plastic* in a base of bovine collagen. Skin testing is required as allergic reactions can result from the bovine collagen. Being made up of tidy spheres, this substance is difficult to remove if there are problems. Two or three sessions are the norm to achieve a good result. At this stage, foreign body type granulomas similar to those seen with liquid silicone occur in one person in a thousand. This material looks promising. Although, being conservative by nature, I would wait another 5 years before using it, to check its long-term effects.

Aquamid
This is another permanent injectable. It consists of a gel made up of 2.5 per cent cross-linked polyacrylamide and 97.5 per cent water. It is suitable for lips and nasolabial folds but not fine lines. This looks promising, but remember that it is permanent. Whilst it has been used in Eastern Europe for 10 years, think very carefully before going ahead with this. There have been some reported problems with its use.

THE PERMANENTS:

Goretex
- Surgically injected into the lips to rejuvenate or produce a pouting look.
- Implants can migrate and may become infected in the long term and require removal which can be difficult.

Artecol
- ❏ Used for filling lines, lip augmentation and filling nasolabial folds.
- ❏ Skin testing required as allergic reactions may occur from the base of bovine collagen.
- ❏ Two or three sessions required to obtain good result.
- ❏ Looks promising, but suggest waiting until long-term effects are known.

Aquamid
- ❏ Suitable for lips and nasolabial folds.
- ❏ Low risk of side effects.
- ❏ Looks promising, but long-term effects not yet known.

LIVE TISSUE FILLERS

They are known as autologous: this means tissue taken from your own body used as injectable fillers. The beauty of autologous implants and injectables is that you don't react to them since your immune system recognises them as part of you. The disadvantage is that the tissue used needs to be obtained from a different part of your body. It is not available 'off the shelf'. The other drawback is the amount of enhancement is not as predictable as with other temporary fillers. You may need more than one treatment to obtain the desired effect.

AUTOLOGOUS FILLERS

Advantages
- ❏ Implants are derived from your own body tissue.
- ❏ No reaction as your immune system recognises the tissue as part of you.

Disadvantages
- ❏ Tissue needs to be harvested from your own body rather than being available 'off the shelf'.
- ❏ Amount of enhancement is not predictable and may require more than one treatment to get the desired result.

'The only parts left of my original body are my elbows.'

Phyllis Diller

Grow Your Own Collagen

Autologen is one autologous alternative. It is simply processed skin taken from your own body – often during a facelift or tummy tuck. Instead of being discarded, the skin is sent to a laboratory which extracts the collagen from it and prepares it to be injected. The processing takes about a month. Three square inches of skin yield about 1ml of collagen – enough to fill several wrinkles in the face three or four times. Autologen filling appears to last slightly longer than bovine collagen and can be stored for up to five years for later use.

Fat Can Be Useful

Autologous fat is as useful as collagen in the right circumstances. Fat transplantation for facial rejuvenation – fat grafting – has gained in popularity over the last 5 years. Fat is harvested from the abdomen or thigh by gentle liposuction under sedation or general anaesthetic. The fat cells are gently washed, prepared and injected into the face to fill lines, augment lips and cheeks and smooth nasolabial folds. Some results obtained have been dramatic. Because fat does best when injected under the skin, and wrinkles occur in the skin itself, many surgeons believe that fat injections used to treat fine wrinkles work less well. I find it an exciting new technique which can produce great results.

'Love yourself first and everything else falls into line. You really have to love yourself to get anything done in this world.'

Lucille Ball

The disadvantage of fat grafting is it is impossible to predict exactly how much of the injected fat will be incorporated successfully. You may require 2 or more treatments to obtain the desired result. Complications include over-filling and occasional lumps caused by fat necrosis – the death of fat cells. Even under the best conditions, fat may shrink by 30 to 50 per cent. Bruising can last a week and there may be some swelling for a month.

FAT GRAFTING

❑ Gaining in popularity.
❑ Fat is harvested from abdomen by liposuction.
❑ Fat cells are washed, prepared and injected as filler to wrinkles, lips, cheeks and nasolabial folds.
❑ Often dramatic results.
❑ The doctor cannot predict accurately how much fat will be incorporated successfully.
❑ Over-filling and lumps caused by necrosis – when fat cells die – are possible complications.

Dermal And Dermal-Fat Grafts

This technique has been used by plastic surgeons for many years to bulk up the upper lip of children with cleft lips, where the lip is thin and underdeveloped. The same technique can be used to augment lips for cosmetic purposes. Under local or general anaesthetic, skin either with or without underlying fat, is taken from the groin, an area with a previous scar or another area undergoing surgery such as skin from a breast reduction or tummy tuck. The top layer of skin, the epidermis, is removed leaving the underlying dermis and fat. Small incisions are made in the corners of the mouth, a tunnel is created in the lip and the graft slipped in. Some shrinkage usually occurs and thus over-correction is commonly aimed for in the first instance. What remains is permanent.

DERMAL AND DERMAL-FAT GRAFTS

- ❑ Used to augment lips.
- ❑ Skin removed from another part of the body such as the groin, then placed in the lips.
- ❑ Result is permanent.
- ❑ As with other autologous options, it is difficult to predict the extent of the ultimate correction.

Isolagen – Live Cell Therapy

Isolagen is a cutting edge approach to facial rejuvenation now being talked about everywhere. It is relatively new technology, not yet available in all countries. The technique involves harvesting your skin's own fibroblasts – the collagen-producing cells in the skin rather than collagen itself – and culturing them in a laboratory from a small tissue sample. In a few weeks these cloned collagen-makers are ready to be injected back into your skin. They can be used to fill soft wrinkles, augment lips and treat acne scarring. The process is repeated every few weeks until the desired result is obtained. Wrinkles improve by approximately 15 per cent when first injected, 35 per cent on the second and 70 per cent at the third treatment. The idea is that living cells implanted will produce their own fresh collagen. It is claimed that effects improve over time and can last for years. Exactly how long a course of treatment will last is not yet known, but it appears that effects on wrinkles tail-off after a few years. Isolagen is not suitable for most people over sixty as their fibroblasts are no longer active enough to do the job. The treatment appears to be safe but is expensive.

ISOLAGEN – LIVE CELL THERAPY

- ❑ Relatively new treatment.
- ❑ Fills soft wrinkles, lips or treats acne scarring.
- ❑ Uses your own fibroblasts instead of collagen.
- ❑ Injected cells start to produce their own collagen.
- ❑ Effects last for several years.
- ❑ Not suitable for over sixties age group.
- ❑ Safe but expensive.

'Isologen has proven to be safe and effective in the multicenter studies that have been underway since 1995. It is a very versatile product that can be used alone or in conjunction with laser resurfacing, chemical peels, bovine collagen, and other nonviable fillers. It appears that Isologen represents the first step in autologous cellular treatment of scars and rhytids [wrinkles] by treating the underlying cause of these conditions, which is the lack of collagen and fibroblasts in the affected areas of the dermis.'

William K. Boss Jr. MD

The benefits of all treatments need to be balanced against the risks involved. Talk to your plastic surgeon and decide on the best approach for you.

POLISHING THE APPLE

the good, the bad and the ugly

Skin resurfacing techniques can be used to clear blotches and blemishes, improve complexion and elasticity, as well as reduce wrinkles. They also stimulate collagen production. The deeper the treatment, the greater the amount of skin tightening, wrinkle improvement and lessening of skin blemishes and scaling. There is even evidence that dermabrasion, deeper chemical peels and laser resurfacing reduce the chances of skin cancers developing in unstable, sundamaged skin.

Blotches And Blemishes

As skin ages, pigmentation can become irregular. These are the easiest blemishes to clear. Skin blotches and blemishes can be caused by either changes in pigment – generally a browning – or blood vessels (red, blue or purple).

'I feel there is something unexplored about a woman that only a woman can explore.'

Georgia O'Keefe

The most common brown blemishes are known as age spots. Not without reason since they tend to increase with age. These are smooth, flat brown patches that respond to bleaching agents like *hydroquinone*. In some countries you can buy lightening creams based on this chemical over the counter. In others, it is by prescription only. Areas that do not respond to this form of skin lightening can often be treated with resurfacing procedures.

Dark, raised and warty looking growths, called seborrhoeic keratoses, are caused by UV damage. After diagnosis, these can be shaved off and cauterised. Vascular blotches – blood vessel related imperfections – are identified by their colour and the fact that pressure on them causes them to disappear. They can be treated with intense pulsed light, electrocautery (but there is a risk of a small scar) or a pulsed dye laser.

See your GP, plastic surgeon or dermatologist to check for any sign of malignancy before considering any kind of treatment for irregular pigmentation.

'It's time we stopped worrying about losing our looks and started celebrating the gifts of age: I feel yummier than ever.'

Sela Ward

CLEARING THE SCALES

Many things, including eczema and psoriasis, cause scaly skin. But as skin ages, particularly when it has been over-exposed to the sun or other environmental hazards, scaliness is usually the result of actinic ketatosis. After years of sun exposure, skin may react by forming patchy scales or horns in sun-exposed areas like the face or backs of the hands. These should be checked by your health professional before having them treated to rule out malignancies. Any patches or areas which continuously scab but never seem to heal are of particular concern. Good moisturisers may help, although freezing with liquid nitrogen, anti-cancer creams containing 5 fluorouracil and resurfacing with chemical peel or laser are all the best methods for severe cases.

Resurface It

Resurfacing can be achieved using a laser, dermabrasion or chemical peels, all of which cause controlled, non-specific wounding of the skin. The more wounding, the more profound the rejuvenating effect but also the higher the risk of scarring, persistent redness and permanent pigmentation changes. Deep peels and CO_2 lasers can produce a ghostly white skin due to loss of all pigment along with a 'tide mark' of demarcation between the treated face and the neck. So beware.

'Youth is happy because it has the ability to see beauty. Anyone who keeps the ability to see beauty never grows old.'

Franz Kafka

DERMABRASION

Some plastic surgeons consider dermabrasion the treatment of choice for upper lip wrinkles and acne scars. It improves both fine wrinkles and dynamic wrinkles – especially when combined with Botox injections – and can be used for the treatment of skin blotches and blemishes, including precancerous skin lesions. Often the procedure needs to be repeated, especially in the case of acne scars, to get the best result. The top layers of the skin are removed either with sandpaper or a special rotating abrasive drum. Large areas require sedation or general anaesthetic.

Healing Takes Time

The face takes 7 to 10 days to heal. Swelling can last 2 weeks. The effect on dynamic wrinkles lasts 1 to 5 years. There is a small risk of pigment changes in the skin. Hyperpigmentation – a complication which turns skin darker – can be treated with bleaching agents like hydroquinone. Hypopigmentation – whiteness in the treated area – is uncommon. If it occurs, it can only be camouflaged with makeup.

'Only time can heal your broken heart, just as only time can heal his broken arms and legs.'

Miss Piggy

CHEMICAL PEELS

These range from superficial 'lunch hour' peels through to medium or deep phenol peels. The deeper the injury, the more profound its effect on wrinkles. The deeper the peel, the higher the risk of scarring and permanent hypopigmentation. However, the more superficial the peel, the more often it needs to be repeated. You only need to have a phenol peel once.

Medium Peels

These offer improvement in skin colour, texture and tone. They can improve fine wrinkles but not dynamic wrinkles. Peels can also improve skin blotchiness and are useful for people with light brown skin. Dark brown skin carries the risk of pigmentation changes. Peels must be carried out by a plastic surgeon or dermatologist making use of pain relief or mild sedation. He paints on a chemical solution, doing one section of the face at a time. You will feel an intense burning during the procedure, which stops as soon as the solution is neutralised. After the peel, the skin appears red. Soon, its superficial layers of skin crack and peel off. This flaking is complete in 4 to 7 days. In contrast to dermabrasion, deep peels and laser resurfacing, neither superficial nor medium peels result in an open wound. Results last from 6 months to 2 years and longevity and improvement can be extended with a good skin care programme. Recovery time is quick and there is a low risk of scarring and of long-term pigmentation problems. However, treatment needs to be repeated periodically to maintain the effect.

'I used to go around looking as frumpy as possible because it was inconceivable you could be attractive as well as smart. It wasn't until I started being myself, the way I like to turn out to meet people, that I started to get any work.'

Catherine Zeta-Jones

GO DEEP

Deep peels are performed with phenol. They are the yardstick against which all other resurfacing techniques are measured. The results of a phenol peel are superior to all other methods of resurfacing be it laser, dermabrasion or medium peels. They can bring dramatic improvement to sun-damaged skin or even eliminate wrinkles in one treatment. Results can last decades. They do not come without risk. Phenol is only suitable for fair skins. Even then with a phenol peel there is always the risk of profound loss of pigment leading to a ghostly pallor, which can be difficult to disguise, even with makeup. The neck cannot be treated with phenol and despite efforts to 'feather' the transition zone between treated and untreated skin, a 'tide mark' is often visible. Your skin will never tan after a phenol peel.

Phenol peels are performed with heavy sedation or general anaesthesia. The heart must be monitored as abnormal heart rhythms (arrhythmias) can be caused by systemic absorption. Afterwards, your face will be swollen, oozing and crusted. Your eyes may even swell shut for a few days. In 7 to 10 days the crusts fall off leaving smooth, healed skin. You will not be presentable in public for 10 to14 days. Redness can persist for up to 3 months. The risk of permanent scarring is higher than with medium peeling, dermabrasion or laser treatment. The skin tightening effect can produce a pulling down of the lower eyelid (ectropion) which requires surgery to correct.

'Beauty is momentary in the mind the fitful tracing of a portal; but in the flesh it is immortal.'

Wallace Stevens

LOWDOWN ON LASERS

Lasers have caught the public's imagination as high-tech, space-age devices, which some think superior to all other treatments. I am not one of them. While laser is by no means the best treatment in all cases, it can have a role in facial rejuvenation. Proponents of lasers for resurfacing argue that they allow more precise removal of the top layers of skin and are more controllable than chemical peels. Advocates of chemical peels argue that they can produce similar results with peeling. Remember, the deeper the injury, the better the improvement in wrinkles and skin tone, but the higher the risk.

Carbon Dioxide Laser

The carbon dioxide (CO_2) laser is essentially a powerful beam of light that vaporises the top layers of skin on contact. It heats the tissue in an attempt to reorganise collagen, improving fine wrinkles and enhancing skin tone. Skin looks smoother, fresher and tighter. It can improve dynamic and to some extent, skin fold wrinkles. But redness can persist for months. And five to ten per cent of patients experience blotchiness. Up to forty per cent of patients may become ghostly white in the areas treated with CO_2 laser. This takes up to five years to develop. Many plastic surgeons no longer use CO_2 laser because of hypopigmentation problems like these. CO_2 laser resurfacing is not something I would have on my own face as I believe the risk of hypopigmentation is too high. There is no chance of looking 'naturally' refreshed if this happens. This treatment is only suitable for fair or olive skin. Scarring can occur, but is less common than with phenol peels. The procedure is performed in an office or hospital under general anaesthetic or sedation. Essentially, what the treatment produces is a controlled graze which weeps as it heals. Healing takes place in seven to ten days and you will have some discomfort during this time. You will be presentable in public in about two weeks. The benefits of CO_2 laser treatment diminish over the years but the procedure can always be repeated.

Erbium Laser

The Erbium laser was developed as a safer alternative to CO_2 resurfacing. It offers the advantage of less downtime and a lower complication risk, although it is not as effective. Darker-skinned people can have Erbium treatment as it has less chance of causing hypopigmentation. You will need local anaesthetic or sedation. It is also less painful than CO_2 both during the procedure and afterwards. The skin will ooze as it heals in 4 to 7 days with redness lasting up to 2 weeks. Erbium laser is more effective than a medium chemical peel with similar recovery time.

'You have to leave the city of your comfort and go into the wilderness of your intuition. What you'll discover will be yourself.'

Alan Alda

SKIN RESURFACING AT A GLANCE

❑ Offers improvement in complexion, skin elasticity and reduction of wrinkles by controlled, non-specific wounding of the skin.
❑ Stimulates collagen production.
❑ May reduce incidence of skin cancer in treated sun-damaged skin.

❑ The deeper the treatment, the more profound the effect but it carries a higher risk of scarring, persistent redness and permanent pigmentation changes.

❑ May leave a 'tide-mark' between face and untreated neck.

Dermabrasion

❑ Improves wrinkles, blotches and acne scars.

❑ Top layers of skin removed.

❑ Need to allow time for healing and reduction of swelling.

❑ Effect lasts 1 to 5 years.

❑ Small risk of pigment changes.

Chemical Peels

❑ Superficial, medium or deep phenol peels.

❑ The deeper the injury, the more profound the effect.

❑ The deeper the peel, the higher the risk of scarring and permanent hypopigmentation.

❑ Allow healing and recovery time.

Carbon Dioxide Laser

❑ Powerful beam of light vaporises top layers of skin.

❑ Laser allows more precise removal of top layers of skin.

❑ Only suitable for fair or olive skin.

❑ Redness, blotchiness or scarring may occur.

❑ Effect reduced over time but can be repeated.

❑ Most plastic surgeons are less keen on CO_2 than they used to be.

Erbium Laser

❑ Less downtime, lower complication risk, and less painful than CO_2.

❑ Not as effective as CO_2.

❑ More effective than a medium chemical peel with similar recovery time.

'If you're able to be yourself, then you have no competition. All you have to do is get closer and closer to that essence.'

Barbara Cook

The benefits of all treatments need to be balanced against the risks involved. Talk to your plastic surgeon and decide on the best approach for you.

SKILLS OF A SURGEON

get the inside story

As skin ages it can become lax. Gravity makes soft tissues slump. When non-invasive techniques do not offer the help you need, surgery may hold an answer. A viable alternative in the hands of a skilled plastic surgeon, it can bring dramatic improvements. It is the profound external method of making skin look younger. Cosmetic surgery is not for everybody. Whether or not it feels right for you, only you can decide.

Cosmetic surgery is on the rise. Between 1996 and 2000, the number of cosmetic procedures carried out in English-speaking countries more than doubled. The increase continues. Some of the major problems in a field where so much growth is taking place are finding a truly competent surgeon, working out what kind of procedure can accomplish the changes that you are looking for, and becoming aware of the risks involved.

'It is sometimes asserted that a surgical operation is or should be a work of art . . . fit to rank with those of the painter or sculptor.'
Wilfred Batten Lewis Trotter 1932

No surgical procedure is without risks. The more you know about all of these things beforehand, the better the results you are likely to get from any procedure. Let's take things step by step.

Is Surgery For You?
Take a look in the mirror and figure out what your goals are before you discuss them with anyone or go looking for a surgeon. It is important to be clear about what you want to change or improve. Never consider cosmetic surgery to please someone else. Don't be dissuaded from it either if you are sure this is what you want. It is equally important to be clear about why you want help from a plastic surgeon. There is no doubt that your physical appearance affects self-esteem and how well you interact with your outside world. But if you look to surgery to heal an ailing marriage, you are likely to be disappointed. In such cases, counselling can be a better way to go.

'If you really want something you can figure out how to make it happen.'

Cher

Be Realistic

The most common cause of disappointment after any surgical proce-dure is unrealistic expectations beforehand about what is possible. This is a far more frequent problem than suboptimal results. It is easy for anyone to understand in their head what surgery can and cannot do for you, but it can sometimes be easier to be driven by emotions and ignore what you know. Become well informed through careful discus-sion with whatever surgeon you choose. Be as clear as you possibly can be about what you want to change, and listen carefully to what your surgeon tells you about what is possible and what is not.

It is important to find a surgeon with whom you feel comfortable, whom you can trust, and to whom you are able to speak openly and honestly about everything – from how much the procedures will cost to what to expect afterwards. The more you know and the clearer you both are with each other, the more smoothly everything runs from start to finish. Any plastic surgeon worth his salt will be clear and honest with you about risks involved.

'We bring back, refashion, and restore to wholeness the features which nature gave but chance destroyed, not that they may charm the eye but that they may be an advantage to the living soul . . . the end for which the physician is working is that the features should fulfil their offices according to nature's decree.'

Gaspare Tagliacozzi, 1597

PRIOR TO SURGERY

❏ Discuss the medical risks with your surgeon. Complications following cosmetic surgery may be less acceptable than those with medically necessary procedures.

❏ When your surgeon is fully qualified and experienced you have the best opportunity of achieving a good outcome.

Qualification Matters

Finding the right surgeon is not always an easy task. You cannot do this by ringing your local hospital or answering one of the advertisements you find in the back of a magazine. Beware of seductive advertising. Often the best surgeons don't advertise at all. Ask your family doctor to refer you to the best plastic surgeon. Personal recommendation from friends or acquaintances who have themselves had surgery and are pleased with the results can also help. You can search for board-certified plastic surgeons in the telephone directory or contact the medical association in the country in which you live. Unfortunately, in many countries, ordinary physicians are permitted to perform cosmetic surgical procedures although they are neither qualified in plastics nor experienced enough to work with optimal skills. You may want to visit more than one surgeon before deciding which you want to go with.

CHECK OUT YOUR SURGEON

A skilled surgeon will make sure you get a good understanding of everything that's involved. He or she should:

❏ Be able to communicate in simple, easy-to-understand language.
❏ Explain clearly what procedures are appropriate for the results you have in mind.
❏ Describe each procedure involved, its limitations, its risks and alternatives.
❏ Make you feel at ease so you are free to discuss all of your needs and concerns fully.
❏ Describe in full both how to prepare for your surgery and what to expect afterwards during the recovery period.
❏ Be clear about what the costs involved will be.
❏ Insist that you come for a second consultation before proceeding with surgery.

'To me, fair friend, you never can be old. For as you were when first your eye I eyed. Such seems your beauty still.'

Marlon Brando

The Consultation

There are a number of things you will want to do when meeting with a surgeon. Whatever your concerns, speak about them. Find out if the procedure will be carried out under a general or local anaesthetic. Let your surgeon know if you have any worries. You can ask how many similar procedures he has carried out in the past couple of years and if he will show you photographs of some of his results on patients who have had the same procedure. Find out what hospital or hospitals he uses or if the procedure can be done in his office. Ask if you will be charged for follow-up appointments or if these are part of the fee you pay for surgery.

EIGHT STEPS TO GOOD RESULTS

1. Make sure plastic surgery is what you want.
2. Locate the right qualified surgeon.
3. Check out the rapport between you.
4. Be clear and honest about everything.
5. Ask the right questions and get full, clear answers.
6. Get clear about risks involved.
7. Plan your timetable around surgery and recovery so it will fit in with your life and work.
8. Get your body in top condition in the weeks before surgery through diet and regular exercise.

'Any change, even a change for the better, is always accompanied by drawbacks and discomforts.'

Arnold Bennett

Drugs And Cigarettes

How well surgery goes depends a lot on how fit and vital your skin and body as a whole are beforehand. So get yourself in the best possible shape in the run-up to any procedure. That way you will be doing the best for your body as well as helping your surgeon to do his best for you. Smoking undermines the body's ability to recover from surgery. Smokers are more prone to infection, wound healing problems and complications from anaesthesia. Some surgeons refuse to carry out cosmetic procedures on smokers. Prescription drugs can also interfere with surgery so make sure you inform your surgeon about anything you are taking and take his advice. Aspirin and ibuprofen make you more prone to the risk of bleeding during an operation and to haematomas afterwards. Many over-the-counter remedies for colds or allergies contain these or similar compounds. Discuss all this with your surgeon and follow his advice to the letter.

The Perfect Facelift

Now let's look at some of the surgical procedures available. The facelift is the plastic surgeon's classic rejuvenation tool. It minimises jowls, defines the jaw line and improves the neck. By removing skin and tightening soft tissues beneath, facelifts decrease skin fold wrinkles. When done well, they can create dramatic rejuvenating effects. A neck lift, usually combined with a facelift, is the only way to significantly improve a neck with lax skin and 'turkey gobbler' (*platysma*) bands. It can give a clearly defined angle between chin and neck and make a huge difference to your appearance.

'Wrinkles should merely indicate where smiles have been.'

Mark Twain

When you think of facelifts, you may get images of a few Hollywood stars whose skin looks so tight that they have to smile to relieve the tension. That is not a good facelift. What happens in Hollywood should stay in Hollywood. A good plastic surgeon aims for a natural look of harmonious balance. He avoids the 'operated' look as far as possible. You don't want to end up with skin that looks like an overstretched piece of leather.

A facelift is most often performed under general anaesthesia, although some surgeons prefer local anaesthetic and sedation. The surgeon makes an incision in the hair at the temple, just in front of the ear, around the earlobe and into the hair behind the ear. Through this incision he lifts up the skin and the layer of fibrous tissue underneath – called SMAS – is tightened. He may also tighten the back edge of the platysma muscle. The skin is then laid gently back down without tension, the extra skin removed and stitches inserted.

A FACELIFT CAN IMPROVE

❑ Sagging cheeks and a deep nasolabial fold between the nose
   and mouth.
❑ Sagging neck.
❑ Firmness.
❑ Facial contour definitions.
❑ Jowls.

IT WILL NOT IMPROVE

❑ Quality of skin.
❑ Forehead.
❑ Eyelids.
❑ Crow's Feet.

A neck lift may also involve an incision under the chin. The surgeon can then free up the skin of the neck and join it to the freed-up skin of the facelift. He tightens or divides the front end of the platysma muscle to remove the turkey gobbler platysma bands.

There is a small risk of developing a blood clot under the facelift requiring another trip to the operating theatre. Weakness of the facial muscles sometimes occurs although this is usually temporary. Most often incisions heal with a fine, almost invisible scar, although it is possible for more prominent scarring to occur.

A Look To The Brow

As a face ages, the eyebrows tend to slump over the top of the eye socket, adding to the bagginess of the upper lid which can become hooded. In order to keep upper eyelids from hanging into the field of vision, forehead muscles work overtime holding the brow up. This produces a furrowed brow full of wrinkles. Heavy upper eyelids can even make people feel tired.

'There's more to life than cheekbones.'

Kate Winslet

Endoscopic Skills

The traditional approach for enhancing a forehead was an open brow lift involving a huge incision across the scalp. Now, thanks to advances in technology and surgical skills, minimally invasive techniques often replace previously large operations. A keyhole endoscopic brow lift is a perfect example. This method has revolutionised the procedure. As a result, demand for the technique has burgeoned. Along with this has come the realisation that much of the bagginess and excess skin in the upper eyelid is actually due to a slumping of the forehead. Addressing this root cause enables a surgeon to create more natural and harmonious results. With an endoscopic forehead lift, much less skin needs to be removed and often an upper *blepharoplasty* is not required. The other benefit of forehead-lifting – as well as raising the brow and improving the upper lids – is weakening or removal of the frown muscles.

To decide whether a brow lift or upper blepharoplasty or both is best to rejuvenate the upper lid, you need to look at the position of the brow and forehead. If the brow is already in a pleasing position but there are baggy upper eyelids, an upper lid or blepharoplasty alone may be enough. But if, taking hold of the brow area and pulling the skin gently up seems to rejuvenate the whole of the upper lid and gets rid of sags and bags, then a brow lift is enough. You don't need a blepharoplasty. If on elevating the brow to a higher position there are baggy upper eyelids, both a blepharoplasty and brow lift can bring the best results.

WHAT A FOREHEAD LIFT CAN ACCOMPLISH

- ❏ A softening of horizontal forehead wrinkles.
- ❏ A reduction in lateral hoods.
- ❏ An elevation of the brows for a younger look.
- ❏ An improvement in scowl lines between the brows.

IT WILL NOT IMPROVE

- ❏ Crow's feet.
- ❏ Puffy eyes.
- ❏ Baggy eyelids.

Under general anaesthetic, five small cuts are made in the hairline. Through these cuts, special instruments and an endoscope – a minute telescope – are introduced to free the forehead tissues from the skull beneath. The endoscope allows frown muscles to be seen on a TV screen. Parts of these muscles are removed to weaken them and improve the frown lines. The freed up forehead is then held in a desired higher position, permanently. Often a surgeon will do a facelift at the same time as he does a forehead lift.

The most common complication of this operation comes from over-doing it. This produces a 'surprised look' because the brow has been placed too high. Fortunately, this happens rarely. In the early days of this operation, overly enthusiastic removal of the frown muscles lead to a hollowing of the glabella region between the brows. This can be avoided by removing less muscle. Other complications include temporary inability to close your eyes if this procedure is carried out at the same time as an upper lid *blepharoplasty*, or small patches of hair loss at the incision sites and changes to the feeling of the forehead and front of the scalp. Studies following up patients over a 5 year period confirm that good results are long lasting.

'The conditions necessary for the surgeon are four: first, he should be learned; second he should be expert; third, he must be ingenious; and fourth, he should be able to adapt himself . . . Let the surgeon be bold in all things, and fearful in dangerous things.'

Guy de Chauliac, 1363

Soul Windows

Eyes are the focal points of any face – windows of the souls. We communicate and register emotions through our eyes. An eyelid lift – blepharoplasty – can have a dramatic effect on facial aesthetics. As we age, the upper eyelids become hooded with excessive skin as well as droopy because of a slumping of fat in the upper lid. The lower eyelids form bags of excess skin and protruding fat. Eyelid lifts to upper and lower lids can have a dramatic freshening effect, removing excess skin and fat to rejuvenate the eyes from a tired, haggard look.

EYELID SURGERY WILL IMPROVE

❑ Baggy eyelids.
❑ Puffy eyelids.
❑ Lax lower lids.

THINGS IT WILL NOT CHANGE

❑ Dark circles.
❑ Crow's feet.
❑ Droopy eyebrows.
❑ Scowl lines.
❑ Hooded lids.

'I have everything I had twenty years ago – except now it's all lower.'
Gypsy Rose Lee

Liposculpture
A plastic surgeon can combine liposuction with fat injections to change the contours of a face, reduce skin fold wrinkles and improve the nasolabial folds, while redefining the jaw line and removing jowls. But liposuction is a relatively new technique for the face and long-term results are not fully known. It is highly operator-dependent. Carried out without sufficient skill, it can lead to unsightly irregularities in facial contours. Many plastic surgeons are not happy offering liposuction to the face. Fat injections (see page 270) can fill and replace facial fat, smoothing lines, plumping lips and filling gaunt cheeks.

From Here To Eternity
Once surgery is finished and your surgeon lets you go home, you begin the recovery process. How much discomfort you experience after surgery varies enormously from one person to another. Virtually every surgical procedure creates some swelling and bruising. As this fades you begin to see the results emerge. It is important to keep your head elevated for two or three days after any kind of face surgery. This minimises swelling and speeds recovery. Your surgeon may suggest an ice pack or cold flannel applied to the area soon after surgery as another means

of minimising swelling. He will remove the bandages at your first visit to his office following surgery and take out the stiches between 3 and 5 days after surgery. Be sure to check with your surgeon about when it is OK for you to shower and bathe. You will be able to return to work sometime between five days and three weeks later depending on the procedure he has used and the kind of work you do.

'There is no me. I do not exist. There used to be a me but I had it surgically removed.'

Peter Sellers

THINGS TO REMEMBER ABOUT RECOVERY

❏ With some procedures, it is usual to spend a night in the hospital – check with your surgeon.
❏ Because almost all cosmetic surgery involves some swelling or bruising, be patient – the results you are waiting for will come when this swelling subsides and bruising fades.
❏ Look after yourself with a nutritious diet.
❏ Take plenty of rest, as you feel the need, and don't feel guilty about taking time out for yourself after elective surgery.
❏ Enjoy the results. You deserve them. You have made your own decisions, and done your best to have everything run smoothly.

'Who we are looking for is who is looking.'

Saint Francis of Assisi

In the hands of a skilled plastic surgeon, cosmetic procedures can achieve remarkable aesthetic results. But it is important to remember that the deepest beauty comes from valuing who you are, looking after your life and giving yourself permission to live from your own authentic values. Only you can make this happen.

PART
SEVEN:

HOLOGRAPHIC
BEAUTY FOR
LIFE

the meeting of the matrices

THE CONSCIOUSNESS MATRIX

charisma and creativity for life

Beautiful skin vibrates with energy. How yours looks and feels, functions and ages – or doesn't – depends on how well the living matrix of your body is nurtured. Hormones and biophotons, lotions and potions, what you eat and don't eat, and how well you protect yourself from toxic overload are the name of the game. But there is another matrix too, out of which beauty continues to be born. I call it the *consciousness matrix*. Explore it. It can reward you with ageless charisma that is priceless.

What I call the consciousness matrix is that collection of thoughts and feelings, values, beliefs and memories which we carry with us always. It is the birthplace within – the point of origin and growth out of which we live and out of which beauty of the highest order emerges.

I believe that at the core, each of us is here on the planet to live out who we are as fully as possible. The more we do that the more beautiful we become. Just as when our skin or body is polluted the highest expression of skin health and beauty are undermined, so it is with the consciousness matrix. When we are filled with fear, with a belief that who we are is not good enough, when we have been taught not to trust ourselves, our consciousness matrix becomes polluted and impinges on our ability to express our unique authentic beauty to the full. In short, we are unable to realise our full potential for charisma.

The Beauty That You Are
Within the individual genetic package which is you is nestled your very own brand of uniqueness that encompasses far greater physical, creative and spiritual potential than any of us could hope to realise in only one lifetime. Our upbringing, our environment – physical, emotional, spiritual, social – can create distortions in all of us. These distortions can produce artificial behaviour – phoney personalities or false images or values into which we try to squeeze ourselves. Most of us carry around a burden of false ideas, notions and habit patterns

which have nothing to do with who we are. They have been imposed upon us by our families, our religion, the cultural norms of our society. They pollute our consciousness matrix and need to be cleared away like rubbish. Real beauty isn't going to come from the outside. It's already within, just waiting to be discovered.

Make Way For Charisma

The word charisma means 'talent, grace, a favour especially vouchsafed by God'. Charisma depends not so much on specifics as on the over-all impression you create – an expression of your personal and idiosyncratic feeling for who you are, what you love most – even what looks best on you. It is something of far greater value than a docile conformity to conventional notions about fashion and beauty. Charisma is bold, assertive and witty. And, contrary to popular opinion, it is *not* the exclusive province of the *special elect* – women with perfect size 10 bodies and not a wrinkle on their faces. Far from it.

Charisma is ageless. It exists in every culture. It is the real icing on the *Skin Revolution* cake – an *external* expression of your unique authenticity. It gives you panache, boldness and humour. It transforms physical limitations like wide hips or giraffe necks into assets. Charisma can make a *statement* out of a nose that by conventional standards is too big. It makes you stand out in a crowd. Developing your own brand of charisma can not only be fun and exert a dazzling effect on your outside world, it can empower you to live more and more of who you are – from your core.

'Between two evils, I always choose the one I never tried before.'

Mae West

CHARISMA TRUE AND FALSE

What gives you charisma? The Chanel suit you wear? The car you drive? The way you have been taught to use your body or speak your words? Not really. For stylish or charming as these things may be they are more often than not chosen without any consideration of whether or not they have a connection with the individuality of the woman who wears them. It is rather like hanging Christmas baubles on a willow tree.

As such they offer little more than the *appearance* of charisma. And like pastiche, appearances never deceive a discerning eye.

Wild, Free And Authentic

Charisma – the real McCoy – has certain characteristics. Expansiveness, for instance, joy, creativity and vitality. The more you trust yourself and allow your own brand of energy to flow from within, the more your own charisma develops naturally. It works the other way round too. The more fun you have exploring different modes of self expression using colour, clothes and makeup, the more you call forth your own brand of this energy of beauty. Then the Chanel suit, the dress from Oxfam, or the wild rastafarian dreadlocks you go for take on a whole new flavour. They are no longer status symbols of acceptability or rebellion but you choose them for the enjoyment and aesthetic pleasure they bring. They become means of expressing whatever you want to express about yourself. As this happens you can break through forever the barrier of exploitation which is so destructive to a woman's sense of personal value and which operates so heavily in our commercial society. Then *you* can be in control of *them* rather than them being in control of you.

Allowing your own charisma to blossom is first a question of acknowledging that you matter. Second, it means making time to care for yourself and to explore who you are and who you want to become. Finally – it means discovering the art of play.

Your unique nature can be expressed in a myriad of ways from the most simple to the most profound: in the colours you like best, the way you wear your hair, the makeup you choose as well as how you think and talk, in the deep values you embody, in the dreams you dream and the things you do – creations of art, intellectual or physical feats, or just being yourself. That is why at its essence, charisma is both disarmingly simple and immeasurably complex – neither more nor less than living day by day from a full and honest outpouring of your individuality – that spirit which is *unique* to you.

'I'm tired of all this nonsense about beauty being only skin-deep. That's deep enough. What do you want, an adorable pancreas?'

Jean Kerr

Narcissism Imprisons

Only when the pursuit of beauty becomes a thing *apart* from the expression of a woman's individual nature does it go all wrong. This is because beauty, treated only as an external, has sad repercussions for your own sense of self-worth. It pollutes the consciousness matrix badly. Like the old mechanistic world-view which has blinded us to what we have been doing to our planet, it imprisons us within false images and feelings of inadequacy that make it hard to live creatively or to bring the joy of your own unique energy to what you do.

THE COURAGE TO BE

Contacting your unique spirit, coming to respect it, and having the courage to live from it – in all of its many manifestations – is what developing charisma is all about. Sometimes challenging, frequently exciting, this process can be a lot of fun too. As it takes place the externals in your life – clothes and makeup, the way you move and relate to your world – cease to be arbitrary, or things picked up uncertainly and carried around or hidden behind. Instead they develop and unfold beautifully and mysteriously – almost organically – from within, as ever more potent expressions of who you are.

Go Against The Rules

Take energy for instance. Being able to live out your energy potential depends on how well you nourish yourself – physically, emotionally and spiritually – day by day. This does not just mean a day-to-day routine which incorporates exercise, good food and restorative sleep. For energy also depends on living from your core – not by other people's rules. It depends on living what you love most, what frees your blood and feeds your spirit. In discovering this and living more and more in this way you not only fulfil your own life more richly than is possible in other ways – after all we can only collect so many PhDs, BMWs and sexy lovers. You also bring the very highest gifts you have to give to your family, your community and the earth as a whole. Live your soul's passion and you call on virtually endless energy – the single most powerful ingredient in charisma.

SOUL SECRETS

Most of us have spent our lives learning not to listen to our inner voice. Our consciousness matrix has been filled with all sorts of rubbish by our parents, our educational system, our bosses, our spouses and the media which teaches us not to trust ourselves but rather to live our lives according to external 'rules'. The kind of internal dialogue which goes through our minds as we are continually bombarded in this way drains our sense of who we are. It also creates a lot of 'static' which obscures that softer voice that comes from deep within about what we really value, what we want or what we are.

'If you don't like something change it; it you can't change it, change the way you think about it.'

Mary Engelbreit

Expanding The Matrix

Leading-edge research has amassed evidence that through our consciousness we are linked via extremely complex energetic interfaces both with other living organisms and with the planet itself. This is the larger matrix – the holographic nature of consciousness which in very real ways changes material reality. Becoming aware of these interfaces – connections which are now being mapped by brain researchers, biologists and high level physicists – can be fascinating. Coming to make use of them is another highly subtle yet tremendously potent and exciting aspect of living with charisma.

Throughout history the basic unity of mind and body has formed an integral aspect of man's belief systems and healing practices – from ancient Egyptian medicine and Ayurvedic medicine (the oldest known system of healing in the world) to Chinese Medicine, homeopathy and spiritual healing. But, during the eighteenth century and especially from the onset of the industrial revolution, this awareness was largely replaced by a dominant paradigm, or world-view, which sees man as a blend of mechanism and egotism. A world-view is a dominant way of looking at reality which remains unconscious in a culture but which tends to govern the judgements one makes whether large or small. Ours holds first that all phenomenon in the universe, even life itself, are nothing more than a complex yet ultimately explainable series of chemical and physical reactions, second that differences between organic and non-organic life are only in degree, and finally that the whole is nothing more than the sum of its parts. This mechanistic paradigm has been useful. It has enabled us to study and organise experience scientifically and it has been responsible for our technological development.

OFF WITH THE BLINKERS

Like the proverbial iceberg, most of us live with the lion's share of our potential for beauty, joy, creativity and power submerged beneath a sea of unknowing. We go about our day-to-day duties and pleasures conscious only of what comes to us through our five senses. How does it taste and feel? What does it sound like? What do we see in front of our eyes? Meanwhile beneath the vast ocean of consciousness that constitutes what it is to be fully human, our greater selves hibernate waiting to be awakened. Too often we live our lives from too narrow a perspective and then wonder why we feel imprisoned.

Shifting Paradigms

But no matter how useful, every dominant paradigm has its limitations. Ours, for instance, has led us to ignore the organic interrelatedness of nature in favour of the notion that it is man's task through science and technology to 'harness nature' for his own ends – the results of which we are having to wrestle with in the increasingly unstable weather conditions, the dangerous thinning of the ozone layer, and unprecedented ecological disruptions so serious that many believe they could herald the end of human life on the planet. Our mechanistic worldview has also contributed to a sense of human alienation which is expressed in our art and our literature and in our destructive social behaviour. Now, however, our dominant paradigms are exploding around us thanks to findings in high level physics, psychoneuroimmunology, and the new biology. Energetic links are being established between the inner and outer world of man and the complex nature of interactions between consciousness and material reality are being mapped. The scientists and the philosophers now know that a mechanistic worldview is nowhere near big enough to explain reality. As a result, new world-views are rapidly evolving which, strange as it may seem, can play a powerful role in the development of charisma. In no small part this is because they enable us to break down the barriers of the self-limiting images each of us hold. (How often do we think thoughts such as, 'Oh I could never do that' or 'I'm too small . . . too stupid . . . too afraid'?) Getting in touch with evolving paradigms is an important part of the skin revolution too. Coming to terms with them may seem a long way from deciding what kind of lipstick you wear or how you look after your hair and skin, yet understanding them can lead to as great an expansion of self-expression in those areas as it can in how you think, dream, behave and choose to direct your ambitions.

BREAKING THE BARRIERS

For to live with charisma is to live in the fullness of your being. Each of us is asked continually to break down barriers, to bring to consciousness the self-imposed limitations we have been living with and to open oneself to new possibilities whether they come in the form of physical beauty – hair, body, skin, nails and all the rest – or new passions and ideals. All these things are part of the revolution too.

'I only answer to two people, myself and God.'

Cher

Transformation Is Real

Transformation is not an empty dream. The ability to transform ourselves has been deeply encoded in our genes, and it's as though every part of us knows how to bring it about. Skin revolution is all about triggering your own powers of transformation to enhance your good looks, regenerate your energy, rejuvenate your body, and help you to come closer to living from the core of your being – with authenticity. Transformation is not simply about change – anyone can change. Transformation is about the kind of change where you go through a doorway, one that you can't go back through – like being born – very like the transformations you see around you in nature: the caterpillar that spins a cocoon and turns into a white jelly in order to turn into a butterfly.

'Habit is habit and not to be flung out of the window by any man, but coaxed downstairs a step at a time.'

Mark Twain

From Caterpillar Into Butterfly

I have written *Skin Revolution* in the hope that it can help trigger your own powers of transformation in order to enhance your good looks, regenerate your energy, rejuvenate your skin and come closer to living your own unique brand of beauty from the core of your being – with authenticity. All of the information you have read within, all the things you have tried – from my 5 Day Facelift Diet, to MSM, Far Infrared Sauna, and cutting edge skincare formulations – are merely the nuts and bolts of transformation. Some are time-tested techniques that work because in one way or another they trigger your own genetic programming for deep change and renewal. Others, like Isologen and pulsed light therapy, are state-of-the-art, up to the minute gems never before available to us. The important thing to remember is: the real magic of transformation comes from you alone.

And magic it is. A programme to detoxify your body using The Living Matrix 21 Day Turnaround will not only remove fine lines from a face beginning to show the wear and tear of life. Because in essence the living matrix of your body and the consciousness matrix are one, believe it or not, three weeks on the programme can help shift your perceptions of reality. You may well find you wake up in the morning feeling more the way a child does, with a sense of excitement about the day ahead instead of having to ply yourself with coffee just to get going.

'To err is human, but it feels divine.'

Mae West

Gifts From The Matrix

The more you nurture your living matrix, the clearer your consciousness matrix will become and the easier you will find it to hear the whispers from your soul and the messages from your body about who you are. As the consciousness matrix is detoxified of false notions, fears and other people's rules, a genuine sense of our own value develops more and more. This carries us towards a way of living in which exercise becomes a natural part of day-to-day life – not something you have to force yourself to do because somebody told you it is good for you. It can also help you recognize some of the beauty intrinsic to your soul – something that happens not in any superficial, narcissistic way but quite naturally and honourably as you learn to care for yourself in simple ways. One good life change attracts others. Altering your diet for instance or learning a technique for deep relaxation brings such benefits in terms of health and beauty that you are likely to find yourself interested in making other changes too – quite naturally over time. You may find yourself taking three steps forward and two back. That's great. For that is the way real transformation happens – not by following some programme slavishly – and it leads you down a path that not only transforms the way you look and feel but also enables you to bring more to life while life brings more to you.

The Power Of Instinct

Each of us has a longing to become what we fully are. Fulfilling it asks that we reconnect with instinct too. Instinct is the voice of the multi-sensory quantum realms. In short, it asks that we come home to ourselves. You can do this without drugs, without gurus, without becoming a disciple or having to belong to any privileged group. You can do it regardless of your age, your physical condition or your religious beliefs. Creativity and charisma become part of your day-to-day experience as soon as you are ready to:

❑ Become a willing explorer of the multi-dimensional universe in which you live.
❑ Learn to recognise, honour and respect the beauty of the individual soul and give it authentic expression in your life.
❑ Allow your world-view to expand until it gets large enough to encompass the *whole* of reality.
❑ Let go of the restrictions imposed on you from childhood, religion and education.
❑ Seek out your individual place within the order of the universe.
❑ Develop a deep and abiding friendship with the inhabitants of the multi-dimensional universe in which we make our homes – from the moles and the stars, the grass and the trees, the rocks and the quasars, to the helping spirits who guide, bless and inform

us, the muses who inspire us, the angels who shine for us and the maggots who eat away decaying matter so that new life may come forth from old.

❏ Learn to build powerful bridges between the rich inner world of consciousness and your day-to-day existence.

❏ Commit yourself to bringing your own unique creations into being.

'I think of life itself now as a wonderful play that I've written for myself, and so my purpose is to have the utmost fun playing my part.'

Shirley MacLaine

Connect With The Greater Hologram

A good thing to do when you are faced with questions you can't answer, or are worried about something you think you can't solve, is to find yourself a tree, lean on it and ask the tree for advice. It may sound strange to you but this is a very old technique used throughout history all over the world. Primitive people believed trees and rocks, the wind and sea, all had wisdom and consciousness. What we know now as a result of leading-edge science, particularly in the area of high level physics, is that there may be a great deal of sense in this. For in addition to the material world that we can reach out and touch with our hands, there is a world of consciousness in which everything is connected. One of the big secrets to transformation is that the more you can begin to experience your connections with the trees, the rocks, the sea, the more you feel safe to allow the transformative process to take place. You can begin to let go of whatever doesn't belong to you, letting the old and unnecessary die in order to bring the new, more authentic you into being.

'A painful time in our life is what I call a "healing crisis". We are letting go of something old and opening to something new.'

Shakti Gawain

GO FOR IT

Transformation is one of the great mysteries of life. It is by no means easy. It always demands that, like a snake, we shed the skin that has become too small to contain us as we grow. That is not an easy thing to do and for a time can leave us vulnerable until the new one grows firm and strong to protect us. But transformation is so exciting and so rewarding that who cares if you have to experience a headache while your body is detoxifying or shed tears over the loss of a relationship. Such events are milestones along the road each one of us walks towards wholeness, authenticity and freedom. They are momentary experiences firmly anchored in space and time, like sights we see looking through the windows of a train on the most exciting journey any of us ever take – the journey of our own unfolding within the magnificent web of life to which we belong. May your own transformative experiences be rich and rewarding. Life needs the unique beauty and energy and charisma you have to bring to the rest of us.

'We can move the entire mountain one piece at a time.'

Chinese Proverb

So forget fears of narcissism and self-indulgence. Each of us is unique and the charisma which celebrates that uniqueness can not only lift us to new levels of joy and energy and accomplishment but also enrich the lives of all who know us. Perhaps most important of all, through the expression of that uniqueness in our feelings, thoughts and actions, it can enable us to play the unique part we have to play in the future of our society and of the planet itself. Sounds revolutionary? It is. Where else would you find such heresy but in the middle of the Perma Youth Revolution. We are entering a new age of intelligence, awareness and interrelatedness. I for one am going to enjoy the exploration even if it means my having to sacrifice a few of my own sacred cows along the way. I hope you will join me. For along with all the horror in our world there is much promise. Has there ever been a more perfect moment for beauty to come into its own?

UNRAVELLING THE MYSTERIES OF THE MATRIX

the tale of obsession ends . . . or does it?

The more I learned about the nature of the living matrix, the more sure I was that for healthy ageless skin we need to support it in the highest possible way – not only *internally* through changes in diet but *externally* too. How? By giving skin direct access to everything it needs to thrive. Do this and the skin itself gets on with the job of beauty making.

I figured that if only we could feed our skin, say twice a day, with a synergistic mixture of matrix substances which it could readily make use of – in the form of a lotion, a cream, a spray, whatever – then we could encourage skin of every age and condition to regenerate itself and help it realise its innate genetic potentials for firmness, smoothness and strength. I believed too that we could drastically slow down degeneration and even reverse many of the signs of ageing at the same time.

Unlocking Skin's Potentials

The genetic materials within your skin's cells, the mitochondria which produce skin's energy, the fibroblasts which make its collagen, and all the skin's other vital constituents, have no way of knowing how old they are. They function for better or worse by simply responding to the quality of the fluid they are bathed in. As biochemist Jeffrey Bland says, 'You can unlock the tremendous potential for good health that is stored within your genes. That potential may not be optimally realised at the present time due to a mismatch between what your genes need and what they are given.' In other words, the way DNA, mitochondria and fibroblasts behave depends on the quality of fluids in which they are suspended. If one can maintain a 'sea' of the right synergistic nutrients, our skin's DNA becomes convinced that nothing has changed and we ensure the finest genetic expression of health and beauty year after year.

I figured we would need to provide the living skin with the wherewithal

to rebalance itself. Then we could encourage it, quite naturally, to eliminate problems as diverse as excessive dryness or oiliness, hyper-reac-
tivity, sallowness, a tendency to broken veins or breakouts, and any
number of other conditions which develop when metabolic balance
becomes disturbed by deficiencies. I knew from long experience in health
that, given what it needs to do the job, the body has an almost infinite
wisdom and the capacity to rebalance itself, restore vitality and thrive.

Toxic Wastes Kill Beauty

What happens when our skin becomes polluted from chemicals in the
environment, high sugar and insulin in the blood, drugs and prolonged
stress, is that the quality of the watery gels and fluids of the living
matrix becomes depleted, low in energy and unable to support health.
It no longer provides the DNA, fibroblasts, cell walls and other vital
components of skin what they need – partly because the pollution itself
uses up the antioxidants and co-factors necessary for enzymes to do
their job and partly because the skin is simply not receiving optimal
quantities of all the biochemicals, substrates and energy it needs to
behave in a youthful way.

In keeping with the principles of functional medicine and integral
biology – for which I have the highest respect – I figured that a product
to help skin realise optimal genetic expression, bring it the highest
possible protection from ageing, and encourage self-repair would need
to do two things: help the living matrix release any toxic burden and
feed it everything it needs.

To create such a product became my goal. It would have to be
absolutely pure and chemical-free. And it would need to supply – in
proper, synergistic, balance and concentration – everything the skin
needs. In addition, the energy aspects of the formula had to be right.

Back To Basics

I am a great admirer of the work of American research scientist James
L. Oschman who wrote the superbly researched paradigm-breaking
book *Energy Medicine . . . The Scientific Basis*. I went back to Oschman's
own description of the living matrix for inspiration. 'Evidence accu-
mulates that the nuclear matrices, cytoskeletons, and extracellular
matrices are mechanically, chemomechanically, electromechanically, and
functionally interconnected throughout the organism . . . Viewed as a
whole, the living matrix is a dynamic solid state communication network
with global systemic regulatory roles. Major components of the network
have semi-conductor properties, a high degree of order (e.g. phospholipid

properties and arrays of cytoskeletal, motor, and connective tissue proteins), tensional integrity (tensegrity), and can produce coherent self-sustaining oscillations with complex harmonics.'

I read his words over and over – at first hardly understanding them. Before long, I was literally getting visions of the living matrix in my dreams.

My Search For Support

While doing the research for *Age Power* and *Skin Revolution* I had hoped to find people who could help me create such a formula. I came across a brilliant chemist on the West Coast of the United States who understood the holographic nature of the body and was as keen as I was. He knew a lot about cell communication. He also felt as passionately as I did that the most powerful and only truly effective way of making skin more beautiful was to provide the body with everything it needs and let the skin's own metabolic processes do the work of regeneration and rejuvenation. But sadly he was untrained in formulating cosmetics, unfamiliar with the living matrix model and had no idea how to create the completely natural preservative system I needed.

Then I sought out Nigel Allan – expert on chirally correct skincare. I learned an enormous amount from him. But Nigel is not a chemist. And although he too saw that my vision of living matrix skin support was far in advance of anything that had been done, there was no way he could work with me on the nuts and bolts of creating it.

A few weeks later a New York ex-merchant banker, who was busy setting up one of the biggest medically-based, anti-ageing projects ever conceived, came to me asking if I would put together a range of anti-ageing products for his corporation. Great. Here was my chance. When I started to tell him about the importance of feeding the living matrix, his eyes glazed over. 'Yes, yes,' he said '. . . that's what I had in mind . . . sort of a cross between Nicholas Perricone and Howard Murad . . . know what I mean?'

Under The Volcano

I have a home in the Southern Hemisphere. It sits on the side of the crater of a 12-million-year-old extinct volcano filled with sea water. I love to spend time there writing, dreaming, just *being* with the land. I love to watch as the sun, rising over the Pacific, floods my home with fire. So much do I like being there that when I am, I avoid going out. I usually find a way of getting somebody else to do the shopping for me.

One Friday morning I was stuck and had to go into town for myself. On the shelves of an organic emporium where I buy vegetables, I noticed a range of skincare products I had never seen before. Giving into my passion for smells and textures and my love of lotions and potions, I put down the basket I was carrying and rubbed some hand lotion from a sample bottle on my arm. I was taken aback by the beauty of it – not only the way it went on my skin but its fragrance which obviously had come from the natural smell of the plants used to formulate it. But there was something else I noticed too – something about the energy it conveyed when you put it on – refreshing, uplifting; it made you feel good all round. I asked my friend Wendy who owned the store what it was. 'Living Nature,' she told me. 'The creation of New Zealand chemist Suzanne Hall.' I bought three or four products, played with them for a couple of days and was impressed. I rang Suzanne Hall, told her how much I admired her range and asked if I could interview her for a book I was going to write – *Skin Revolution.*

A Meeting Of Mind And Spirit

We met. She described herself to me as somebody who had really wanted to go to art school but ended up doing chemistry by mistake. I saw immediately that she was a rare combination of artist and scientist. It turned out to be one of those meetings where you feel you have known somebody forever. The interview never did get done. Instead we spent the evening talking about what we loved most, what we believed about the skin, about the body, about life itself – about the dreams we had and the frustrations we wrestled with. I found myself telling her about my vision of creating a single holographic skin nutrient product – a true source of nourishment and energy for the living matrix which everybody from 15 to 115 could use – something that could supply what skin needed to resist ageing, repair itself, and live out its potential for health and beauty. Within two hours I was sure that I wanted to work with her to create it. Having grasped fully what I was wanting to do, Suzanne became as excited about it as I was. Despite her workload, which would have defeated a herd of elephants, she agreed to help me.

Back To The Books

For months we exchanged ideas and information. I went back to textbooks on biochemistry and physiology. I traced the metabolic pathways involved in collagen synthesis and DNA repair. I charted all of the nutrients and substrates involved. I also learned everything I could about the living matrix itself and became ever more fascinated by this amazing mechanical, energetic, biochemical and informational network which regulates all the physiological processes in our body. Suzanne delved into chirality, made list after list of natural ingredients and analysed their components. In formulating the product we were aiming to create a kind of living matrix itself in which each ingredient synergistically supported the other to enhance the energetic and biochemical order of living skin. Together we worked out what would create the most perfect synergy.

We wanted to make sure that what we ended up with would be metabolically active and that it would contain every key ingredient – all those biological and energetic agents needed to empower skin's highest genetic expression. Since the surface of cell membranes control the flow of essential nutrients and oxygen into the cells as well as the removal of wastes, we had to make sure we could establish the right kind of ionic communications for this to happen smoothly. Because the extra-cellular matrix of skin is made up of water, negatively charged molecules of proteoglycans, and fibrous proteins like collagen and elastin, we had to work out exactly what components were needed to support this too. Next we had to work out how to get all this into the skin – how to create an active delivery system that would deliver the goods, yet still protect the integrity of the stratum corneum and leave its protective barrier intact.

Pure And Chemical-Free

Both Suzanne and I were determined we would use nothing in the formula which is foreign to the body itself and nothing that could in any way pollute the living matrix or undermine the skin's health – no chemicals, none of the paraben preservatives, no artificial fragrances. And whatever we made, it had to work as well on the skin of a 19-year-old boy with a tendency to acne as it did on a menopausal woman whose hormones were in flux and whose skin therefore needed all the help it could get.

We decided to create the product as a fine mist – something you could spray on each morning and night – which would be easily taken up by skin and could refresh the spirit as it regenerated the flesh. It would need to work as well on naked skin as it did under or over makeup. We wanted it to be something you could decant into a small atomizer, slip into your purse or pocket and use throughout the day when the skin is exposed to computers, wind or weather or is in any way under stress. The formula would have to be as useful to a woman who loved using masses of creams and lotions as well as to a man who did nothing at all for his skin.

The mist began to evolve. It even started to take on a life of its own.

We discovered some remarkable things while developing the prototypes: two teenagers who had long struggled with acne and tried just about everything to get rid of it reported that our Mist was the only thing that had ever made a significant difference. Women who had for years experienced reactions to virtually every skincare product they used reported their skin thrived on Living Matrix Mist™ and that it gave no reactions. The skins of men and children responded positively – from that of a two-year-old with remnants of German measles to a 72-year-old carpenter with severe sun damage. One after another reports came in: 'my skin has never looked better.' 'Right from the beginning my skin seemed to drink up the spray as though it was hungry for it.' 'I spray it over my makeup to give me energy when I feel myself flagging.'

They were encouraging. It felt good to know that our holographic approach to nurturing skin by giving it what it needs and letting its own metabolic processes do the rest could deliver. But still we were not satisfied. We wanted to know how it would behave when fed to living skin cells in the laboratory. We wanted to have its actions measured by government laboratories using flow cytometry to find out if it would protect DNA and prevent inflammation. We wanted to know if it would encourage fibroblast activity – necessary for the production of new collagen as well as a dozen other things.

The Consciousness Equation

Once we had established the product's effectiveness on a biochemical level, once we had worked out the biophoton to support it, I addressed the subtler aspects of how it could be used to uplift the consciousness of the person using it. I wanted it to enhance skin beauty, not only chemically and physically, but to uplift the spirit as well. For help with this I turned to people working at the leading edge of sound and focused intention techniques. I wanted the experience of using the mist to be one that was not only refreshing and uplifting. I intended on a spiritual level for the product to carry a very clear intention: to help call forth the authentic beauty and creative power of the person using it.

I turned to the work of Kate Rossetto in the United States for help with this. Kate is one of the most skilled and gifted healers I have ever come across and I knew that she could provide this important element. I knew too that Kate was highly skilled in how to use essential oils, not only for their therapeutic properties, but to create a powerful synergy between the vibrational energies of these plant essences and the more than fifty natural ingredients we had used to create the biochemistry of the matirx. Then I began to explore what emerging paradigm sound research had to offer us and how the use of specific sound in the manufacturing might be used to enhance the formula and a man or woman's experience of using it.

Blessing for Authentic Beauty

I asked Kate to work with prayer and blessings – spiritual energy which can not even be quantified in biochemical or physical terms – so that every bottle would carry blessings to those using it. First and foremost the product needed to be excellent and effective biochemically. I knew we had accomplished this but I wanted more: in relation to its subtle energies and consciousness uplifting intentions it had to be right also. I believe that the expression of authentic beauty is not just holistic – that is a *whole body* experience – it is truly *holographic* – a *whole being* experience. In the end we had a product that was truly created with the help of scientists, aestheticians, and healers from through out the world – something in which the whole turned out to be far greater that the sum of its parts.

With An Ending, New Beginnings

Before long I began to dream about the possibility of creating a sister product to go with Living Matrix Mist™ – a nutraceutical supplement that would support and strengthen skin from inside out as Living Matrix spray could through the skin's surface, even further strengthening the energetic and biochemical order of the living matrix. That, too, is on its way.

The process of making things that are beautiful or which can help create beauty has always fascinated me. It demands a strange combination of imagination, vision, trial and error, discipline and plain hard slog – which for me is always a large part of making anything happen. And, although I hate the frustration and difficulties along the way, I would rather create things that fascinate me more than anything else I can think of.

I have always believed that to create anything, you have to love it enough to be willing to do whatever is necessary to bring it into being. What has been great about creating Living Matrix Mist™ is being able to share the frustration, the slog and all the excitement with Suzanne, whose love and fascination with the task at hand not only matches but further inspires my own.

So this is where my tale of obsession with beauty has brought me. At least for the moment. I suspect that this may not be the end of the story. For beauty is a magnificent and infinitely seductive thing to become obsessed by. You never know where it will take you next. Wherever, in my case, that turns out to be, I hope I will be ready for it.

APPENDICES:

FURTHER READING

Allan, Christian B., Lutz, Wolfgang, *Life Without Bread: How a Low-Carbohydrate Diet Can Save Your Life*, New York, McGraw Hill, 2000

Andes, Karen, *A Woman's Book of Strength*, Perigee Books, 1995

Antczak, Dr. S & G., *Cosmetics Unmasked*, London, Thorsons, 2001

Audette, R., Gilchrist T., *Neanderthin: Eat like a Caveman to Achieve a Lean, Strong, Healthy Body*, New York, St. Martin's Press, 2000

Baechle, Thomas & Westcott, Wayne, *Strength Training Past 50*, Leeds, Human Kinetics, 1997

Balch, James F., *The Super Antioxidants: Why They Will Change The Face of Healthcare in the 21ˢᵗ Century*, New York, M. Evans & Co. Inc., 1998

Bank, David MD., & Sobel E., *Beautiful Skin: Every Woman's Guide to Looking Her Best At Any Age*, MA, Adams Media Corporation, 2000

Batmanghelidj, Dr. F., *Your Body's Many Cries for Water: You Are Not Sick, You Are Thirsty*, Global Health Solutions, 1995, 1997

Becker, R.O., & Marino, A., *Electromagnetism and Life*, Albany, NY, State University of New York Press, 1982

Becker, Robert O., & Selden, Gary., *The Body Electric: Electromagnetism and the Foundation of Life*, New York, William Morrow & Co., 1985

Bennett, Peter ND, Barrie, Stephen ND, Faye, Sara, *7-Day Detox Miracle: Revitalize Your Mind and Body with this Safe and Effective Life-Enhancing Program*, Roseville, CA, Prima Publishing, 2001

Benson, Herbert MD, & Proctor, William, *Beyond the Relaxation Response: How to Harness the Healing Power of Your Personal Beliefs*, New York, Berkley Pub Group, 1994

Berkson, Burton, M.D., Challem, Jack, Smith, Mellissa Diane, *Syndrome*

X: The Complete Nutritional Programme to Prevent and Reverse Insulin Resistance, Canada, John Wiley & Sons, 2000

Bircher, Ralph, *'A Turning Point in Nutritional Science'*, Lee Foundation for Nutritional Research, Milwaukee, Wisconsin reprint, n.d.

Bircher-Benner, M.O., *Food Science for All*, London, C.W. Daniel, 1928

Bircher-Benner, Max, *The Prevention of Incurable Disease*, unpublished translation by Hilda Martin

Bircher-Benner, Max, *The Meaning of Therapeutic Order*, unpublished translation by Hilda Martin

Brand-Miller, Jennie, et.al. *The Glucose Revolution*, New York, Marlowe, 1999, 2000

Brekhman, I.I. *Man and Biologically Active Substances*, Oxford, Pergamon Press, 1980, Franklin Book Company, 2nd edition (July 1980)

Burkitt, Denis, *Refined Carbohydrate Foods and Disease: Some Implications of Dietary Fibre* , New York, Academic Press, 1975

Carson, Rachel, *Silent Spring*, London, Penguin, 1962, 2000

Challem, Jack, Burt Berkson, M.D., Ph.D & Melissa Diane Smith, *Syndrome X: The Complete Nutritional Programme to Prevent and Reverse Insulin Resistance*, Canada, John Wiley & Sons, Inc., 2000

Cichoke, Anthony J. *Enzymes & Enzyme Therapy: How to Jump Start Your Way to Lifelong Good Health*, New Canaan, Connecticut, Keats Publishing Inc., 1994

Colburn T., Dumanoski D., & Myers J.P., *Our Stolen Future: Are we Threatening our Fertility, Intelligence and Survival? A Scientific Detective Story*, New York, Plume 1997

Colgan, Michael, with Colgan, Lesley, *The Flavonoid Revolution, Grape Seed Extract and Other Flavonoids Against Disease*, Apple Publishing Company, Canada, 1997

Colgan, Michael, *Hormonal Health: Nutritional & Hormonal Strategies for Emotional Well-Being & Intellectual Longevity*, Vancouver, Canada, Apple Publishing, 1996

Cordain L., PhD., *The Paleo Diet*, New York, Canada, John Wiley & Sons Inc., 2002

Crile, George, *The Bipolar Theory of Living Processes*, New York, Macmillan, 1926

Crile, George, *The Phenomenon of Life: Toward a Philosophical Biology*, New York, W.W. Norton, 1936

Dadd, Debra Lynn, *Nontoxic, Natural and Earthwise: How to Protect Yourself from Harmful Products and Live in Harmony with the Earth*, Los Angeles, LA, Jeremy P. Tarcher Inc., 1990

Dadd, Debra Lynn, *The Nontoxic Home and Office, Protecting Yourself and Your Family from Everyday Toxins and Health Hazards*, Los Angeles, LA, Jeremy P. Tarcher Inc., 1990

Erickson K., *Drop Dead Gorgeous: Protecting Yourself from the Hidden Dangers of Cosmetics*, USA, Contemporary Books, 2002

Evans W., *Biomakers: The 10 Keys to Prolonged Vitality*, Fireside, August 1992

Fagan D., & Lavelle M., *Toxic Deception: How the Chemical Industry Manipulates Science, Bends the Law, and Endangers Your Health*, Secaucus, NJ, Common Courage Press, 1999

Fairley J., & Stacey S., *Feel Fabulous Forever: The Anti-Ageing Health and Beauty Bible*, Penguin Books Australia Ltd., 1999

Fallon, Sally, Mary Enig, PhD., & Pat Connolly, *Nourishing Traditions: The Cookbook that Challenges Politically Correct Nutrition and Diet Dictocrats*, New Trends Publishing, 1999

Fisher, J.A. MD, *The Plague Makers: How we are Creating Catastrophic New Epidemics – And What we Must Do to Avert Them*, New York, Simon & Schuster, 1994

Frankel, P., & Madsen F., *Stop Homocysteine Through the Methylation Process: The Key to Controlling Homocysteine and SAM and their Effect on Heart Disease, Aging, Cancer, Osteoporosis, Depression, AIDS and Other Diseases*, Thousand Oaks, California, TRC Publications, 1998

Green, Lawrence MD., *The Dermatologist's Guide to Looking Younger: An Essential Guide from A to Z*, CA., Crossing Press, 1999

Hayflick L., *How and Why We Age*, New York, Ballantine Books, 1994

Hampton A., *What's in Your Cosmetics?: A Complete Consumer's Guide to Natural and Synthetic Ingredients*, Tucson, Odonian Press, 1995

Hoffer, Abram, & Walker, Morton, *Orthomolecular Nutrition: New Lifestyle for Super Good Health*, New Canaan, Conn., Keats Publishing, 1978

Howell, Edward, *Enzyme Nutrition*, Lotus Press, 1986

Kenton Leslie, *The New Joy of Beauty*, London, Vermilion, 1995, 2000

Kenton, Leslie, *The New Ageless Ageing*, London, Vermilion, 1995

Kenton, Leslie, *The X Factor Diet: For Lasting Weight Loss and Vital Health*, London, Vermilion, 2002

Kenton, L. & S. *The New Raw Energy*, London, Vermilion, 1995, 2001

Kenton, Leslie, *Age Power: A Revolutionary Path to Regeneration, Creativity and Fulfilment*, London, Vermilion, 2002

Kenton, Leslie, *Passage to Power: Natural Menopause Revolution*, London, Vermilion, 1998

Krimsky, Sheldon, & Goldman, Lynn, *Hormonal Chaos: The Scientific and Social Origins of the Environmental Endocrine Hypothesis*, Baltimore, MD, The Johns Hopkins University Press, 1999

Krimsky, Sheldon, *The Science and Politics of Endocrine Disrupters*, John Hopkins University Press, November 18, 1999

Lee J.R., MD., *Natural Progesterone: The Multiple Roles of a Remarkable Hormone*, Jon Carpenter Publishing, 1999

Lee J.R., MD., & Hopkins, Virginia, *What Your Doctor May Not Tell You About Pre-menopause: Balance Your Hormones and Your Life from Thirty to Fifty*, New York, Warner Books Inc., 1999

Lee J.R., MD., & Hopkins, Virginia, *What Your Doctor May Not Tell You About Menopause: The Breakthrough Book on Natural Progesterone*, New York, Warner Books Inc., 1996

Lees, Mark et al., *Skincare: How to Save Your Skin*, NY, Delmar, 2001

Lees M., *Skin Care: Beyond the Basics*, NY, Milady Publishing Co. Inc., 2001

Lewis W., *The Lowdown on Facelifts and Other Wrinkle Remedies*, London, Quadrille Publishing Ltd., 2001, 2002

Liberman, Jacob O.D. PhD., *Light: Medicine of the Future*, Bear & Company, 1992

Lininger, Schuyler W., et.al. editors, *The Natural Pharmacy*, Rockland CA, Prima Publishing, 1999

Loftus J.M. MD., *The Smart Woman's Guide to Plastic Surgery: Essential Information from a Female Plastic Surgeon*, Illinois, Contemporary Books, 1999

Lowe N., Prof. & Sellar P., *Skin Secrets*, London, Collins & Brown Ltd., 1999

Meyerowitz S., *Sproutman's Kitchen Garden Cookbook: 250 Flourless, Dairy-less, Low Temperature, Low Fat, Low Salt, Living Food Vegetarian Recipes*, Mass., Sproutman Publications, 1999

Meyerowitz S., *Sprouts the Miracle Food: The Complete Guide to Sprouting*, Mass., Sproutman Publications, 1998

Murray, Michael ND, *Encyclopedia of Nutritional Supplements: The Essential Guide for Improving Your Health Naturally*, Rocklin CA., Prima Publishing, 1996

Murray, Michael T. *Dr. Murray's Total Body Tune-Up: Slow Down the Aging Process, Keep Your System Running Smoothly, Help Your Body Heal Itself,* Bantam Books, 2001

Perricone N. MD., *The Perricone Prescription,* New York, Harper Collins, 2002

Perricone N. MD., *The Wrinkle Cure: the Formula for Stopping Time,* London, Vermilion, 2001

Price, W., *Nutrition and Physical Degeneration,* 6th ed., New York, McGraw Hill, 2002

Roberts, Arthur J. MD., O'Brien, Mary E. MD., & Subak-Sharpe, Genell MS, editors, *Nutraceuticals: The Complete Encyclopedia of Supplements, Herbs, Vitamins and Healing Foods,* USA, Penguin Putnam, 2001

Schmidt, Michael A., *Smart Fats: How Dietary Fats and Oils Affect Mental, Physical and Emotional Intelligence,* Berkeley, California, Frog Ltd, 1997

Seigel, Bernie S. MD., *Peace, Love & Healing: Bodymind Communication & the Path to Self-Healing: An Exploration,* New York, Harper & Row, 1988

Stauber J.L., & Rampton S., *Toxic Sludge is Good For You: Lies, Damn Lies and the Public Relations Industry,* Monroe, Maine, Common Courage Press, 1995

Steingraber, Sandra Dr., *Living Downstream: An Ecologist Looks at Cancer and the Environment,* Perseus Publishing, 1997

Toxic Toy Story, Greenpeace, USA, available at www.greenpeaceusa.org

Vance, Judi, *Beauty to Die For: The Cosmetic Consequence,* New York, To Excel Inc., 1999

Weil, Andrew MD., *Spontaneous Healing: How to Discover and Enhance Your Body's Natural Ability to Maintain and Heal Itself,* New York, Ballantine Books, Random House Inc., 1996, 2000

'What's Wrong with the Body Shop?' *London Greenpeace,* 21 March 1998

REFERENCES

One – The Living Matrix

Al-Abed Y., Liebich H., Voelter W., Bucala R., 'Hydroxyalkenal formation induced by advanced glycosylation of low density lipoprotein', *J Biol Chem* 271 (6), Feb 9 1996

Antczak Dr. S & G., *Cosmetics Unmasked*, London, Thorsons, 2001

Bank, David, MD. & Sobel E., *Beautiful Skin: Every Woman's Guide to Looking Her Best at Any Age*, MA., Adams Media Corporation, 2000

Becker R.O., *Cross Currents: The Promise of Electromedicine, the Perils of Electropollution*, Los Angeles, Jeremy P. Tarcher, Inc., 1990, 1991

Becker, Robert O., 'Electromagnetic forces and life processes', *Technological Review*, Dec 1972

Berridge M.J., Rapp P.E., and Treherne J.E., Eds. 'Cellular oscillators', *J. Exp. Biol.* 81, Cambridge University Press, Cambridge, 1979

Berrry M.N., Gregory R.B., Grivell A.R., Henly D.C., Phillips J.W., Wallace P.G., & Welch G.R., 'Linear Relationships between Mitochondrial Forces and Cytoplasmic Flows Argues for the Organized Energy-coupled Nature of Cellular Metabolism', *FEB* 224, 1987

Bitter, Patrick, 'Non-invasive Rejuvenation of Photodamaged Skin using Serial, Full-Face Intense Pulsed Light Treatments', *American Society for Dermatologic Surgery Inc.*

Bruce E., *Living Foods for Radiant Health*, London, Thorsons, December 2003

Bircher-Benner M., '*The Meaning of Therapeutic Order*', unpublished translation by Hilda Martin

Bland J.S., *The 20-Day Rejuvenation Diet Program*, New York, McGraw Hill, 1996

Brand-Miller, Jennie et al. *The Glucose Revolution*, New York, Marlowe, 1999, 2000

Breithaupt H., 'Biological Rythyms and Communications' in *Electromagnetic*

Bio-Information, 2nd Ed. (F.A.Popp, R. Warnke, H.L. Konig and W. Peschka, Eds.), Urban Schwarzenberg, Munich, 1979

Bucala R., Makita Z., Koschinsky T., Cerami A., Vlassara H., 'Lipid advanced glycosylation: pathway for lipid oxidation in vivo', *Proc Natl Acad Sci*, USA, 90 (14): July 15 1993

Carson, Rachel, *Silent Spring*, London, Penguin, 1962, 2000

Challem, Jack, Berkson, B., MD., & Smith MD., *Syndrome X: The Complete Nutritional Programme to Prevent and Reverse Insulin Resistance*, New York, John Wiley & Sons, Inc., 2001

Coats C., *Living Energies: Viktor Schauberger's Brilliant Work With Natural Energy Explained*, Bath, Gateway Books, 1996

Colborn, et al., *Our Stolen Future: Are We Threatening our Fertility, Intelligence and Survival? A Scientific Detective Story*, New York, Plume, 1997

Davydov A.S. 'Energy and Electron Transport in Biological Systems', in *Bioelectrodynamics and Biocommunication* (M.W. Ho, F.A. Popp and U. Warnke, eds.), World Scientific, Singapore, 1994

Dilman, V., and Dean W., *The Neuroendocrine Theory of Aging and Degenerative Diseases*, Pensacola, Florida, The Center for Bio-Gerontology, 1992

Fagan D., & Lavelle, M., *Toxic Deception: How the Chemical Industry Manipulates Science, Bends the Law and Endangers Your Health*, Secaucus, N.J., LPC, 1999

Farlow C.H., *Dying to Look Good*, USA, Kiss for Health Publishing, 2000

Harold F.M., *The Vital Force: A Study of Bioenergetics*, New York, W H Freeman, 1987

Hicks M., Delbridge L., Yue D.K., Reeve T.S., 'Increase in crosslinking of nonenzymatically glycosylated collagen induced by products of lipid peroxidation', *Arch Biochem Biophys* 268 (1), Jan 1989

Ho M.W., and Knight D., 'Collagen Liquid Crystalline Phase Alignment, the DC Body Field and Body Consciousness'

Ho M.W., and Popp F.A., 'Biological Organization, Coherence and Light Emission from Living Organisms', *Thinking About Biology* (W.D. Stein and F, Varela., Eds.), New York, Addison-Wesley, 1993

Hume E.D., *Bechamp or Pasteur? :A Lost Chapter in the History of Biology*, London, The C.W. Daniel Co., 1932, RA Kessinger Publishing Co., 1996, print on demand

Jackson S.M., Williams M.L., Feingold K.R., Elias P.M., 'Pathobiology of the stratum corneum', *West J Med* 158 (3), Mar 1993

Knight D. and Feng D., *Collagens as Liquid Crystals* – paper presented at British Association for the Advancement of Science Molecular Self-Assembly in Science and Life, Keele, 1993

Lowe N. Prof., & Sellar, P., *Skin Secrets*, London, Collins & Brown Ltd., 1999

MacDonald S.M., *Detoxification and Healing*, New York, McGraw Hill, 1998

Mooradian A.D., and Thurman J.E., 'Glucotoxicity – potential mechanisms', *Clinics in Geriatric Medicine*, 1999

Neel J., 'Diabetes mellitus. A "thrifty" genotype rendered detrimental by progress', *American Journal of Human Genetics*, 1963

Oschman J.L., *Energy Medicine – The Scientific Basis of Bioenergy Therapies*, New Hampshire, USA, Churchill Livingstone, 2000

Oschman J.L., 'Structure and Properties of Ground Substances', *American Zoologist* 24, 1984

Pederson K., et al., 'The Preservatives Ethyl, Propyl, and Butylparaben Are Oestrogenic in an In Vivo Fish Assay', *Pharmacological Toxicology* 86, March 2000

Pizzorno J.P., and Murray M., *Encyclopaedia of Natural Medicine*, London, Century Hutchinson, 1990

Price W., *Nutrition and Physical Degeneration*, 6th ed. New York, McGraw Hill, 2002

Rattemeyer M., and Popp F.A., 'Evidence of Photo Emission from DNA in Living Systems', *Naturwissenschaften* 68, 1981

Rauch E., *Health Through Inner Body Cleansing: The Famous Mayor Intestinal Therapy from Europe*, Karl F. Haugverlag, 1998

Rogers L., 'Top Perfumes Linked to Cancer Scare in Chemicals', *Sunday Times*, Nov 24 2002

Sevanian A., Wratten M., McLeod L.L., Kim E., 'Lipid peroxidation and phospholipase A2 activity in liposomes composed of unsaturated phospholipids: a structural basis for enzyme activation,' *Biochem Biophys Acta* 961, Aug 12 1988

'Skin Permeation: Fundamentals and Application', *Cosmetics & Toiletries*, IL, Allured Publishing Corporation, 1996

'The Chemistry and Manufacture of Cosmetics', *Cosmetics & Toiletries*, IL, Allured Publishing Corporation, 1996

Swerdlow Joel, 'Unmasking Skin', *National Geographic*, November 2002

Tsong T.Y., and Gross C.J., 'The Language of Cells – Molecular Processing of Electric Signals by Cell Membranes', *Bioelectrodynamics and Biocommunication* (M.W. Ho., F.A. Popp and U Warnke, eds), World Scientific, Singapore, 1994

'What's Wrong with the Body Shop?' *London Greenpeace*, Mar 21 1998

Two – Unlocking The Power

Allan, Christine B., and Lutz, Wolfgang, *Life Without Bread: How a Low Carbohydrate Diet Can Save Your Life*, New York, McGraw Hill, 2000

Ames B.N., 'Paleolithic diet, evolution, and carcinogens', *Science*, 1987

Ames B.N., 'Micronutrients prevent cancer and delay aging', *Toxicol Lett*, 1998

Araneo B., et al. 'DHEAS as an effective vaccine adjuvant in elderly humans', *Annals of the New York Academy of Sciences*, 1995

Arlt W., et al. 'Dehydroepiandrosterone replacement in women with adrenal insufficiency', *New England Journal of Medicine*, Sep 30 1999

Audette R., Gilchrist T., *Neanderthin: Eat like A Caveman to Achieve a Lean Strong, Healthy Body*, New York, St. Martin's Press, 2000

Baker, Valerie L., 'Alternatives to oral estrogen replacement: Transdermal methods of delivery', *Obstetrics and Gynecology Clinics of North America*, June 1994

Balch, James F., *The Super Antioxidants: Why they will Change the Face of Healthcare in the 21ˢᵗ Century*, New York, M. Evans & Co. Inc., 1998

Beales P.E., Burr L.A., Webb G.P., Mansfield K.J., Pozzilli P., 'Diet can influence the ability of nicotinamide to prevent diabetes in a non-obese diabetic mouse: a preliminary study', *Diabetes Metab Res Rev*, 1999

Becker, Robert O., 'Electromagnetic forces and life processes', *Technological Review*, December 1972

Beutler, Jade and Murray, Michael, *Understanding Fats and Oils: Your Guide to Healing with Essential Fatty Acids*, Vancouver, Apple Publishing Co., 2000

Bircher-Benner M., *The Essential Nature and Organization of Food Energy and the Application of the Second Principle of Thermo-Dynamics to Food Value and its Active Forces*, London, John Bale & Sons & Curnow, 1949

Bounous G., et al., 'Endocrine response to animal and vegetable protein', Barth C.A. and Schlimme E., editors, *Milk Proteins*, New York, Springer Verlag, 1989

Boyce N., 'How to defy death – stay thin', *New Scientist*, 1999

Bower B., 'The two million year old meat and marrow diet resurfaces', *Science News*

Budwig, Johanna, *Flax Oil as a True Aid Against Arthritis, Heart Infarction, Cancer and Other Diseases*, Vancouver, Apple Publishing Co., 1996

Budwig, Johanna, *The Oil-Protection Diet*, Vancouver, Apple Publishing Co., 1996

Bukowieki L.J., et al., 'Insulin resistance and defective thermogenesis', *Obesity: Dietary Factors and Control*, edited by Rosmos et al., Tokyo, Japan Scientific Societies Press, 1991

Cahill G.F., 'Physiology of insulin in man', *Diabetes*, 1971

Cermani et al., 'Glucose and aging', *Scientific American*, May 1987

Chakmakjian Z.H., and Zachariah N.Y., 'Bioavailability of progesterone with different modes of administration', *Journal of Reproductive Medicine*, June 1987

Challem, Jack et al. *Syndrome X – The Complete Nutritional Program to Prevent and Reverse Insulin Resistance,* New York, Wiley & Sons, 2001

Chang K.J., 'Influences of percutaneous administration of estradiol and progesterone on human breast epithelial cell cycle in vivo', *Fertility and Sterility,* 1995

Claustrat B., et al. 'Melatonin and Jet Lag: confirmatory result using a simplified protocol', *Biol Psychiatry,* 1992

Colgan, Michael, *The Right Protein for Muscle and Strength,* One in the Progressive Health Series, Colgan Institute, Vancouver, Apple Publishing Co., 1999

Cooper A., et al. 'Systemic absorption of progesterone from Progest cream in post-menopausal women', *Lancet,* Apr 25 1998

Cowan L.D., Gordis J.A., Tonascia J.A., Jones G.S., 'Breast cancer incidence in women with a history of progesterone deficiency', *J Epidemiol,* 1981

Cromer B.A., 'Effects of hormonal contraceptives on bone mineral density', *Drug Safety,* Mar 1999

Crowley C.L., Payne C.M., Bernstein H., Bernstein C., Roe D., 'The NAD precursors nicotinic acid and nicotinamide protect cells against apoptosis induced by a multiple stress inducer, deoxycholate', *Cell Death Differ,* Mar 7 2000

DeWees, Allen A., *The Glycemic Index: Glycemic Impact of Food,* at www.anndeweesallen.com/dal.gly2.htm

Dilman V., and Dean W., *The Neuroendocrine Theory of Aging and Degenerative Disease,* Pensacola, Florida, The Center for Bio-Gerontology, 1992

Eaton S.B., et al., 'Stone Agers in the fast lane: Chronic degenerative diseases in evolutionary perspective', *American Journal of Medicine,* 1988

Eaton S.B., Eaton S.B.III and Konner M.J., 'Paleolithic Nutrition Revisited: A twelve year retrospective on its nature and implications', *European Journal of Clinical Nutrition,* 1997

Eaton S.B., et al., 'An evolutionary perspective enhances understanding of human nutritional requirements', *Journal of Nutrition,* 1996

Eaton S.B., Shostak M., and Konner M., *The Paleolithic Prescription: A Program for Diet and Exercise and a Design for Living*, New York, Harper Collins, 1988

Elliott R.B., Pilcher C., Stewart A., Fergusson D., McGregor M.A., 'The use of nicotinamide in the prevention of type 1 diabetes', *Ann NY Acad Sci*, 1993

Fallon, Sally, *Nourishing Traditions: The Cookbook that Challenges Politically Correct Nutrition and the Diet Dictocrats*, Washington DC, New Trends Publishing Inc., 1999

Fitzpatrick L., and Good A., 'Micronized progesterone: clinical indications and comparison with current treatments', *Fertility and Sterility*, Sept 1999

Foidart J., et al. 'Estradiol and progesterone regulate the proliferation of human breast epithelial cells':, *Fertility and Sterility*, May 1998

Guarente, 'SIR2 links chromatin silencing, metabolism and aging', *Genes and Development*

Heinrich, Richard L., *Starch Madness: Paleolithic Nutrition for Today*, Nevada City, California, Blue Dolphin Publishing, 1999

Holman R.T., 'The slow discovery of the importance of omega-3 essential fatty acids in human health', *Journal of Nutrition*, 1998

Holman R.T., 'Significance of essential fatty acids in human nutrition', *Lipids 1*, 1976: 215

Ilipkiss A., 'Carnosine, a protective, antiaging peptide?' *Int J Biochem Cell Biol*, 1998

Ilipkiss A., et al., 'Protective effects of carnosine against MDA-induced toxicity towards cultured rat brain endothelial cells', *Neuroscience Letters*, 1997

Ilipkiss A., et al., 'Protective effects of carnosine against protein modification mediated by nialondialdchyde and hypochlorite', *Bioch Biophys Acta*, 1998

Ilipkiss A., Ghana H., 'Carnosine protects proteins against methylglyoxal-mediated modifications', *Biochem Biophys Res Comm*, 1998

Imai S.I., Armstrong C.M., Kaeberlein M., Guarente L., 'Transcriptional silencing and longevity protein Sir 2 as an NAD dependant histone deacetylase', *Nature*, 403:795–800, 2000

Kaeberlein, McVey, Guarente, 'The SIR2/3/4 complex and SIR2 alone promote longevity in Saccharomyces cerevisiae by two different mechanisms', *Genes and Development*, 1999

Katahn, Martin, *The Tri-Color Diet: A Miracle Breakthrough in Diet and Nutrition for a Longer and Healthier Life*, New York, W.W. Norton, 1996

Kaunitz H., 'Medium Chain Triglycerides (MCT) in Aging and Arteriosclerosis', *Journal of Environmental Pathology, Toxicology and Oncology*, 1986

Kenton, Leslie and Kenton, Susannah, *The New Raw Energy*, London, Vermilion, 1994, 1995

Kenton, Leslie, *Age Power: A Revolutionary Path to Rejuvenation, Creativity and Fulfilment*, London, Vermilion, 2002

Kenton, Leslie, *The X Factor Diet: for Lasting Weight Loss and Vital Health*, London, Vermilion, 2002

Kenton, Leslie, *Passage to Power: Natural Menopause Revolution*, London, Vermilion, 1998

Klatz R., and Goldman R., *Stopping the Clock*, New Canaan, Conn., Keats Publishing, 1996

Klurfeld D.M., and Kritchevsky D., 'The Western Diet: An examination of its relationship with chronic disease', *Journal of American College of Nutrition*, 1986

Krantz S., Lober M., & Henschel L., 'The nonenzymatic glycation of proteins and nucleic acids, their importance for the development of diabetic complications, possible molecular basis of aging and autoimmunological processes', *Exp Clin Endocrinol*, 1986

Lee B.M., & Wolever, T.M.S., 'Effect of glucose, sucrose and fructose on plasma glucose and insulin responses in normal humans; comparison with white bread', *European Journal of Clinical Nutrition*, 1998

Lee, John R., & Hopkins, Virginia, *What Your Doctor May Not Tell You about Menopause: The Breakthrough Book on Natural Progesterone*, New York, Warner Books, 1996

Lee, John R., 'Sleep, Surviving and Breast Cancer', *The John R Lee MD Medical Letter*, Apr 2000

Lee, John R., 'Women's heart disease, heart attacks and hormones', *The John R Lee MD Medical Letter*, Aug 1998

Lemon H.M., 'Oestriol and prevention of breast cancer', *The Lancet*, Mar 10 1973

Licastro F., Walford R.L., 'Modulatory effect of nicotinamide on unscheduled DNA synthesis in lymphocytes from young and old mice', *Med Ageing Dev.*, 1989

Lininger, S.W., Jr. DC, et.al., eds., *The Natural Pharmacy*, Rockland, C.A. New York, Prima Publishing, 1999

Maichuk I.F., Formaziuk V.E., Sergienko V.I., 'Development of carnosine eye drops and assessing their efficacy in corneal disease', 1997

Matuoka et al., 'Rapid reversion of aging phenotypes by nicotinamide through possible modulation of histone acetylation', *Cellular and MolecularLife Sciences*, 2001

McFarland G.A., Holliday R., 'Further evidence for the rejuvenating effect of the dipeptide L-carnosine on cultured human diploid fibroblasts', *Exp Gerontol*, 1999

Micheli V., Simmonds H.A., Sestini S., Ricci C., 'Importance of nicotinamide as an NAD precursor in the human erythrocyte', *Arch Biochem Biophys*, Nov 15 1990

Modan M, et al., 'Hyperinsulinemia: A link between hypertension, obesity and glucose intolerance', *Journal of Clinical Investigation*, 1985

Mooradian A.D., & Thurman J.E., 'Glucotoxicity – potential mechanisms', *Clinics in Geriatric Medicine*, 1999

Morgenthaler J., & Simms M., *The Smart Guide to the Low-Carb Anti-Aging Diet*, Petaluma, California, Smart Publications, 2000

Mullokandov E.A., Franklin W.A., & Brownleee M., 'DNA damage by the glycation products of glyceraldehydes 3-phosphate and lysine', *Diabetologia*, 1994

Murray, Michael T. MD., *Encyclopedia of Nutritional Supplements – The Essential Guide for Improving Your Health Naturally*, Rocklin, CA., Prima Publishing, 1996

Olsson A.R., Sheng Y., Pero R.W., Chaplin D.J., Horsman M.R., 'DNA damage and repair in tumor and non-tumor tissues of mice induced by nicotinamide trials in pre-type 1 diabetes', *J. Pediatr Endocrinol Metab*, 1996

Papoulis A., al-Abed Y., and Bucala R., 'Identification of N2–(1–carboxyethyl) guanine (CEG) as a guanine advanced glycosylation end product', *Biochemistry*, 1995

Peat R., 'Coconut Oil', *Townsend Letter for Doctors and Patients*, 1995

Pierpaoli, Walter and Regelson, William, '*The Melatonin Miracle': Nature's Age-Reversing Disease-fighting, Sex Enhancing Hormone*, New York, Pocket Books, 1995

Plu-Bureau G. et al. 'Percutaneous progesterone use and risk of breast cancer: results from a French cohort study of premenopausal women with benign breast disease.' *British Journal of Cancer*, 1994

Poullain M.G., et al., 'Effect of whey proteins: Their oligopeptide hydrolystates and free-amino acid mixtures on growth and nitrogen retention in fed and starved rats', *Journal of Parenteral and Enteral Nutrition*, 1989

Preston J., et al., 'Toxic effects of B-amyloid on immortalised rat brain endothelial cell: protection by carnosine, homocarnosine and B-alnine', *Neurosciencce Letters*, 1998

Price W., *Nutrition and Physical Degeneration*, 6th edition, New York, McGraw Hill, 2002

Pushkarsky T., Rourke L., Spiegel L.A., Seldin M.F., & Bucala R., 'Molecular characterization of a mouse genomic element mobilized by advanced glycation endproduct modified-DNA (AGE-DNA)', *Mol Med*, 1997

Quinn P.J., Boldyrev A.A., Formaziuk C.E., 'Carnosine: its properties, functions and potential therapeutic applications', *Mol Aspects Mod*, 1992

Radack K., et al., 'The effects of low doses of n-3 fatty acid supplementation on blood pressure in hypertensive subjects: A randomised controlled trial', *Archives of Internal Medicine*, June 1991

Rattan, 'Repeated mild heat shock delays ageing in cultured human skin fibroblasts', *Biochemistry and Molecular Biology International* 45(4), 1998

Reaven G., 'Role of insulin resistance in human disease', *Diabetes*, 1988

Reaven G., 'Syndrome X', *Clinical Diabetes*, 1994

Reaven G., 'Syndrome X: 6 Years Later', *Journal of Internal Medicine Supplement*, 1994

Reiss, Uzzi., *Natural Hormone Balance for Women: Look Younger, Feel Stronger, and Live Life with Exuberance*, New York, Pocket Books, 2002

Riklis E., Kol R., Marko R., 'Trends and developments in radio protection: the effect of nicotinamide on DNA repair', *Int J Radiol Biol*, Apr 1990

Roberts, Arthur J., et al., editors, *Nutraceuticals: The Complete Encyclopedia of Supplements, Herbs, Vitamins and Healing Foods*, New York, Penguin Putnam, 2001

Roberts P.R., Black K.W., Santamauro J.T., 'Dietary peptides improve wound healing following surgery', *Nutrition*, 1998

Rudin, Donald, & Felix, Clara, *Omega-3 Oils: To Improve Mental Health, fight Degenerative Diseases, and Extend Your Life*, Garden City Park, New York, Avery Penguin Putnam, 1996

Sadler R., 'The benefits of dietary whey protein concentrate on the immune response and health', *South African Journal of Dairy Science*, 1992

Seidel W., and Pischetsrieder M., 'Immunochemical detection of N2[1-(1-carboxy)ethyl] guanosine, an advanced glycation end product formed by the reaction of DNA and reducing sugars or L-ascorbic acid in vitro', *Biochim Biophys Acta*, 1998

Tanny J.C., Dowd G.J., Huang J., Hilz M., Moazed D., 'An enzymic activity in the yeast Sir 2 protein that is essential for gene silencing', *Cell*, 1999

Tarnha M., et al., 'Hydroxyl radical scavenging by carnosine and Cu (ii)-carnosine complexes', *Int J Radiat Biol*, 1999

Thorpe S.R., Baynes J.W., 'Role of the Maillard reaction in diabetes mellitus and diseases of aging', *Drugs Ageing*, 1996

Torjeson P.A., et al., 'Lifestyle changes may reverse development of the insulin resistance syndrome', *Diabetes Care*, 1997

Trevisan M., et al., 'Syndrome X and mortality: A population-based study', *American Journal of Epidemiology*, 1998

Wade N., 'Scientist at work: Dr Leonard Guarente searching for genes to slow the hands of biological time', *The New York Times*, Sept 26 2000

Wanagat J., Allison D.B., Weindruch R., 'Caloric intake and aging mechanisms in rodents and a study in nonhuman primates', *Toxicol Sci* 52, Dec 1999

Wright, Jonathan V., and Morgenthaler, John, *Natural Hormone Replacement for Women over 45*, Petaluma, Cal., Smart Publications, 1997

Yen S.S., et al. 'Replacement of DHEA in aging men and women. Potential remedial effects.' *Annals of the New York Academy of Sciences*, 1995

Yudkin J., 'Medical problems from modern diet', *Journal of the Royal College of Physicians of London*, Jan 1975

Three – Mapping The Minefields

Adair R.K., 'A Flaw in the Universal Mirror', *Scientific American*, 1988

Antczak, Dr. Stephen and Gina, *Cosmetics Unmasked*, Thorsons, 2001

'A Two Decade Drop in Sperm Counts', *Sci News*, 25 Feb 1995

Bazzato G., et al. *Lancet*, 1981

Beasley J., and Swift J., eds., *The Kellogg Report: The Impact of Nutrition, Environment and Lifestyle on the Health of Americans*, Anandale-on-Hudson, NY: The Institute of Health Policy and Practice, The Bard College Centre, 1990

Begley S., & Glick D., 'The Estrogen Complex', *Newsweek*, 21 March 1994

Bennett P., Barrie S. & Faye S., *7-Day Detox Miracle: Revitalize Your Mind and Body with This Safe and Effective life-Enhancing Program*, California, Prima Health, 2001

Bland J., *The 20-Day Rejuvenation Diet Program*, New York, McGraw Hill, 1996

Block N.J., 'Why do Mirrors Reverse Right/Left but Not Up/Down?' *Journal of Philosophy*, vol.71, May 16 1974

Bradley D., 'A new twist in the tale of nature's asymmetry', *Science*, 1994

Brant et al., 'The final report on the safety assessment of TEA, DEA, MEA', *Journal of the American College of Toxicology*, 1983

Bremer J., *Physiol Rev*, 1983

Bridges B., 'Fragrance: emerging health and environmental concern', *Flavour and Fragrances Journal* Vol.17 Issue 5, 2002, http://www.fpinva.org/Fragrances Review.htm

Burton G.W., Traber M.G., 'Vitamin E – Antioxidant activity, biokinetics and bio-availability', *Annu Rev Nutr* 10, 1992

Cairns-Smith A.G., 'Chirality and the common ancestor effect', *Chemistry in Britain*, 1986

Casdorph H. Richard, MD., and Morton Walker MD., *Toxic Metal Syndrome: How Metal Poisonings Can Affect Your Brain*, NY., Penguin Putman, 1995

Cohen J., 'Getting all turned around over the origins of life on earth', *Science* 267

Dadd, Debra Lynn, *The Nontoxic Home and Office: Protecting Yourself and Your Family from Everyday Toxins and Health Hazards*, rev.ed., Los Angeles, CA., Jeremy P Tarcher Inc., 1992

Dadd, Debra Lynn, *Nontoxic, Natural and Earthwise: How to Protect Yourself from Harmful Products and Live in Harmony with the Earth*, Los Angeles, CA., Jeremy P Tarcher Inc., 1990

De Groot A.C., and Frosch P.J., 'Adverse reactions to fragrances: A clinical view', *Contact Dermatitis*, 1997

'Denaturation of Epidermal Keratin by Surface Active Agents', *Journal of Invest. Dermatology*, 1959

Dougherty R.C. et al., 'Negative Chemical Ionisation Studies of Human and Food Chain Contamination with Xenobiotic Chemicals', *Environ Health Perspect* 36, 1980

Dufty, William, *Sugar Blues*, New York, Warners, 1993
Earman, John, 'Kant, Incongruous Counterparts and the Nature of Space and Space-Time', *Ratio*, vol. 13, June 1971

'Editorial, Intestinal Endotoxins as Mediators of Hepatic Injury: An Idea Whose Time Has Come Again', *Hepatology* 10, 1989

Erickson, Kim, *Drop Dead Gorgeous: Protecting Yourself From The Hidden Dangers of Cosmetics*, Contemporary Books, Toronto, 2002

FDA, *Division of Colours and Cosmetics, Progress Report on the analysis of cosmetic products and raw materials for nitrosamines*, Washington DC. GPO, 1988'

'Final report on the safety assessment of Methylparaben, Ethylparaben, Propylparaben and Butylparaben' *Journal of the American College of Toxicology* Vo.3 No.5, 1984

'Final report on the safety assessment of Isobutylparaben and Isopropylparaben', *Journal of the American College of Toxicology* 14 (5):364372, Lippincott-Raven Publishers, Philadelphia, 1995, Cosmetic Ingredient Review

Fox M.A., Whitesell J.K., 'Chemical Perspectives. Thalidomide: Disastrous Biological Activity of the 'Wrong' Enantiomer', *Organic Chemistry* 2nd ed., Jones and Bartlett, Boston, 1997

Fox, Maggie, 'Cosmetics full of suspect chemicals, group says', *Reuters*, July 11 2002

Frey W., 'Intranasal Delivery: Bypassing the Blood-Brain Barrier to Deliver Therapeutic Agents to the Brain and Spinal Cord', *Drug Delivery Technology* (5), July/Aug 2 2002

Fritsch, Vilma, *Left and Right in Science and Life*, London, Barrie and Rockliffe, 1968

Gardner M., *The New Ambidextrous Universe: Symmetry and Asymmetry, from Mirror Reflections to Supershings*, New York, W.H. Freeman & Co., 1991

Hershoff R.J., and Bradlow H.L., 'Obesity, Diet, Endogenous Estrogens and the Risk of Hormone Sensitive Cancer', *Am J Clin Nut* 45, 1987

Hegstrom R.A., Kondepudi D.K., 'The Handedness of the Universe', *Scientific American*, 1990

Heuberger E, Hongratanaworakit T., Bohm C., Weber R., & Buchbauer G F., 'Effects of chiral fragrances on human autonomic nervous system parameters and self-evaluation', *Chem. Senses*, Apr 26 2001

Horwitt M.K., 'Vitamin E – A re-examination'. *Am J Clin Nutr*, 1976

http://www.answersingenesis.org/docs/3991.asp

http://www.chiral.com

http://www.leffingwell.com/chirality/chirality.htm

http://www.rod.beavon.clara.net/chiralit.htm

Ingold, K.U., et al., 'Biokinetics of and discrimination between dietary RRR- and SRRR- alpha-tocopherols in the male rat', *Lipids* 22, 1987

Komiyama K., et al., 'Studies on the biological activity of tocotrienols', *Chem Pharm Bull*, 1989

Main D.M., and Hogan T.J., 'Health Effects on Low-Level Exposures to Formaldehyde', *J Occup Med* 25, 1983

'Makeup Kit Holds Hidden Danger of Cancer', *The Observer* July 4, 2002

McCarty M.F., *Med Hypotheses*, 1982

McFadden S.A., 'Phenotypic Variation in Xenobiotic Metabolism and Adverse Environmental Response: Focus on Sulfur-Dependant Detoxification Pathways', *Toxicology* 111, 1996

Manahan S.E., *Toxicological Chemistry and Biochemistry* [3rd edition], Chelsea, MI: Lewis Publishers, 2002

Mislow K., Bickart P., 'An Epistemological Note on Chirality', *Israel J. Chem* 15, 1976

Prelog, Vladimir, *Chirality in Chemistry*, Nobel Lecture, Dec 12, 1975

Raloff J., 'Beyond Estrogens: Why Unmasking Hormone-Mimicking Pollutants Proves So Challenging', *Sci News* 148, 1995

Raloff J., 'That Feminine Touch: Are Men Suffering from Prenatal or Childhood Exposure to 'Hormonal' Toxicants?' *Sci News* 145, 1994

Raloff J., 'The Gender Benders: Are Environmental "Hormones" Emasculating Wildlife?' *Sci News* 145, 1996

Rogers, Sherry A., MD, 'Chemical Sensitivity: Breaking the Paralyzing Paradigm', *Internal Medicine World Report*, Feb 1–14 1992

Saifer, Phyllis MD., *Detox: A Successful & Supportive Program for Freeing Your Body from the Physical and Psychological Effects of Chemical Pollutants*, Los Angeles, CA., Jeremy P Tarcher, 1984 (Out of Print)

Salam A., 'The Role of Chirality in the Origin of Life', *Journal of Molecular Evolution*, 1991

Schneider J., et al., 'Effects of Obesity on Estradiol Metabolism: Decreased Formation of Nonuterotropic Metabolites', *J Clin Endocrinol Metab* 56, 1983

Schreier, Peter et al. *Analysis of Chiral Organic Molecules: Methodology and Applications*, Walter deGruyter, 1995

Silver, Helene, *Body Smart System: The Complete Guide to Cleansing and Rejuvenation*, rev.ed., Sonora, CA., Healthy Healing, 1995

Stehlin, Duri, 'Cosmetic Safety: More Complex Than at First Blush', *USDFA Consumer*, May 1995

Steinberg D.C., *Cosmetics and Toiletries: Preservatives for Cosmetics*, IL, Allured Publishing Corporation, 2000

Steingraber S., *Living Downstream: An Ecologist Looks at Cancer and the Environment*, Reading, MA, Addison-Wesley, 1997

Streitweiser A., Heathcock C.H., Kosower E.M., *Introduction to Organic Chemistry*, 4th ed. New York, Prentice Hall, 1998

Steinman D., and Epstein S., *The Safe Shoppers Bible: A Consumer's Guide to Nontoxic Household Products*, New York, John Wiley & Sons Inc., 1995

Stirling, Pamela, 'Skin Deep', *NZ Listener*, July 13 2002

Testa B., Carrupt, P.A. Gal, J. 'The So-Called 'Interconversion' of Stereoisomeric Drugs: An Attempt at Clarification', *Chirality*, 1993

Thaxton C.B., Bradley W.L., Olsen W.L., *The Mystery of Life's Origin: Reassessing Current Theories*, New York, Philosophical Library Inc., 1984

Vance, Judi, *Beauty to Die For: The Cosmetic Consequence*, New York, To Excel Inc., 1999

Wright, Camille, 'Shampoo Report', *Images International Inc.*, 1989

Yoffe, Emily, 'Chemical Good Looks', *US News*

Four – Tapping The Elements

Abergel R.P., MD., Lyons R., MD., Castel, J., MS, S Dwyer R., MD., and Uitlo I., MD., PhD, 'Cultures', Harbor UCLA Medical Centre, CA., *J Dermatol. Surgery Oncol.* 13:2, Feb 1987

Ainsleigh H.G., 'Beneficial effects of sun exposure on cancer mortality', 1993

American Journal of Clinical Dermatology, 2001

American Journal of Clinical Dermatology, June 2000

Archives of Dermatology, December 2000

Bajpai R.P., 'Coherent nature of the radiation emitted in delayed luminescence of leaves', *J.Theor., Biol 19,* 1999

Belkin M.I., Schwartz U., 'New Biological Phenomena Associated with Laser Radiation, Tel-Aviv University', *Health Physics, Vol. 56 No.5,* May 1989

Beral V. et al. 'Malignant melanoma and exposure to fluorescent lighting at work',. *Lancet,* Aug 7 1982

Beral V., Ramchara S., and Faris R., 'Malignant melanoma and oral contraceptive use among women in California', *The Walnut Creek Contraceptive Drug Study US National Institutes of Health, vol 111,* 1986

Bergold Dr. Orm MD., 'The Effect of Light and Colour on Human Physiology', *Raum & Seit, Vo. 1 No. 4,* 1989

Bitter P.H., 'Noninvasive rejuvenation of photodamaged skin using serial, full-face intense pulsed light treatments', *Dermatol Surg,* 2000

Black H.S. et al., 'Relation of antioxidants and level of dietary lipids to epidermal lipid peroxidation and ultraviolet carcinogenesis', *Cancer Research,* 1985

Bland J.S., *Func Med Update,* Mar 2000

Bohn, David, 'The Implicate Order and the Super-implicate Order', *In Weber,*

R. (ed.) *Dialogues with Scientists and Dosages: The Search for Unity*, London and New York, Routledge and Keagan, 1986

Braverman B., PhD.,McCarthy R., Pharmd., Lyankovich A., MD., Ford D., BS, Overfield M., BS and Bapna M., PhD., 'Effect of Helium-Neon and Infrared Laser Irradiation in Wound Healing in Rabbits', Rush-Presbyterian-St Lukes Medical Centre, University of Illinois, *Lasers in Surgery and Medicine*, 1989

British Journal of Dermatology, Nov 2001

British Journal of General Practice, Oct 1999

Broad W. and Wade N., *Betrayers of the Truth*, NY, Simon Schuster, reprint 1983

Bykov V.J., et al., 'Ultraviolet B-induced DNBA damage in human skin and its modulation by a sunscreen', *Cancer Res*, July 1998

Ceder K., *Healthy office lighting: A bright idea*. Healthy Office Rep, 1992

Chang J.J.,. Fisch J., & Popp F.A., (eds) *Biophotons*, Kluwer Academic Publishers, 2002

Chien C.H., Tsuei J.J., Lee S.C., Huang Y.C., Wei Y.H., 1991 'Effect of emitted bioenergy on biochemical functions of cells', *American Journal of Chinese Medicine*

Clinical Experimental Dermatology, Oct 2001

Colburn T., Dumanoski D., & Myers J.P., *Our Stolen Future: Are we Threatening our Fertility, Intelligence and Survival? A Scientific Detective Story*, New York, Plume, 1997

Cunnane S.C. et al. 'Nutritional attributes of traditional flax-seed in healthy young adults', *Am J Clin Nutr, 1995*

Dadd, Debra Lynn, *The Nontoxic Home and Office*, Jeremy P. Tarcher Inc., 1992

Dadd, Debra Lynn, *NonToxic, Natural and Earthwise How to Protect Yourself from Harmful Products and Live in Harmony with the Earth*, Los Angeles, CA, Jeremy P. Tarcher Inc., 1990

Dilman V., and Dean W., *The Neuroendocrine Theory of Aging and Degenerative Disease*, Pensacola: Center for Bio-Gerontology, 1992

Douglass W.C., *Second Opinion*, Feb 1994

Environmental Health Perspective, Mar 2001

Fisher J.A., MD., *The Plague Makers: How we are Creating Catastrophic New Epidemics – And What we Must Do to Avert Them*, New York, Simon & Schuster, 1994

Garland F.C. et al. *Occupational sunlight exposure and melanoma in the US Navy*, Arch Environmental Health, 1990

Glasgow P.D., Hill I.D., McKevitt A.M. et al., 'Low intensity monochromatic infrared therapy: a preliminary study of the effects of a novel treatment unit upon experimental muscle soreness', *Lasers Surg Med*, 2001

Goldberg D.J., and Samady J.A., 'Intense Pulsed light and Nd:YAG laser non-ablative treatment of facial rhytids', *Lasers Surg Med*, 2001

Goldberg D.J., and Cutler K.B., 'Nonablative treatment of rhytids with intense pulsed light', *Lasers Surg Med*, 2000

Goldberg D.J., 'New collagen formation after dermal remodelling with an intense pulsed light source', *J Cutan Laser Ther*, 2000

Grimes D.S., 'Sunlight, cholesterol and coronary heart disease', *Quarterly Jour Applied Nutr*, 1995

Hattersley J.G., 'The negative health effects of chlorine', *Journal Orthomolecular Med.*, 2000

Hernandez-Perez E., and Ibiett E.V., 'Gross and microscopic findings in patients submitted to nonablative full-face resurfacing using intense pulsed light: a preliminary study', *Dermatol Surg*, 2002

Hobday, Richard, *The Healing Sun: Sunlight and Health in the 21st Century*, Findhorn, Scotland and Tallahassee, Florida, The Findhorn Press, 1999, 2000

Horowitz L.R., Burke T.J., Carnegie D., 'Augmentation of wound healing using monochromatic energy', *Adv. Wound Care*, 1999

Hunter, Linda Mason, *The Healthy Home: An Attic-to-Basement Guide to Toxin-Free Living*, Universe.Com, 2000

Journal of the American Academy of Dermatology, July 2001

Journal of Chromatography, BioMedical Applications

Journal of Epidemiology, Dec 1999

Journal of Ethnopharmacology, Dec 1999, Free-Radical Biology and Medicine, January 2000

Journal of Photochemistry and Photobiology, Nov 2001

Justus E.D., Lehmann F. MD., *Therapeutic Heat and Cold*, 4th edition, Lippincott, Williams and Wilkins, 1990

Kawadda A., Shiraishi H., Asai M., Kameyama H., Sangen Y., Aragane Y., and Tezuka T., 'Clinical improvement of solar lentigines and ephelides with an intense pulsed light source', *Dermatol Surg*, 2002

Kennedy A.R. et al., 'Fluorescent light causes malignant transformation in mouse embryo cell', *Science*, 1980

Kime Z., *Sunlight*. Penryn, CA, World Health Publ, 1980

Kitchen S., MSCMCSP, Partridge C., PhD, 'A Review of Low Level Laser Therapy, Centre for Physiotherapy Research', *Kings College London Physiotherapy*, Vol. 77, No. 3, March 1991

Krimsky, Sheldon and Goldman Lynn, *Hormonal Chaos: The Scientific and Social Origins of the Environmental Endocrine Hypothesis*, Baltimore, MD, The Johns Hopkins University Press, 1999

Krimsky, Sheldon, *The Science and Politics of Endocrine Disrupters*, John Hopkins University Press, November 18, 1999

Kripke D.F., 'Light treatment for nonseasonal depression: Speed, efficacy and combined treatment'. *J Affective Disorders*, 1998

Lee J.R., MD., *Natural Progesterone: The Multiple Roles of a Remarkable Hormone*, Jon Carpenter Publishing, 1999

Lee J.R., MD., & Hopkins, Virginia, *What Your Doctor May Not Tell You About*

Pre-menopause: Balance Your Hormones and Your Life from Thirty to Fifty, New York, Warner Books Inc., 1999

Lee J.R., MD., & Hopkins, Virginia, *What Your Doctor May Not Tell You About Menopause: The Breakthrough Book on Natural Progesterone*, New York, Warner Books Inc., 1996

Leske M.C., and Chylack L.T. Jr, et al. 'Antioxidant vitamins and nuclear opacitie', *Ophthalmology*, 1998

Liberman, Jacob O.D. PhD., *Light: Medicine of the Future*, Bear & Company, 1992

Lieberman B., *Doomsday déjà vu: Ozone depletion's lessons for global warming*, Working paper, The European Science and Environment Forum, Cambridge, November 1998

Life Extension Foundation, *Life Extension Update*, June 1993

London W.P., 'Full-spectrum classroom light and sickness in pupils', *Lancet*, Nov 21 1987

Mandel, Peter, *Esogetics: The Sense and Nonsense of Sickness and Pain*, Sulzbach/Taunus, Germany, Energetik Verlag, 1993

McKibbin L.S., DVM., Paraschak D., BSc.MA;Mod, *Use of Laser Light to Treat Certain Lesions in Thoroughbreds*

Mieg C., Mei W.P., and Popp F.A., 'Technical Notes to Biophoton Emission, Recent Advances in Biophoton Research and its Applications', *World Scientific*, Singapore, 1992

Moan J. and Dahlback A., 'The relationship between skin cancers, solar radiation and ozone depletion', *British Journal of Cancer*, 1992

Murray F., '*The Murray Report*', *Let's Live*, Oct 16 1997

Muehsam D.J., Markov M.S., Muehsam P.A., Pilla A.A., Shen R., Wu Y., 'Effects of Qigong on cell-free myosin phosphorylation: preliminary experiments', *Subtle Energies*, 1994

Negishi K., Wakamatsu S., Kushikata N., Tezuka Y., Kotani Y., & Shiba K., 'Full face photorejuvenation of photodamaged skin by intense pulsed light with integrated contact cooling: initial experiences in Asian patients', *Lasers Surg Med*, 2002

Negishi K., Wakamatsu S, Kushikata N., and Tezuka Y., 'Photorejuvenation for Asian skin by intense pulsed light', *Dermatol Surg*, 2001

Niggli H.J., 'Kinetics of excision repair in human skin', *J.Invest.Dermatol* 92

Niggli H.J., (1993a) 'Artifical Sunlight irradiation induces ultraweak photon emission in human skin fibroblasts', *J. Photochem.Photobiol.B.Biol.* 18

Niggli H.J., (1996) 'The cell-nucleus of cultured melanoma cells as a source of ultraweak photon emission', *Naturwissenschaften* 83

Niggli H.J., *Ultraweak photon emission in differentiated fibroblasts*, IIB Conference, 1999

Norrell, Johannes et al., *The Sunscreen Octyl Methoxycinnamate Binds to DNA*, Department of Physics, University of Alabama, Birmingham

Ohshiro T., *Low Reactive-Level Laser Therapy: A Practical Application*, New York, John Wiley & Sons, 1991

Oschman J.L., *Energy Medicine: The Scientific Basis of Bioenergy Therapies*, Churchill Livingstone, 2000

Oschman J.L., *The Connective Tissue and Myofascial Systems*, Dover, NH, M.O.R.A. Press, 1981

Oschman J.L. and Oschman N., *New evidence on the nature of healing energy, Part I: Communication in the living Matrix*, Dover, NH, N.O.R.A. Press, 1994

Ott J.N., *Light, Radiation and You: How to Stay Healthy*, Greenwich, CT; Devin-Adair Publishers, 1985

Ott J.N., *Interview by Bland JS*, Jan 1991

Ott J.N., *Lecture to Society for Clinical Ecology*, 1974

'Oxidation strongly linked to aging', *Sci News*, Aug 14 1993

Pearce F., 'Ozone hole innocent of Chile's ills', *New Scientist*, Aug 21 1993

Peat R., 'Coconut oil, In *Mercola J Healthy News You Can Use*, Mar 24 2001

Peat R., *Ray Peat's Newsletter*, 1995

Peat R., *Sunlight: Using it to sustain life*, From Female Hormones preprint, PO Box 5764 Eugene, 1995

Phoenix, OR, A.Z., *Anodyne Infrared Therapy, Anodyne Therapy System* [website] Fasterhealing.com, 1998

Photodermatalogy, Photoimmunology & Photomedicine, Dec 2000

Photodermatoloty, Photoimmunology & Photomedicine, Feb 2001

Popp F.A., Gu Q., & Li H.I., 'Biophoton Emission: Experimental Background and Theoretical Approaches', *Mod.Phys.Lett.B* 8 21 and 22, 1994

Popp F.A., Ruth B., Bahr W., Bohm J., Grass P., Grolig G., Rattemeyer M., Schmidt H.G, & Wulle P., 'Emission of visible and ultraviolet radiation by active biological systems', *Collective Phenomena 3*, 1981

Dualibe Carlos, *Integrative Biophysics: Biophotonics*, Dordrecht, Kluwer Academic Publishers, 2003

Prieto V.G., Sadrick N.S. Lloreta J., Nicholson J., & Shea C.R., 'Effects of intense pulsed light on sun-damaged human skin, routine and ultrastructural analysis', *Lasers Surg Med*, 2002

Rampen F.H., Nelewans R.T. & Kerbeek A.L.M., 'Is water pollution a cause of cutaneous melanoma?', *Epidemiology*, 1992

Recer P., 'Sun may prevent breast cancer', *Seattle Post-Intelligencer*, Nov 4 1997

Ridley M., 'Taking the sting out of the sunshine myth', *The Sunday Telegraph*, Apr 3 1994

Robbins, John, *Reclaiming Our Health: Exploding the Medical Myth and Embracing the Source of True Healing*, Tiburon, California, H J Kramer, Inc., 1998

Rochkind S, MD., Rousso M, MD., Nissan M., PhD, Villarreal M, MD., Barr-Nea L. MD., Rees D.G. MD., 'Burns', *Lasers in Surgery and Medicine* 9, 1989

Schein O.D., Vicencio C., & Muoz B., et al. 'Ocular and dermatologic health effects of ultraviolet radiation exposure from the ozone hole in southern Chile', *Amer Jour Public Health*, Apr 1995

Schneider, Dona and Freeman, Natalie, *Children's Environmental Health: Reducing Risk in a Dangerous World,* American Public Health Association, 2000

Shwartz S.A., DeMattei R.J., Brame K.G., Spottiswoode S.J.P., 1990 'Infrared spectra alteration in water proximate to the palms of therapeutic practitioners', *Subtle Energies*

Seddon J.M., Ajani U.A. et al. *Dietary carotenoids, vitamins A,C, and E, and advanced age-related macular degeneration,* Eye Disease Case-Control Study Group, JAMA, 1994

Short R.V., 'Melatonin; Hormone of Darkness', *Brit Med J,* 1993

Smith K.C., 'The Photobiological Basis of Low Level Laser Radiation Therapy, Stanford University School of Medicine', *Laser Therapy,* Volume 3, No. 1, Jan-Mar 1991

Sternberg S., 'Breathing freely threatens seeing clearly', *Sci News* 1997 (Mar 8): see also JAMA, Mar 5 1997

'Sunlamp use linked to melanoma', *Sci News,* 1994

Surinchak J., MA., Alago M., BS., Bellamy R. MD., Stuck B., MS., and Belkin, M., MD., 'Effects of Low-Level Energy Lasers on Healing of Full-Thickness Skin Defects, Lettennan Army Institute of Research. Presido of San Francisco, CA', *Lasers in Surgery and Medicine,* 1983

Thalen B.E. et al. 'Light treatment in seasonal and nonseasonal depression', *Acta Psychiatr Scand,* 1995

The Politics of Sunlight,. What Doctors Don't Tell You, 1995

Thomassoi D.D.S., *Effects of Skin-Contact Monochromatic Infrared Irradiation of Tendonitis, Capsulitis and Myofascial Pain,* 19th Annual Scientific Meeting, American Academy of Neurological and Orthopaedic Surgeons, Aug 1995, *Facial Pain,* TMJ Centre, Denver, CO

Thomasson T.L., 'Effects of skin-contact monochromatic infrared radiation on tendonitis, capsulitis and myofascial pain', *J Neurol Orthop Med Surg,* 1996

Valerian V., *'Leading Edge International Research Group', Release,* Dec 21 1998

Walker M., 'The healing powers of QiGong (Chi Kung) in 4 parts', *Townsend Letter for Doctors,* Jan, Feb/Mar, Apr and May issues

Wang Z.Y., Huang M.T., & Lou Y.R., et al. 'Inhibitory effects of black tea, green tea, decaffeinated black tea, and decaffeinated green tea on ultraviolet B light-induced skin carcinogenesis in 7, 12-demethylbenz[a]anthracene-initiated SKH mice', *Cancer Res*, 1994

Weil, Andrew, M.D., *Spontaneous Healing: How to Discover and Enhance Your Body's Natural Ability to Maintain and Heal Itself*, New York, Ballantine Books, Random House Inc., 2000

Westerdahl J., Olosson H., Masback A. et al. 'Use of sun lamps and malignant melanoma in southern Sweden', *Am J epidem*

Whelan, Harry, *Physical Therapy* 72 (7), Jul 1992 (60 ref)

Young S., PhD, Bolton P., BSc, Dyson U., Phd, Harvey W., PhD, Diamantopoulos C., BSc, 'Macrophage Responsiveness to Light Therapy', London, *Lasers in Surgery and Medicine*, 9, 1989

RESOURCES

Leslie Kenton's Website: www.lesliekenton.com Here you will find a mass of helpful tools, techniques, inspiration and resources for practitioners and products as well as links to other websites which Leslie has found valuable. The website is highly active. Information changes weekly including messages from Leslie, herbs of the week, recipes of the week, news about forthcoming events and workshops Leslie is doing throughout the world. There too you have the opportunity to *become a friend* and submit your questions. Those chosen each month are answered personally by Leslie.

Jesse Kenton-Smith's Website: www.cosmeticsurgerynz.com Jesse Kenton-Smith BSc(Hons), MBBS, FRCS, FRACS (Plast) – Jesse's passion for plastic surgery centres around the high level of its technical demands and the satisfying results it can bring. Apart from aesthetic medicine and cosmetic procedures, Jesse's main area of interest is rebuilding the faces of children with cleft lips and palates and doing work on hands.

Living Matrix Mist™: Leslie's nutrient spray for skin, took her more than three years to research and then formulate with the help of scientists from all over the world. Use the mist twice a day, morning and night, and whenever skin needs refreshment or extra support – especially when using computers or on an aircraft. It is designed to supply skin of every age and type what it needs to carry out essential functions – from DNA repair and protection from free radical damage to making new collagen and strengthening cell walls in optimal ways. Use Living Matrix Mist™ with moisturisers and night treatments if you like. It works both under and over makeup. Many find, after a week or two, they prefer Living Matrix Mist™ on its own because it addresses so completely the needs of living skin. Completely natural and absolutely pure, the product contains no chemical fragrances, parabens or other substances to pollute the living skin. It relies on Hall's celebrated natural preservative system and is packaged in specially made dark violet medical bottles to prolong life and enhance biophoton energy. For how to order:
Living Matrix
Freephone: 0800 0975612
Freefax: 0800 0975613
Telephone: 01794 324 982
www.livingmatrix.org
www.livingmatrix.co.uk
email: info@livingmatrix.co.uk

SKIN REVOLUTION SPECIFICS

NB – If a website address is not shown for any product you are interested in, type in the name of the company or product on www.google.com

Air-Care Portable Ioniser
Air Ion Technologies
13b Queensway
Stem Lane
New Milton
Hampshire BH25 5NN
UK
Tel: +44 (0) 1425 638169
E-mail sales@airiontechnologies.com
Website: www.airiontechnologies.com

Flaxseeds (Linseeds)
Vacuum-packed whole flaxseeds (linseeds) are available in most health-food stores. I use Linusit Gold as they are well packed and fresh. They are available from The Nutri Centre. Organic flaxseeds are also available from Higher Nature Limited. Keep them refrigerated. See suppliers of good quality natural supplements.

Flaxseed Oil (Linseed oil)
Organic Flaxseed Oil is available from:
Savant Distribution Ltd
FREEPOST NEA 12027
Leeds LS16 6YY
UK
Order line (UK): 08450 606070. Tel: +44 (0) 113 388 5248
Fax: +44 (0) 113 274 5777
E-mail: info@savant-health.com
Website: www.savant-health.com

Far Infrared Sauna
Physiotherm® Infrared Saunas – In Europe and USA:
Physiotherm®
B.Köllensperger Strasse 1
A-86065 THAUR/Innsbruck
Austria
Tel: +43 (0) 5223 54 777
Fax: +43 (0) 5223 54777 22

E-mail: infrarot@physiotherm.com
Website: www.physiotherm.com

In the Asia Pacific Region:
MagMed Ltd
100 Munro Road
Te Puna
RD5 Tauranga
New Zealand
or
PO Box 14283
Tauranga, New Zealand
Tel: +64 (7) 552 4877
Fax: +64 (7) 552 4850
E-mail: sales@magmed.co.nz or info@4sauna.co.nz
Website: www.4sauna.co.nz or www.magmed.co.nz

Hormone Creams: In most countries hormone creams are available only through a doctor's prescription. You can purchase progesterone cream from:

Wellsprings Trading Ltd
PO Box 322
St Peter Port
Guernsey GY1 3TP
Channel Islands
UK
Tel: +44 (0) 1481 233370
Fax: +44 (0) 1481 235206
Website: www.progesterone.co.uk

You can purchase Progest and other hormone creams by post from:

Women's International Pharmacy
5708 Monova Drive
Madison WI 53716
USA
Tel: ++(1) 608 221 7800
Fax: ++(1) 608 221 7819

For information on the multiple uses of natural progesterone for women's health contact:

Natural Progesterone Information Service (NPIS)
PO Box 24
Buxton SK17 9FB
UK
Tel (UK): 07000 784849

For information about natural health developments including information on progesterone products and other hormone creams, contact:

Well Woman's Information Service
BCM 1212
London
WC1N 3XX
UK
Tel (UK): 08707 651212
Fax (UK): 08707 650305
E-mail: info@wwis.com

Microfiltered Whey Protein
Solgar produce Whey To Go Protein Powder in vanilla, chocolate, honey nut and mixed berry flavours, I prefer the vanilla and chocolate. However, the chocolate contains artificial sweetener. BioPure Pure Protein by Metagenics or Twinlab Super Whey Powder are also good sources of micro-filtered whey protein. Whey To Go and BioPure can be purchased from the Nutri Centre. See suppliers of good quality natural supplements below.

MSM Max
These MSM tablets are the purest and most potent form of MSM available – fast-acting and 100% pure with no additives or binders.
Website: www.richdistributing.com

MSM Rich 'n Pure Lotion
Only natural ingredients are used in Dr Rich's hydrating lotions. Designed specifically to help repair damage to your skin, they may be used by men and women alike. Your skin gradually develops a new softness and elasticity. This lotion contains 17% Methyl Sulfonyl Methane (MSM) produced through distillation to ensure highest quality.
PO Box 33830, Portland or 97292, USA
Tel: ++(503) 761 7450
Fax: ++(503) 761 5383
Website: www.richdistributing.com

Also available from:
The Naturally Curious Company
PO Box 46, Pukekohe
Auckland 1800
New Zealand
Tel: +64 (9) 239 0496.
Fax +64 (9) 239 0936
Website: www.naturalchoices.co.nz

Multi Vitamin & Mineral Supplement: Vita Synergy for women and Vita Synergy for men is the first truly 100% all natural vitamin, mineral and herbal supplement made entirely from food source nutrients and is available from Xynergy Health Products. It is highly bioavailable and is my favourite. Solgar also do excellent multiple vitamins and minerals such as Omnium, so do Nature's Plus and Higher Nature. See suppliers of good quality natural supplements.

SKIN REVOLUTION NUTRACEUTICALS

The following three shops are an excellent source for good quality vitamins, minerals and nutraceutical supplements mentioned in *Skin Revolution*. They also do efficient mail order service.

The Nutri Centre
7 Park Crescent
London
W1B 1PF
Tel: +44 (0) 207 436 5122
E-mail: customerservices@nutricentre.com
Website: www.nutricentre.com
The best suppliers of nutritional supplements and information, unique in the world. The Nutri Centre is not only the UK's leading supplier of supplements, it also has one of the finest collections of books on holistic health and nutrition including spiritual and psychological books related to health. This small shop in the basement of The Hale Clinic is always at the cutting edge of what is happening in holistic health. Their products can be ordered easily online or by telephone. The Nutri Centre carries more than 20,000 health and natural beauty care products including those which are available in health food stores as well as those sold only through practitioners. What you order is dispatched within 24 hours throughout the world. They have become Britain's largest supplier of complementary medicine

textbooks to British colleges and universities. They print an interesting newsletter on holistic health with extracts printed on line. The centre is dedicated to service. No order is too small or too large. Almost all of what you need for natural health and beauty you will find here. I can't recommend them highly enough.

Oliver's Wholefood Store
Another excellent place which offers a full range of supplements and natural remedies with an efficient nationwide mail order service is Oliver's Wholefood Store. They are winners of 'Organic Community Shop of the Year 99' and 'Health Food Store of the Year 99'. Full organic grocer with off-licence, specialising in excellent quality organic food – vegetables, fish, meat etc. Opening Times Monday – Sunday 9am-7pm. Oliver's organise regular health lectures.
5 Station Approach
Kew Gardens
Richmond
Surrey
TW9 3QB
Tel: +44 (0) 208 948 3990
Fax: +44 (0) 208 948 3991
E-mail: info@oliverswholefoods.co.uk

Fresh & Wild
Tel (UK): 0800 0323 456
E-mail: mailorder@freshandwild.com or homeshop@freshandwild.com
Website: www.freshandwild.com
Good both for supplements and for natural skincare ranges.

Manufacturers and Importers
The following companies supply a selection of good quality vitamins, minerals and nutraceutical supplements mentioned in *Skin Revolution*.

Solgar Vitamin & Herb
Beggar's Lane
Aldbury
Tring
Herts
HP23 5PT
Tel: +44 (0) 1442 890 355
Fax: + 44 (0) 1442 890 366

E-mail: solgarinfo@solgar.com
Website: www.solgar.com

Higher Nature Ltd
The Nutrition Centre
Burwash Common
East Sussex
TN19 7LX
Tel: +44 (0) 884 668
Fax: +44 (0) 1435 883720
E-mail: info@higher-nature.co.uk or nutrition@higher-nature.co.uk
Website: www.higher-nature.co.uk

SKIN REVOLUTION FOOD SUPPLIERS

ORGANIC FOODS: The Soil Association publishes a regularly updated national directory of farm shops and box schemes called *Where to Buy Organic Foods* that costs £5 including postage from:
The Soil Association
Bristol House
40–56 Victoria Street
Bristol
BS1 6BY
UK
Tel: +44 (0) 117 929 0661
Fax: +44 (0) 117 925 2504
E-mail: info@soilassociation.org
Website: www.soilassociation.org.

Organics Direct
Offers a nationwide home delivery service of fresh vegetables and fruits, delicious breads, juices, sprouts, fresh soups, ready-made meals, snacks and baby foods. They also sell the state-of-the-art 2001 Champion Juicers and the 2002 Health Smart Juice Extractor for beginners. They even sell organic wines – all shipped to you within 24 hours.
Organics Direct
1–7 Willow Street
London EC2A 4BH
UK
Tel: +44 (0) 207 729 2828
Fax: +44 (0) 207 613 5800

Website: www.organicsdirect.com
You can order online.

Clearspring
Supply organic foods and natural remedies as well as macrobiotic foods by mail order. They have a good range of herbal teas, organic grains, whole seeds for sprouting, dried fruits, pulses, nut butters, soya and vegetable products, sea vegetables, drinks and Bioforce herb tinctures. Write to them for a catalogue:
Clearspring
Unit 19a, Acton Park Estate
London W3 7QE
UK
Tel: +44 (0) 208 749 1781
Fax: +44 (0) 208 746 2249.
Website: www.clearspring.co.uk.
You can order by telephone, fax, post or shop online

Organic meat: A UK Guide to where to buy organic meat
www.organicbutchers.co.uk
Organic Butchers
Crescent Consulting
1 The Crescent
Northampton, NN1 4SB
UK
Tel: +44 (0) 1604 459962
Fax: +44 (0) 01604 459963
E-mail: butcher@touchstoneconsultants.co.uk

Eastbrook Farms Organic Meat
This is my favourite supplier of all sorts of organic meat because they take such care over every order.
Eastbrook Farms Organic Meats
The Calf House
Cues Lane
Bishopstone
Swindon
Wiltshire, SN6 8PL
UK
Mail order: +44 (0) 1793 790460
Helpline: +44 (0) 1793 790340
Fax: +44 (0) 1793 791239

E-mail: info@helenbrowningorganics.co.uk
Website: www.helenbrowningorganics.co.uk

Longwood Farm Organic Meats
Good-quality organic beef, pork, bacon, lamb, chicken, turkey, duck and
geese, a variety of types of sausage, all dairy products, vegetables and
organic groceries (2000 lines), are available mail order from:
Longwood Farm Organic Meats
Tuddenham St Mary
Bury St Edmunds
Suffolk IP28 6TB
UK
Tel: +44 (0) 1638 717120
Fax: 01638 717120 or +44 (0) 1638 717120

Stevia
In most countries, not in the UK alas, stevia is readily available in health
food stores in many forms. It comes as clear liquid extract in distilled
water, powdered stevia leaf, as full strength (very sweet) stevioside extract.
In shaker form you can use stevia as you would sugar to sprinkle on foods
and drinks. It even comes in tiny single serving packets which you can
carry around with you in your pocket or handbag. From the UK, where
stevia is unfortunately no longer available, you may be able to order it
direct from abroad by looking on the web or asking a friend who lives in
the US to send you some. Stevia is unquestionably the best form of sweetener in the world. Far from doing harm it actually has many beneficial
properties. Keep an eye on my website as the friends of the website often
post updates on how to order stevia from abroad if you live in the UK or
EU where it is no longer available.

Water
Getting pure water can be difficult. One in ten of us drink water which
is contaminated with poisons above international standards. I have finally
found a water purifier which I think is good – the Fresh Water 1000 Water
Filter System. It removes more than 90 per cent of heavy metals, pesti-
cides and hydrocarbons such as benzene, trihalmethanes, chlorine,
oestrogen and bacteria without removing essential minerals like calcium.
Available from:
The Fresh Water Filter Company Ltd
Gem House
895 High Road
Chadwell Heath

Essex, RM6 4HL
UK
Tel: +44 (0) 208 597 3223
Fax: +44 (0) 870 0567 264
E-mail: mail@freshwaterfilter.com
Website: www.freshwaterfilter.com

SKIN REVOLUTION HERBS

For all the herbs mentioned in *Skin Revolution* the following companies below supply a selection of good quality products.

Phyto Products Ltd
An excellent company originally set up to supply herbalists with high-quality herbs and plant products. Every plant and herb they sell states the source of origin. All Phyto Products' plants are purchased only from recognisable sources. They do a full range of tinctures, herbal skin creams (including Calendula Cream, Comfrey Cream, Arnica Ointment and St John's Wort Oil), fluid extracts, herbs and the Schoenenberger plant juices. Virtually all the herbs mentioned in this book are supplied by this company in both tincture form and the loose dried herb. They do not supply herbs in capsules but they now do some herbs in tablet form. Write to them for their price list. They have a minimum order of £20 (before VAT) plus carriage.
Phyto Products Ltd
Park Works
Park Road
Mansfield Woodhouse
Mansfield
Nottinghamshire NG19 8EF
UK
Tel: +44 (0) 1623 644 334
Fax: +44 (0) 1623 657 232

Specialist Herbal Supplies
This company has been supplying high-quality additive-free herbal aids to health practitioners in the UK and abroad since 1982. They now do a range of good-quality products for the general public as well, offering single herbs and mixtures as capsules, tinctures or extracts. Write to them for their catalogue:

Specialist Herbal Supplies
Freepost (BR1396)
Brighton
East Sussex BN41 1ZZ
UK
Freephone (UK): 0800 542 5212
Fax: +44 (0) 1273 424 345
E-mail: feedback@specialist-herbal.com
Website: www.herbalsupplies.com

Bioforce (UK) Ltd
Suppliers of herbal extracts, tinctures, homeopathic remedies and natural
self-care products and foods, Bioforce is a Swiss company started by the
Swiss expert in natural health, Alfred Vogel. The company always use fresh
herbs in preparing their products at the Bioforce factory in Roggwil. They
do over 100 different herbal and homeopathic preparations, all of which
are very high quality. They can be ordered by post but are often also avail-
able in good healthfood stores and pharmacies carrying herbal products.
Bioforce (UK) Ltd
2 Brewster Place
Irvine
Ayrshire KA11 5DD
UK
Tel: +44 (0) 1294 277 344
Fax: +44 (0) 1294 277 922
E-mail: enquiries@bioforce.co.uk
Website: www.bioforce.co.uk

Bio-Health Ltd
Bio-Health do an excellent range of single herbs, ointments and multi-
herb compounds in tablet and capsule form which you can purchase from
good healthfood stores or order by post. Write to them for a catalogue.
Bio-Health Ltd
Culpepper Close
Medway City Estate
Rochester
Kent ME2 4HU
UK
Tel: +44 (0) 1634 290 115
Fax: +44 (0) 1634 290 761
E-mail: info@bio-health.co.uk
Website: www.bio-health.co.uk

Herbal Apothecary

The Herbal Apothecary manufactures and supplies the largest range of medicinal herbs in the UK, and for nearly 20 years has been the single largest supplier of herbal medicines to medical herbalists. They provide a wide range of plant and herbal products ranging from cut herbs to powders, tinctures, fluid extracts, creams, capsules and tablets together with essential oils.

The Herbal Apothecary Ltd
103 High Street
Syston
Leicester LE7 1GQ
UK
Tel: +44 (0) 116 260 2690
Fax: +44 (0) 116 260 2757

Solgar Vitamin & Herb

An American company founded in 1947 which produces good quality nutritional supplements and standardised single herbs and formulas under strict pharmaceutical standards of manufacture – in many cases stricter than USA government requirements. These include standardised full potency Herbal Female Complex (containing soy isoflavones), Feverfew Willow Complex, Milk Thistle Dandelion Complex, Ginger Fennel Complex, Olive Leaf Echinacea Complex, and Herbal Male Complex. Solgar products are available from top healthfood stores, some chemists, and The Nutri Centre.

Solgar Vitamins Ltd
Beggars Lane
Aldbury
Tring
Herts HP23 5PT
UK
tel: +44 (0) 1442 890 355
fax: +44 (0) 1442 890 366
E-mail: solgarinfo@solgar.com
Website: www.solgar.com

SKIN REVOLUTION SKINCARE

THE NATURAL-ETHICAL-POTENTS

Barefoot Botanicals Ltd

This is an excellent small range of highly ethical natural products:

Barefoot Botanicals Ltd.,
P.O Box 343
Brighton BN2 1XW
UK
Tel (UK): 0870 220 2273
Fax: (UK): 0845 330 1768
US: 1–800 Rosehip
Rep. of Ireland: 1 219 6980
E-mail: salesuk@barefoot-botanicals.com
Website: www.barefoot-botanicals.com

Living Nature and Living Nature Professional
Biologically active, natural skincare and body care. These products are free
of chemical preservatives or additives. They are organic, or wild-crafted,
contain no synthetic chemicals, no parabens and no genetically modified
substances. Living Nature and Living Nature Professional are two of the
purest skincare ranges in the world.

UK – for stockist and mail order:
Living Nature UK
Unit 6, Gardeners Business Park
Sherfield English Road
Plaitford
Hants SO51, 6EJ
UK
Tel: +44 (0) 1794 323 222
Fax: +44 (0) 1794 323 555
E-mail: uk@livingnature.com
Website: www.livingnature.com

Australia – for nearest stockist and mail order:
Destination Health
PO Box 88 Mason Street
Newport
Victoria 3015
Australia
Tel: +61 (0) 3 9399 4799
Fax: +61 (0) 3 9398 0274
E-mail: sales@desthealth.com or diane@desthealth.com

New Zealand – for nearest stockist or mail order:
PO Box 193
Kerikeri
New Zealand
Freephone (NZ): 0508 548 464
Tel: +(64) 9 407 7895
Fax: +(64) 9 407 4056
E-mail: enquiries@livingnature.com
Website: www.livingnature.com

Scents of Balance
Kate Rossetto's unique American range of products includes a light-as-air Rose Silk Face Cream and 'Take Me There' emotional healing mists. These are high frequency sprays unique in their mood shifting and personal empowerment properties. Completely natural in formulation, they have also been infused with prayer and come in six varieties for different purposes: Forgiveness, Freedom, Power and Grace, Sweet Dreams, I AM and JOY.
Kate Rossetto
Scents of Balance
2055 Andromeda Lane
Billings, MT 59105
USA
Tel: +1 (406) 2445 9182
E-mail: kate@scentsofbalance.com
Website: www.scentsofbalance.com

The Green People Company Ltd
Brighton Road
Handcross
West Sussex RH17 6BZ
UK
Mail order/enquiries: +44 (0) 1444 401 444
Fax: +44 (0) 1444 401011
www.greenpeople.co.uk or www.greenpeople-organic-health.co.uk

THE NATURALS

These products are formulated primarily from natural ingredients. Most of them still contain parabens and other chemicals used as preservatives or for other purposes. However, these manufacturers are committed to producing cosmetics which are environmentally aware and as ecologically responsible as they can manage.

AD®skin synergy Nourishing Night Treatment
A wonderful nourishing gel which I like to use not only at night but as a base for mineral makeup application around the eyes.
AD®skin synergy
PO Box 25595
London NW7 1WT
UK
Tel (UK): 0870 240 3350
E-mail: amanda@amandadenningpr.co.uk

Annemarie Börlind
C/O Simply Nature
Unit 7, Old Factory Buildings
Battenhurst Road
Stonegate
Wadhurst
East Sussex TN5 7DU
UK
Tel: +44 (0) 1580 201687

Aubrey Organics
4419 North Manhattan Avenue
Tampa FL 33614
USA
Tel: +1 (800) 282 7394
Fax: +1 (813) 876 8166
Website: www.aubrey-organics.com

Aveda
Aveda Environmental Lifestyle Store
28–29 Marylebone High Street
London W1U 4PL
UK
Tel: +44 (0) 207 224 3157
or
174 High Holborn
London WC1 7AA
Tel: +44 (0) 207 759 7350
Website: www.aveda.com

Decléor UK Ltd
59a Connaught Street

London W2 2BB
UK
Tel: +44 (0) 207 262 0403
Fax: +44 (0) 207 262 1886
Website: www.decléor.co.uk

Dr. Hauschka Skin Care Inc.
59 North Street
Hatfield
MA 01038
USA
US Freephone: 800 247 9907
US Fax: +1 413 247 0680
Mail order (UK): +44 (0) 1386 792 622
Australia: +61 (2) 9818 6119
Can: +1 514 286 9146
E-mail: enquiries@drhauschka.co.uk
Website: www.drhauschka.co.uk and www.drhauschka.com

Jurlique
Naturopathic Health & Beauty Co
West Quay Drive
Yeading
Middlesex UB4 9TB
UK
Mail order/enquiries: +44 (0) 181 841 6644
Fax: +44 (0) 181 841 7557
E-mail: sue.pierce@jurlique.co.uk
Website: www.jurlique.com.au

Liz Earle
Union
22 Union Street
Ryde
Isle of Wight PO33 2DT
UK
or
PO Box 50
Ryde
Isle of Wight PO33 2YD
UK
Customer Care Line: +44 (0) 1983 813999

Tel: +44 (0) 1983 813913
Fax: +44 (0) 1983 813912
Website: www.lizearle.com or www.lizearle.net/lizearle/

Neways International UK Limited
Harvard Way
Kimbolton
Huntingdon
Cambridgeshire PE28 0NN
UK
Tel: +44 (0) 1480 862700 or +44 (0) 1480 861764
Fax: +44 (0) 1480 861769
E-mail: info@neways.co.uk
Website: www.neways.com or www.neways.co.uk

Origins
Stockists (UK): 0800 731 4039
Australia: +61 (2) 9238 9111 or +61 (2) 9904 8920
Can: +1 (613) 721 4537 or +1 (514) 282 4537
Website: www.origins.com

Ren Ltd
43 Crawford Street
London W1H 1JR
UK
Tel: +44 (0) 207 724 2900
Fax: +44 (0) 207 724 2678
E-mail: info@ren.ltd.uk
Website: www.ren.ltd.uk

Simplicite
This is good range of ethical natural products made from pure plants.
New Zealand, United Kingdom and Ireland, Singapore
Belangel Ltd
Website: www.belangel.com
Address: P.O. Box 36–572,
Christchurch
New Zealand
Tel: +64 (3) 377 0753

Australia – Simplicite (Head Office)
34 Commercial Rd

Newstead
Brisbane QLD
Australia 4005
Tel: +61 (7) 3852 1081
Website: www.simplicite.com.au

Weleda

Weleda grew out of the work of Rudolf Steiner and have been making medicines and body care products for 75 years. Weleda UK grow over 400 species of plants organically and biodynamically for use in their medicines and body care range. They do an excellent arnica cream and a delightful skincare range. Available from good health stores and pharmacies or order direct:
Weleda (UK) Ltd
Heanor Road
Ilkeston
Derbyshire DE7 8DR
UK
Tel: +44 (0) 115 944 8200
Fax +44 (0) 115 944 8210
Mail order/information: +44 (0) 115 9448 222
Websites: www.weleda.co.uk www.weleda.com www.welda.com.au www.weleda.co.nz www.welda.ca

CHIRALLY CORRECT COSMETICS

These products have been formulated using chirally correct ingredients – either 'left-handed' or 'right-handed' molecules – to create biologically active, effective skincare products.

Kyra

These are my favourites of the chirally correct skincare products. It is a small, simple to use collection, great for travel, sold by a company with integrity. They will ship anywhere in the world.
SuperNatural Alternatives
PO Box 74110
RPO Strathcona
Calgary, AB T3H 3B6
Canada
Toll free (USA): 1 866 424 4725 (North America-wide)
Fax: +1 (866) 242 2550
Tel: +1 (403) 242 6583

Fax: +(1) 403 242 9670
E-mail: taylore@supernatural.com or info@supernatural.com
Website: www.supernatural.com

Cosmetic Surgery
Website: www.interfacegroup.com

Isocare
Website: www.isocare.net

THE BIOLOGICAL ACTIVES

This group of products contains nutraceuticals. They belong to the new wave of skincare which attempts to use vitamins and supplements like DMAE, alpha lipoic acid, Co Q10 and ALA to treat skin from the outside in. These products all contain chemical preservatives and conventionally formulated emulsions. Many of these are considered cosmeceuticals instead of cosmetics. In truth, there is no difference between the two. The name 'cosmeceuticals' is very often used to identify the kind of products you buy from a dermatologist or salon rather than what you buy over the counter in a store or pharmacy, but there is no legal definition of 'cosmeceuticals'.

Advanced Skin Therapy
My favourite collection in this category, this range has been formulated in the United States by Nuala Briggs – the woman who probably knows more about high-tech treatments for skin than anyone else in Britain. It is a large range, so you will need to pick and choose, depending on what your skin needs. They will ship anywhere.
Advanced Skin Therapy
42 Harley Street
London W1G 9PR
UK
Tel (UK): 07000 560 821
And
58 Weston Road
Brighton
East Sussex BN3 1JD
UK
E-mail: hq@advancedskintherapy.co.uk
Website: www.advancedskintherapy.co.uk

Environ
Environ products are specially formulated by South African plastic surgeon Dr. Des Fernandes, a man who knows more about the use of vitamin A and vitamin C than anyone else. Most of his Environ products are fragrance free and all are free of colorants.

ENVIRON® Skin Care
G11 Accesspark
Kenilworth
Cape Town
South Africa
or
PO Box 36057
Milnerton 7435
South Africa
Tel: +27 (21) 552 3499
Fax: +27 (21) 552 3699
E-mail: info@cosmotech.co.za

Distributed by:
Wholeview Ltd
Suite 29, Unit 1
1000 North Circular Road
London NW2 7JP
UK
Tel: +44 (0) 208 450 2020
Fax: +44 (0) 208 450 0901
E-mail: environuk@aol.com

Environ Skin Care Ltd
62 Ladies Mile
Remuera
Auckland
New Zealand
Tel: +64 (9) 524 2005
Fax: +64 (9) 524 7042
E-mail: environnz@xtra.co.nz

Environ's Cosmetic Roll-Cit
Developed by Dr. Des Fernandes, this is a revolutionary device in skincare treatments. The Roll-Cit is a roller riddled with minute needles which

barely open the surface of the skin to allow deeper penetration of active ingredients. It is designed to help restore skin tightness, thicken the skin, soften facial lines, cause scarring to be less obvious and to speed up the disappearance of pigmentation marks.

N. V. Perricone
A pioneer in the nutraceutical-based skincare, Nicholas Perricone, author of *The Perricone Prescription*, has a good range of skincare products you can order online. The range is huge, with each product based on one or two active ingredients such as DMAE and ALA as well as internal supplements.
N.V. Perricone M.D. Cosmeceuticals-Europe
4th Floor, 60 Cheapside
London EC2V 6AX
UK
Tel: +44 (0) 207 329 2000
Fax: +44 (0) 207 248 0668
Website: www.nvperriconemd.com or www.nvperriconemd.co.uk

Ultraceuticals
Founded by Australian doctor Geoffrey Heber, who specialises in aesthetic medicine, and his wife Deborah Davis, the Ultraceutical range is well formulated and biologically active. Their Ultra C Treatment cream, containing 23% micronised Vitamin C in an oil base, is an excellent product and one of the few on the market that delivers what it promises without damaging the skin. Their Dark Circle Eye Cream based on Retinol and vitamin K is also first rate.
Ultraceuticals Pty Ltd
PO Box 238
Glebe NSW 2037
Australia
Tel: +61 (0) 2 9660 3066
Fax: +61 (0) 2 9660 3166
In Australia Freecall: 1800 355 890
In New Zealand Freecall: 0800 445 684
Website: www.ultraceuticals.com.au

Art A Face
A favourite of plastic surgeons, this range is based on colostrum which has wonderful healing properties after surgery or peels. Their fragrance is not great but they work well and are unique in the world. Their revolutionary Overnight Cream is first rate.

Suite 332
63 Remuera Road
Remuera
Auckland 1005
New Zealand
Tel: +64 (9) 309 0992
Fax: +64 (9) 309 0992
E-mail: info@artaface.com
Website: www.artaface.com

SKIN REVOLUTION MAKEUP

Makeup Artist Valentine Gotti

My friend Valentine Gotti is a great makeup artist with the rare ability to create both fascinating, highly-eccentric faces for the covers of magazines as well as taking any woman's face and making it an even more beautiful expression of who she really is. Valentine can be booked for an appointment
Tel: 00 33 610 612 678 (mobile)
The current price is £250 per session (approximately 90 minutes) with a personal theme and portrait.

Jane Iredale

My favourite mineral makeup comes from Jane Iredale. Jane began her career as a casting director for television commercials, working with models and actors who wear a lot of makeup for long periods under harsh lighting. Jane has created a range of natural-looking mineral-based products which can be used by all skin types. There are some new products on the market – cream colours for eye and cheeks. The range keeps getting better and better.
Distributed in the UK by
Landmark Distributors Ltd
Unit 1, 1000 North Circular Road
London NW2 7JP
UK Freephone: 0800 328 2467
Tel: +44 (0) 208 450 7111
Fax: +44 (0) 208 450 0901
E-mail: janeireladeuk@aol.com
Website: www.janeiredale.com
Canada: +1 (800) 661 7025
Website: www.stogryn.ca

Australia: +61 (0) 2 9660 3066
E-mail: susanf@ultraceuticals.com.au

M.A.C. Cosmetics
Mail order (UK): +44 (0) 207 534 9222
Website: www.maccosmetics.com

Shu Uemura
Great brushes and eyelash curlers.
Mail order (UK): +44 (0) 207 240 7635
Website: www.shu-uemura.co.jp

PARAMEDICAL TREATMENTS

The Advanced Harley Street Clinics
42 Harley Street
London W1G 9PR
UK
Tel (UK): 07000 560 821
E-mail: hq@advancedskintherapy.co.uk
Website: www.advancedskintherapy.co.uk
Also at:
85 Main Road
Gidea Park
Essex RM2 5EL
UK
and:
58 Weston Road
Brighton
East Sussex BN3 1JD
UK

Prescription Skincare
Under the direction of Stephen Gilbert FRCS, FRACS and Margaret Gilbert
243 Remuera Road
Remuera
Auckland
New Zealand
Tel: +64 (0) 9 524 7039
Fax: +64 (0) 9 524 6043
E-mail: theinstitute@nzipcs.co.nz

SKIN REVOLUTION MEDICAL HELP

Who to contact for help in finding a plastic surgeon or guidance in the use of natural hormones.

Australian Society of Plastic Surgeons
Tel: +61 (0) 9437 9200
Australasian College of Dermatologists
Tel: +61 (0) 2987 98177
Fax: +61 (0) 2981 61174
E-mail: admin@dermcoll.asn.au
Website: www.dermcoll.asn.au
British Association of Aesthetic Plastic Surgeons
Information: +(44) 207 405 2234
E-mail: info@baaps.org.uk
Website: www.baaps.org.uk
British Association of Plastic Surgeons
Information: +44 (0) 207 831 5161
E-mail: secretariat@baps.co.uk
Website: www.baps.co.uk
British Association of Dermatologists
Information: +44 (0) 207 383 0266
Fax: +44 (0) 207 388 5263
E-mail: admin@bad.org.uk
Website: www.bad.org.uk
Canadian Society of Plastic Surgeons
Tel: +1 (514) 843 5415
Fax: +1 (514) 843 7005
E-mail: Csps-sccp@symtatico.ca
Website: www.plasticsurgery.ca

Dr Shamim Daya
Expert in use of natural hormones.
57 Harley Street
London W1G 8QS
UK
Tel: +44 (0) 207 580 7537
E-mail: sdaya@ndirect.co.uk

FUNCTIONAL MEDICINE

If you want help in implementing the living matrix programme into your life you can work with a doctor or other health practitioner specifically trained in functional medicine. This is a cutting-edge science-based health-care approach to help a person establish the very highest level of health and vitality. It concerns assessing and treating underlying causes of illness using individually tailored therapies to restore and enhance health natu-rally, as well as to improve whole-person functioning. I suggest that you use these companies direct and request from them a list of healthcare profes-sionals in your area whom you may consult. In Britain Thorne Research and Metagenics products are also available from The Nutri Centre in London as well as by mail order from them and their website (see below).

Here is a list of Thorne Research distributors in various countries:

AUSTRALIA
Graeme H Wallace
Unit 1 13 Elizabeth Street
PO Box 230
Bulleen
VIC 3105
Tel: +61 (0) 3 984 87890
Fax: +61 (0) 3 984 87839

NEW ZEALAND
FX Med
2 Dunlop Road
PO Box 19033
Onekawa Napier
Tel: +64 (0) 6 843 9370
Fax: +64 (0) 6 843 9260

USA HEAD OFFICE
Thorne Research, Inc
PO Box 25
Dover, ID 83825
USA
Tel: +1 (0) 208 263 2337
Fax: +1 (0) 208 265 2488
Website: www.thorne.com

Here is a list of Metagenics importers in various countries:

AUSTRALIA
Health World Limited
Tel: +61 (0) 7 3260 3300
Fax: +61 (0) 7 3260 3399
Website: www.metagenics.com.au

NEW ZEALAND
J.M. Marketing Limited
2/15 Parkway Drive
Mairingi Bay
Auckland
New Zealand
Tel: +64 (0) 9 478 2540
Fax: +64 (0) 9 478 2740
E-mail: info@metagenics.co.nz
Website: www.metagenics.co.nz
or
PO Box 35–383
Brown's Bay
Auckland
New Zealand

REPUBLIC OF SOUTH AFRICA
Amipro Advanced Development Products (pty) Ltd
Tel: +27 (0) 11 608 0280
Fax: +27 (0) 11 608 0299
E-mail: info@amipro.co.sa

UNITED KINGDOM
Nutri Limited
Tel: +44 (0) 166 374 6559
Fax: +44 (0) 166 375 0590

Metagenics UK
Tel: +44 (0) 149 833 243
Fax: +44 (0) 149 833 254
E-mail: info@metagenics.co.uk

USA AND OTHER COUNTRIES
Visit the Metagenics website www.metagenics.com

INDEX

disease, causes of 49–50
disodium EDTA, and skin ageing 110–11
DL- (racemic) mixture of molecules 121
DL-alpha-tocopherol 123
DMAE (dimethylaminoethanol) 65, 134, 142–3
DMDM (hydantoin) 115
DNA
    and biophotons 36
    glucose binding with 61
    and the Human Genome Project 51
    protection of 24, 29, 88
DNA damage 115
    and parabens 34
    and UVA rays 169
    by X-rays and gamma rays 156
DNA repair
    and light energy 155, 160, 162
    measurement of 36
    and nicotinamide 84
    time of day 159
Dong Quai (Chinese angelica)
    for menopausal problems 96
    for PMS skin 92
Dr Hauschka 141
dressings and dips 237–45
drugs
    chiral orientation of 120, 121
    effects on skin 44–5
dynamic wrinkles 256–7
dysbiosis (leaky gut) 82

early humans, diet 68–9
Easy Mayonnaise (and variations) 238–40
eccrine glands 43
eczema 45
EDTA, and skin ageing 110–11
elastin 48
emotions, reflected in the skin 32
enantiomers 121
endocrine system, effects of light 158
endogenous toxins 112
endometriosis 110
energy
    and the living matrix 35
    for the skin 20–1
    and water intake 20
energy-based skin treatments 38–9
energy swings 56, 58
Environ 136, 143, 186
enzymes
    and protein 24
    from raw foods 21–2, 76
epidermis 44, 45
    structure and function 46–7

erbium laser treatment 286, 287
Estée Lauder 143
EU, ban on phthalates 109, 111
exercise 60
    and free radicals 85
exfoliation, excessive 45
exogenous toxins 112
extrinsic ageing 184–6
    causes of 170–1
    as deficiency disease 186
    effects on the skin 168
    process of 256
    susceptibility to 171–2
    and The Living Matrix 21 Day Diet 184–5
eyebrows, signs of ageing and treatments 259
eyes
    dark circles 24
    signs of ageing and treatments 259–60
    soft pillows around 61

face
    ageing process 259–61
    assessing the need for medical treatment 263
facelift 293 see also cosmetic surgery
fake tanning products 183–4
far infrared sauna 192–7
fat burning
    and infrared saunas 195–6
    and omega-3 fats 77
fat grafting 277–9
fatigue 56, 59
fats
    for ageless skin 76–8
    essential 20
    to help lower cholesterol 77–8
    to help shed body fat 77–8
    which do harm 76
FD&C colour pigments 115
female reproductive disorders, and chemical hormone mimics 110
Fernandes, Dr Des 34–5, 135–6, 186
    Roll-Cit instrument 136–7
fibre 71, 75–6
fibroblasts 36, 48, 83, 137
fibroid tumours 110
fillers 257, 270–80
fine lines 14, 24
fish, as protein source 78, 79
Fish Dip 216, 243–4
fish oil 20, 24
Five Day Facelift Diet 14–27
    menus 16–17

hormone creams, nature-identical 90
hormone mimics 110
hormone supplements
    nature-identical 90, 98–100, 103
    herbal 90
hormones
    effects of light 157, 158, 159
    functioning of 90–1
    pharmaceutical 101
    production 158, 159
    receptor sites 90–1
    regulation 43, 44, 157, 158
    and the skin 89–105
HRT 99, 182
Human Genome Project 51
hunter-gatherer diet 68–9
hyaluronic acid (HA) 38
hyaluronic fillers 273
hydroelectric energy 20
Hylaform filler 257, 273
hypothalamus, effects of light impulses
    on 160

Imedeen 10
immune functions of skin 14, 22
    and antioxidants 86
    support from phytonutrients 60, 70
    support from raw foods 76
individuality, learning to express 301–11
infertility 110
inflammation 14, 15, 24
    and antioxidants 86
    causes of 61, 62, 64–5
    and reactive skin 63
    and skin ageing 20
infrared radiation 187–97
    benefits of 189, 191
    and cardiovascular fitness 189–90
    and cell communication 188
    far infrared sauna 192–7
    from the body 190
    healing properties 188
    new technologies 191–7
    penetration into the body 188, 189
infrared sauna 192–7
Instant Omelette 216
instinct, reconnecting with 309–10
insulin
    and ageing 57
    and protein in the diet 20
    receptor sites 58
    secretion by pancreas 58
    transport of glucose into cells 58
insulin balance
    and coffee 102
    and diet 19

and glucose 56, 57–9
and MSM 81–2
and skin ageing 24–5
insulin resistance syndrome 57, 58–9
    and extrinsic ageing 171
    and low glycaemic foods 75
insulin sensitivity
    and ALA 88
    and omega-3 fats 77
intense pulsed light (IPL) therapy 164–5
intracellular oxidative stress see free
    radical damage
intrinsic ageing process 186, 256
ionisers 134
ionising radiation, effects on skin 46
Iredale, Jane 145–8, 149, 151–2
Isolagen, live cell therapy 39, 271,
    279–80
isopropyl alcohol (SD-40) 115

Jane Iredale Cosmetics 145–8, 149,
    151–2
jaw line, signs of ageing and treatments
    261
jetlag 195
jowls, treatments for 261
Juelique 141
junk fats 76
Just Pure 141

keratin 46
keratinocytes 46, 137
kinetin 134
Kyra 141

L- (laevulo) form of a molecule 121
L- series amino acids 122
lactic acid, forms used in skincare 125
Lancaster 143
Lancome 143
Langerhans cells 47
laser treatments 163–4, 258, 285–6, 287
Lauder, Estée 63
Lauder, Leonard 6–7, 8–9
L-carnitine see carnitine
leaky gut 82
legumes, as protein source 78–9
LEPT (low energy photon therapy)
    194–5
licopene 74, 76, 87
light
    beneficial effects on the body 155–67
    biophoton energy in raw foods 22–3
    effects on brain and body 160
    effects on endocrine system 158
    emitted from body cells 155, 157